Techniques of Anaesthesia

Techniques of Anaesthesia

WITH MANAGEMENT OF THE PATIENT AND INTENSIVE CARE

J. A. THORNTON

Professor and Head of University Department of Anaesthetics, Sheffield

and

C. J. LEVY

Consultant Anaesthetist, Sheffield Regional Hospital Board

with special chapters by

H. G. SCHROEDER
D. S. ROBERTSON
W. N. C. McCLEERY

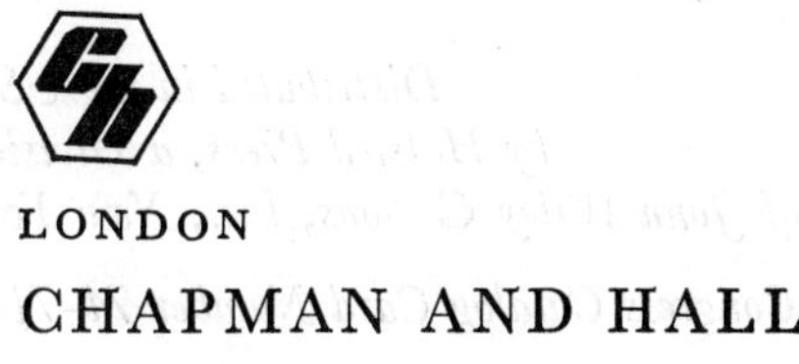

LONDON
CHAPMAN AND HALL

First published 1974
by Chapman and Hall Ltd
11 New Fetter Lane, London EC4P 4EE

Printed in Great Britain by
Willmer Brothers Limited, Birkenhead

ISBN 0 412 12280 4

Distributed in the USA
by Halsted Press, a Division
of John Wiley & Sons, Inc., New York

Library of Congress Catalog Card Number 74–7149

Contents

Preface

In spite of the many excellent textbooks on anaesthesia, very few specifically concentrate on the practical aspect of the art. This has often been brought to our notice by the questions posed by new entrants to the specialty. The basic pharmacology and physiology related to anaesthesia are covered in detail in the standard works, and in monographs; this book therefore is aimed at guidance on practical techniques of day to day anaesthesia with less emphasis on background theory. Its purpose is not only to assist the newcomer but also the established practitioner who is faced with a problem outside his familiar field. It is hoped that the young surgeon or physician who assists in the pre- and post-operative care of patients and the management of the acute medical emergency may find guidance in this book. Finally the doctor preparing for the higher examinations in anaesthesia will find much which is relevant to his purpose.

We wish to express our thanks to the numerous colleagues who have willingly given constructive criticism and advice, in particular Drs. W. J. Patterson, A. M. Wilson, A. D. G. Nicholas, and R. E. Atkinson.

J.A.T.
C.J.L.

Sheffield
1974

The Authors

J. A. THORNTON, M.D. (Lond)., F.F.A.R.C.S., D.A.
Professor and Head of the Department of Anaesthetics
University of Sheffield.
Honorary Consultant Anaesthetist United Sheffield Hospitals
and Sheffield Regional Hospital Board.
Examiner for Final F.F.A.R.C.S. (England).

C. J. LEVY, M.B., B.Ch.(Rand)., F.F.A.R.C.S., D.A.
Consultant Anaesthetist North Sheffield University Hospital.
Honorary Clinical Lecturer University of Sheffield.

H. G. SCHROEDER, M.B., Ch.B. (Birmingham),
F.F.A.R.C.S., D.A.
Honorary Clinical Lecturer in Anaesthetics and
Part-time Lecturer in Resuscitation and Intensive Therapy
University of Sheffield.
Consultant Anaesthetist United Sheffield Hospitals.

W. N. C. McCLEERY, M.B., B.Ch., B.A.O. (Belfast).,
F.F.A.R.C.S., D.A.
Honorary Clinical Lecturer in Anaesthetics University of Sheffield.
Consultant Anaesthetist United Sheffield Hospitals.

D. S. ROBERTSON, M.B., B.S. (Lond)., F.F.A.R.C.S., D.A.
Honorary Clinical Lecturer in Anaesthetics University of Sheffield.
Consultant Anaesthetist United Sheffield Hospitals.

1 *Assessment and Preparation of Patients for Anaesthesia*

Factors affecting operative risk

Certain operative procedures carry with them a much higher rate of mortality and morbidity than others. Pre-existing respiratory disease, obesity, malnutrition, anaemia, and electrolyte disturbances are all features that are well recognized as predisposing to morbidity during and after anaesthesia. Special consideration should be given to patients receiving therapeutic agents and those at the extremes of life. Certain anaesthetic procedures have recognized complications, such as the injudicious use of thiopentone in the 'shocked' patient. The anaesthetist should in all cases take a full history and make a thorough examination. Full records must be available of any past and current drug therapy, dose of drugs, route of administration and untoward reactions (page 447).

Elective surgery should allow time for the correction of such conditions as dehydration, electrolyte abnormalities, anaemia, malnutrition, obesity, dental caries, chest and cardiovascular disease. Use can be made of the anaesthetic outpatient clinic, provided that the patients do not have the inconvenience of having to attend at a separate time to the surgical appointment. The value and success of such a clinic depends upon close co-operation between the anaesthetist and the surgical team.

The accuracy of prediction of operative mortality is so poor that anaesthesia cannot be considered contraindicated in any patient who requires surgery. Emergency anaesthesia and surgery may not allow preparation of the patient beyond the control of bleeding (where it exists), the establishment of adequate pulmonary ventilation, and the treatment of 'shock'. Whenever possible, steps should be taken to ensure that the stomach is empty prior to general anaesthesia and a start should be made to the correction of any fluid and electrolyte imbalance. The medical evaluation of the patient should concern itself with providing optimal conditions for the surgical therapy, and not with the estimation of risk.

Quite apart from the condition of the patient, other factors, such as the skill and the experience of the anaesthetist and surgeon, and the organization of the hospital services, can have an important bearing on the successful outcome of a particular operation.

Despite the fact that the patient may have an uneventful operative phase, post-operative complications may arise. Prolongation of recovery may occur as a result of cerebral hypoxia, particularly in the elderly and those who have been in the upright posture. Other complications may arise from spinal anaesthesia and from chest and cardiovascular incidents. However much care is taken during operation and in the post-operative period there is a small but significant mortality from pulmonary embolism.

In the immediate post-operative period, respiratory and cardiovascular inadequacy, the Fink effect, cyclopropane shock, pain and shivering, may all contribute to hypoxaemia and hazard the patient's recovery.

Detailed assessment of the patient

In the evaluation of a patient for general anaesthesia, a detailed history of past illnesses, disabilities, previous anaesthetics and operations should be obtained. Discreet enquiry may reveal a history of adverse reaction to general anaesthesia such as nausea and vomiting, smoking and alcohol. A thorough examination should include inspection of the teeth, veins and nose, and of movement of joints, particularly the jaw. The haemoglobin content of the blood and blood pressure should be determined, urinalysis carried out, and the chest X-rayed where possible.

The common cold. Opinions vary regarding the management of a patient suffering from the common cold. Whenever possible the operation should be postponed, but when it cannot be deferred the patient should be given antibiotic cover. It should, however, be borne in mind that the presence of an upper respiratory tract infection is likely to increase the chance of the patient developing a post-operative chest infection.

Smoking. Where the patient is in the habit of smoking, sudden withdrawal is unlikely to improve the chest and indeed may increase the chances of sputum retention. In addition, sudden withdrawal at a time when stress is likely to be considerable, will in no way help to calm the patient. A gradual reduction in the quantity smoked should be encouraged, but abrupt cessation can serve no useful purpose.

Alcohol. Excessive alcohol intake over long periods of time may well lead to damage and impairment of functions of the liver.

The patient may be resistant to narcotic agents and have an altered response to neuro-muscular blocking agents. Restlessness and confusion may characterize the post-operative period and call for special handling.

In view of this, consideration should be given to the administration of alcohol during the post-operative period.

Drugs

Monoamine oxidase inhibitors

Some of these (see Table 1.1) have been widely used for the treatment of patients with depressive illness. The possible dangers to patients receiving monoamine oxidase inhibitors when subjected to a general anaesthetic are:

Exaggerated response to some sympathomimetic drugs, e.g. methylamphetamine and phenylephrine but not with adrenaline, noradrenaline, nor isoprenaline.

Exaggerated response to pethidine, pentazocine, phenazocine, and possibly morphine.

Table 1.1 *Monoamine oxidase inhibitors*

Approved name	*Proprietary name*
isocarboxazid	Marplan
mebanazine	Actomol
pheniprazine	*Cavodil*
phenoxypropazine	*Drazine*
pargyline*	Eutonyl
iproniazid	Marsilid
phenelzine	Nardil
nialamide	Niamid
tranylcypromine*	Parnate
tranylcypromine* and trifluoperazine	Parstelin
pivhydrazine	*Tarsavid*
eryptamine	*Monase*

* All the drugs listed except those marked with an asterisk are hydrazine derivatives. Those shown in italic are not available in the United Kingdom.

It has been suggested that if patients are coming to anaesthesia, the monoamine oxidase inhibitors should be stopped at least two weeks prior to surgery. If this course of action is not adopted the following regimen may be instituted:

Premedication. Atropine in reduced dosage, e.g. 0.4 mg and a barbiturate or a phenothiazine derivative if desired.

Anaesthesia. All general anaesthetics should be used with care, with constant observation of the blood pressure. Induction with an ultra-short-acting barbiturate is probably safe if the usual caution is observed and muscle relaxants are not contraindicted, but pethidine, morphine, phenazocine, and pentazocine should not be used. Churchill-Davidson (1965) has suggested that possible adverse reactions to pethidine may be detected by employing a pre-operative test. Pethidine 10 mg is given at half-hourly intervals intramuscularly, up to a total dose of 50–100 mg, and pulse rate, blood pressure, and respiration rate are carefully recorded; any untoward deviation from the normal resting level may indicate an adverse reaction. Vasopressors should not be given. Chlorpromazine (up to 50 mg) or phentolamine (up to 5 mg) given continuously intravenously are suggested should a hypertensive episode occur, following the inadvertent administration of any of the above agents. The intravenous injection of β-adrenergic blocking agents may be considered. Should coma and respiratory depression occur with morphine or pethidine, no attempt should be made to reverse the action with analeptics or drugs such as nalorphine. Ventilation should, however, be supported mechanically if necessary while blood pressure fall should be treated very cautiously, avoiding, if at all possible, pressor agents. Large doses of intravenous hydrocortisone may have a place in the treatment of such hypertensive crisis.

Liver damage has been reported following the use of these drugs, especially those containing the hydrazine group. The liver damage is rare but may be fatal. Episodes of hypertension are sometimes related to the eating of food containing amines (e.g. cheese). Hypotensive episodes, ataxia, paraesthesia and ocular palsies have also been reported.

Tricyclic antidepressants

In subjects receiving therapy with tricyclic antidepressants, such as imipramine, amitryptyline, desipramine, nor-triptyline, potentiation of the pressor effect of phenylephrine, noradrenaline and adrenaline has been noticed.

Lithium

This agent is now well established in the treatment of many forms of mental illness. It is not surprising therefore that many patients presenting for anaesthesia are receiving therapy with this agent. Recently there have been reports of prolonged action of non-depolarising muscle relaxants given to patients receiving lithium carbonate. The possibility of this adverse reaction must therefore be borne in mind when giving neuromuscular blocking agents to such patients.

Oral Contraceptives

It appears that the risk of postoperative thrombo-embolism is increased several-fold in patients taking the oral contraceptive over those not receiving this medication. This risk is obviously increased with intra- and post-operative immobilisation. Some authorities advocate cessation of the medication for 4 weeks preoperatively. As a result of this action the patient would be at risk of conceiving for four weeks preoperatively and an indeterminate time post-operatively. The risk of pregnancy and its attendent complications must thus be balanced against the relatively small risk of thrombo-embolism.

Steroids

It must be remembered that many patients for surgery may have been receiving steroid therapy (e.g. for asthma, rheumatoid arthritis and skin diseases). There have been many reports of the lack of normal response to stress in patients who have been receiving steroid therapy by any route. For instance, adrenal suppression has been noticed three to five days after a single intra-articular injection of 50 mg triamcinolone. Variable depression has also been reported after application of cortico-steroids to the skin. Although many have assumed that some degree of adrenal suppression may exist for as long as two years after cessation of therapy, recent work suggests that this is unlikely to occur if two months have elapsed since the cessation of therapy (Plumpton *et al.*, 1969).

The regimen of management varies. Most anaesthetists have been in the practice of administering additional steroids in an empirical fashion to patients who have received or are receiving steroids. A steady level of blood hydrocortisone is best obtained by providing intramuscular depots; for this purpose 200 mg of cortisone acetate may be injected intramuscularly the day before operation, the same dose to be repeated the morning of operation and again repeated the day following operation. This dose is gradually reduced in the subsequent few days, with the patient reverting to his normal steroid therapy on about the fifth post-operative day. Alternatively:

the normal dose of steroids may be given until the day of operation
on the day of operation treble the patient's normal dose and give this in three divided doses over 24 hours, one dose being given with premedication, one during operation (100 mg hydrocortisone hemisuccinate i.v.) and one in the evening
give double the normal dose on each of the three days following the operation
give one and one-half times the normal dose for the following three days
thereafter give the normal dose

In order to avoid giving extra doses of steroids the following regimen may be adopted as a further alternative. To help with the premedication of patients likely to have an impaired cortical response to surgery, a rapid screening test has been devised (Wood *et al.*, 1965). This test depends upon the rise in plasma cortisol to a single intramuscular injection of 250 μg of a synthetic polypetide – β^{1-24} corticotrophin (Synacthen). This substance, because of its purity, carries little danger of allergy. If the adrenal response is present, then only minutes after the injection of Synacthen the plasma cortisol level has risen above the level existing before the test. The ability of the pituitary/adrenal axis to react to stress may be challenged by the administration of 0.15 u/kg soluble insulin to the patient following an overnight fast. A 3-4 fold increase of plasma cortisol associated with a fall of blood sugar to approx 40 mg/100 ml indicates a satisfactory response to stress. It is suggested that the logical approach would be as follows (Pooler, 1968):

Synacthen test: positive
- No steroid cover
- Ordinary monitoring
- Out-patient surgery allowable

Synacthen test: negative
- Major surgery – steroid cover
- Minor surgery – steroid cover may be withheld but out-patient surgery is not allowable. All patients need careful and continuous monitoring for 24 hours

No Synacthen test:
- Major surgery – steroid cover
- Minor surgery on seriously ill patient – steroid cover. In both cases careful and continuous monitoring for 24 hours
- Minor surgery on fit patients – steroid cover may be withheld but careful, continuous monitoring will be essential for some hours

All patients must be admitted overnight.

β-adrenergic receptor blockade

β-adrenergic blocking agents are being increasingly used in a variety of circumstances, such as for the management of angina pectoris, hypertension, thyrotoxicosis, phaeochromocytoma, and anxiety states. In some ways the use of β-adrenergic blockade is a more effective treatment for the pre-operative alleviation of stress and the cardiovascular consequences induced by fear in patients with hypertensive heart disease, than sedation by opiates, hypnotics and tranquillizers. Care should be exercised when using agents such as diethyl ether, halothane, and cyclopropane, in patients receiving β-adrenergic blocking agents, as severe reduction of cardiac output may occur. Work in animals suggests that β-adrenergic blocking agents may be beneficial in patients suffering blood loss. However, lack of the normal warning increase in pulse rate may be associated with lack of overall response to reduction in circulating blood volume.

Antihypertensive drugs

This subject has been admirably reviewed by Dingle (1966), and the problem has recently been considered in detail by Prys-Roberts *et al.* (1971a, b. 1972, 1973) and Foëx *et al.* (1971) (See Table 1.2).

Table 1.2 *Anti-hypertensive drugs*

Drug	*Limits of action*	*Recommended delay*
methyldopa	4–6 days	7 days
reserpine	10–20 days	14 days
guanethidine	7–21 days	10 days
guanoxan	2–3 days	3 days
debrisoquine	24–48 hours	2 days
bethanidine	24–48 hours	2 days

Rauwolfia: It is unnecessary to discontinue rauwolfia therapy before elective surgery; indeed withdrawal of therapy, of itself, does not assure circulatory stability. However, treatment with rauwolfia and related alkaloids is usually for very mild hypertension and withdrawal is unlikely to harm the patient. It takes about 10 days to eliminate reserpine from the body.

One of the major factors during the administration of an anaesthetic to a hypertensive patient is the possibility of a sudden change of blood pressure, whether the hypertension is treated or not. Should the anaesthetist then recommend the withdrawal of drugs pre-operatively? As the untreated high arterial pressure constitutes a serious risk, the treatment should *not* be withdrawn unless there is a compelling reason. If intravenous agents are to be employed a neuroleptic technique is probably best (see page 381) (Prys-Roberts *et al.*, 1971a, b). Induction should continue with 70% nitrous oxide following pre-oxygenation. As endotracheal intubation is likely to be associated with a hypertensive crisis in treated or untreated cases, prior β-adrenergic blockade has been advocated by Prys-Roberts *et al.* (1971a, b, 1972, 1973). However, the authors believe that adequate topical anaesthesia to the larynx and trachea should suffice provided that enough time is allowed to elapse between spraying and intubation. Halothane is best avoided. Artificial ventilation should be adjusted to avoid hypercapnia or hypocapnia. An intravenous infusion should be established and any fall in BP managed by rapid infusion and reference to the central venous pressure. Pressor agents should be avoided.

If it is thought that anti-hypertensive drugs are putting the patient at risk, their temporary withdrawal must be considered, bearing in mind the fact that in very severe cases of hypertension withdrawal of therapy might itself prove catastrophic. It is possible, however, that the treated hypertensive under anaesthesia is less vulnerable than the untreated (Prys-Roberts *et al.*, 1971 a, b, c). Some anaesthetists, therefore, would leave the patients on their normal regimen. The blood pressure and E.C.G. particularly should be carefully monitored during the operative and post-operative periods.

If it is decided that a drug should be withdrawn, sufficient time must be allowed for the full restoration of sympathetic function. The action of the following drugs is at an end within 24 hours, in patients with normal kidney function: drugs acting by competitive ganglionic blockade; clonidine (half-life 6-8 h) – severe hypertension may occur within 4h of cessation of treatment; hydrallazine; adrenergic α-receptor and β-receptor blockers. Some drugs with a prolonged action are shown in Table 1.2.

Levodopa. Recently, levodopa has been employed in the treatment of Parkinsonism. In this condition the symptoms are due to a deficiency of dopamine in the basal ganglion. Levodopa crosses the blood/brain interface and is converted to dopamine in the brain. Levodopa, which has a short half-life in the body, is usually given in a dose of 2–8 g daily, in four or more divided doses for optimal results. Major adverse reactions associated with levodopa therapy are abnormal movements, psychic and cardiovascular disturbances (dysrhythmias and hypotension), associated with increased catecholamine output. To reduce these complications, levodopa may be prescribed with a decarboxylase inhibitor such as a hydrazine derivative (MK 486 or RO 4-460). Therapy with levodopa is contraindicated in patients receiving butyrophenone derivatives such as haloperidol and droperidol which antagonize the action of dopamine. It should be borne in mind that patients with Parkinson's disease may be receiving tricyclic antidepressants, sedatives, anticholinergics, and digitalis preparations. In patients requiring anaesthesia, therapy with levodopa may be continued until the night prior to operation and continued as soon as possible post-operatively. It is probably advisable to avoid the use of halothane and cyclopropane, and to consider the use of intravenous β-adrenergic blocking agents or lignocaine should dysrhythmias occur during anaesthesia.

Rubber dermatitis and sensitivity to synthetic materials

This is a well-recognized condition. Rubber dermatitis is said to occur with both natural and synthetic products. It is thought that it is rarely due to rubber itself, but to one or more of the organic chemicals used in the conversion of the raw material into the finished product, e.g. mercaptiobenzothiazole (MBT), an accelerator used in the manufacture of rubber. Certain red rubber surgical and anaesthetic equipment contains MBT. In view of the severe reactions that may occur, particularly the reaction of the larynx to an endotracheal tube, exhaustive precautions should be taken that no rubber material comes into contact with a sensitive patient. Endotracheal tubes and connectors should be of plastic or similar synthetic material, and care should be taken with sphygmomanometer cuffs and connections, rubber drains and snares used by the surgical team and with rubber mattresses and cushions.

It must be remembered that some synthetic materials used for endotracheal tubes, drains, etc., can also produce reactions (Guess and Stetson, 1968). Sterilization either by gamma irradiation or ethylene oxide may produce toxic substances, so it is recommended that plastics sterilized by ethylene oxide should be stored for at least one week before being used for procedures entailing prolonged contact with body tissues.

Drug addiction (drug dependence)

Although drug addiction as a social problem is endlessly discussed, the literature on the subject of the drug addict and anaesthesia is very limited. Nevertheless, it is apparent that such patients have a high degree of tolerance to morphine, phenothiazines and barbiturates (Adriani and Morton, 1968). The abstinence syndrome is also well recognized and it would seem advisable to maintain drugs pre-operatively and for the patients to be allowed to continue their drugs in the post-operative period. It should be borne in mind that many of these patients, because of their social and economic status, are malnourished and therefore their general health may be poor.

Patients dependent upon alcohol and the barbiturate drugs manifest marked excitement during the induction of general anaesthesia. The need for an increased amount of agents, due to tolerance and cross-tolerance, may lead to overdosage and technical difficulties during anaesthesia. Cross-tolerance is common between the barbiturates, the alcohol type drugs, and the aliphatic inhalational anaesthetics. Hypotension has been reported during anaesthesia in narcotic addicts and may be treated in some instances by intravenous morphine. The presence of LSD within the tissues at the time of anaesthesia may be a matter of concern, because the drug manifests a certain degree of anticholinesterase activity, which potentiates narcotic activity and inhibits destruction of suxamethonium.

If a patient is receiving narcotics it may be necessary to increase the usual narcotic dose in the premedication. The withdrawal syndrome for alcohol and barbiturates can be serious and terminate fatally if not properly managed. This is in contradistinction to the morphine type where withdrawal is uncomfortable but not fatal. Pentazocine should not be used in the presence of opiate addiction because of the danger of causing sudden withdrawal symptoms.

Premedication

It has been routine practice in the past to give patients certain drugs before they undergo anaesthesia. The main reasons for this therapy have been:

- to allay anxiety
- to reduce secretions resulting from the irritant properties of certain anaesthetic agents
- to counter side-effects of anaesthetic agents on the cardiovascular system
- to potentiate the narcotic effects of general anaesthetic agents
- to counter certain other side effects of general anaesthetic agents, e.g. nausea and vomiting

Sedation

The old system of premedication appeared to assume that patients suddenly become anxious one or two hours prior to operation, yet the fear of anaesthesia and surgery exists in the patient's mind well before this, and logically, treatment should begin long before the patient comes into hospital. Management of anxiety will begin with a careful explanation to the patient of what is likely to take place, and reassurance to allay unnecessary fears.

Management of the pre-anaesthetic state

Assessment of the patient's attitude towards the operation and of his underlying mental makeup should begin when the doctor first comes into contact with him. The aged generally have a philosophical approach toward such episodes in their lives and will probably need little additional help with drugs. It is important that all patients receive adequate sleep whilst they are in hospital and some will need hypnotics to assist them if they are unaccustomed to the noise of hospitals and have to sleep amongst other patients. The immediate pre-operative sedation is a matter for the anaesthetist's judgement, but in many cases if the patient has been carefully handled during his stay in hospital it may be unnecessary to give him additional drugs. Both the surgeon and the anaesthetist will do their best to inspire confidence, and against this background they will only use drugs to assist them in their objective – namely to have the patient in a tranquil state of mind.

Some authorities have laid less emphasis upon immediate pre-operative sedation, and instead have used tranquillizing agents in the few days immediately prior to operation in an attempt to produce tranquillity. However, if light levels of anaesthesia are likely to be employed, it is perhaps worth considering relatively heavy sedation in the immediate pre-operative period in order to reduce the chances of consciousness during anaesthesia. One of the disadvantages of heavy sedation in the immediate pre-operative period is that if the opiates or similar agents are employed there is the likelihood of respiratory depression, particularly if the operation is of short duration.

The anaesthetist must also bear in mind that certain patients are likely to be sensitive to opiates, in that they may develop nausea and vomiting in the post-operative period as a result of the use of these drugs in the pre-medication. In this context it is perhaps worth remembering that certain patients exhibit all the signs of acute circulatory collapse after an average dose of pethidine. A careful enquiry before anaesthesia may elicit details of such reactions.

Drugs. Certain of the drugs which will produce tranquillity of mind are anaesthetic potentiating, including some of the phenothiazines. They not only produce sedation of varying degrees and potentiate anaesthesia, but in certain circumstances are vasomotor depressants (e.g. chlorpromazine). However, the phenothiazines have other properties which are of help to the anaesthetist. They may reduce the incidence of post-operative nausea and vomiting, and have an antisialogogue action. Prothipendyl, meprobamate, diazepam and chlordiazepoxide can be considered amongst the tranquillizing group of drugs.

Another family of drugs which has been introduced into anaesthetic practice is often referred to as the neuroleptic group. These drugs, of which haloperidol and droperidol are perhaps the best known, produce a peculiar state of tranquillity in patients, some of whom become withdrawn from their surroundings. They also potentiate general anaesthetic agents and may produce a Parkinson-type rigidity, particularly when used alone. Table 1.3 lists some of the drugs which may be used for premedication.

Antanalgesia

Certain agents used in relation to premedication and anaesthesia have been found to lower the pain threshold (see table 1.3 and page 376). The barbiturates, promethazine and hyoscine have all been shown to do this. If these drugs are used to produce sedation in patients suffering with pain, they may lead to a state verging on delirium with restlessness and uncontrollable excitement.

Route of administration. Some authorities prefer the oral route because it avoids the pain of an injection. However, this route is unreliable, as the drug may be vomited, or may be very poorly absorbed, particularly in patients with gastro-intestinal disease.

Time of administration. The administration of drugs as a premedication

Table 1.3 *Drugs that may be used for premedication*

All doses apply to a fit 70 kg adult man unless otherwise stated

Drugs	*Dose*	*Comments*
Phenothiazines:		
pecazine (Pacatal)	50–100 mg orally	Antanalgesic
promethazine (Phenergan)	25–50 mg orally or i.m.	Antanalgesic Fails to relieve anxiety in many patients Antisialogogue Antiemetic
promethazine-8-chlorothiophllinate (Avomine)	25 mg orally	Predominant action anti-emetic
promazine (Sparine)	25–50 mg orally or i.m.	Hypotension and tachycardia can occur Some mild analgesic activity Good sedative Poor anti-emetic
trimeprazine tartrate (Vallergan)	3–4 mg/kg	A good sedative for children Some mild analgesic activity
chlorpromazine (Largactil)	25–50 mg orally or i.m.	Raises pain threshold Sedative properties depend on dose Markedvaso-depression with large dose Adrenergic blocker Some mild analgesic activity
trifluoperazine (Stelazine)	2 mg orally or i.m.	Nine times more potent than chlorpromazine Powerful anti-emetic
perphenzine (Fentazine)	up to 5 mg or 2 mg/8h orally	Given mainly for anti-emetic properties
prothipendyl (Tolnate)	20–40 mg orally or i.m.	
Sedatives with a marked analgesic action:*		
morphine†	10–20 mg orally or i.m.	Fairly good sedative properties May cause vomiting
papaveretum	10–20 mg orally or i.m.	As morphine
pethidine†	100 mg orally or i.m.	Alone, sedative properties poor Can cause vomiting
phenoperidine (Operidene)	1·0 mg i.m. can be given	
fentanyl (Sublimaze)	0·1–0·2 mg i.m.	100 times more potent than morphine
pentazocine (Fortral)	30–60 mg i.m.	

Table 1.3—*continued*

Drugs	*Dose*	*Comments*
Barbiturates:‡		
phenobarbitone	15–30 mg orally or i.m.	Antanalgesic Degree of sedation depends on dose and frequency
pentobarbitone (Nembutal)	60–180 mg orally or i.m.	As for phenobarbitone
quinalbarbitone (Seconal)	60–180 mg orally	As for phenobarbitone
butobarbitone (Soneryl)	60–180 mg orally	As for phenobarbitone
amylobarbitone (Sodium Amytal)	60–180 mg orally or i.m.	As for phenobarbitone
Tranquillizers (other than phenothiazines):		
chlordiazepoxide (Librium)	20 mg/8h orally	Produces effective tranquillity
nitrazepan (Mogadon)	5 mg orally	As chlordiazepoxide
lorazepam (Ativan)	3 mg orally	
diazepam (Valium)	10–20 mg orally or i.m.	Can be given intravenously in doses up to 20 mg Give slowly in divided doses of 5 mg Useful to control muscle spasms (tetanus and status epilepticus) When given i.v. useful for shocked patients and post-operative excitement
flurazepam (Dalmane)	15–30 mg orally	
oxazepam (Serenid-D)	10–15 mg orally	
medazepam (Nobrium)	5–10 mg orally	
methylpentynol (Oblivon)	·75–1·0 g orally as capsules or elixir	Small doses particularly valuable in children
glutethamide (Doriden)	250–500 mg orally	One hour pre-operatively
hydroxyzine (Atarax)	25 mg/6h orally	
meprobamate (Equanil; Milltown)	400 mg/6h orally	

* Respiratory depression occurs with all these drugs and is a function of dose. In doses usually employed it is probably more likely with phenoperidine and fentanyl. For further sedatives with a marked analgesic action see page [378]

† The sedative effects of 10 mg morphine and 100 mg pethidine are similar and are unaffected by the addition of atropine. Pre-operative nausea and vomiting and dizziness would seem to be more common after pethidine. The vomiting may be reduced by adding atropine to the pre-medication

‡ phenobarbitone is long acting: the other barbiturates shown above are medium acting

Table 1.3—*continued*

Drugs	*Dose*	*Comments*
amitriptyline (Tryptizol)	25–75 mg orally or i.m.	Caution with monoamineoxidase inhibitors
chloral hydrate	1·0–2·0 g orally	Effective sedatives but gastric irritant
triclofos (Tricloryl)	0·5–2·0 ng orally as tablets or syrup	Less gastric irritation than chloral hydrate
dichloralphenazone (Welldorm)	0·65–1·3 g as tablets or elixir	
hyoscine	0·3–0·6 mg orally or i.m.	A poor sedative, but produces amnesia Good anti-sialogogue Has antanalgesic properties
bromethol (Avertin)	80–100 mg/kg given rectally	Must be freshly prepared
paraldehyde	2–8 ml orally and i.m.	
methaqualone (Melsed)	250 mg as capsules	Give 15–30 minutes before sleep required
ethclorvynol (Serenesil)	500 mg orally	
Neuroleptics: (see page 381)		
haloperidol (Serenace)	2·5 mg i.m.	Good anti-emetic
droperidol (Droleptan)	2·0–4·0 mg may be combined with 1·0 mg phenoperidine or 0·1 mg fentanyl	

should be so timed that the peak effect should have passed just prior to the induction of anaesthesia, particularly the peak effect on respiratory depression.

Antisialogogues

In the days when irritant inhalational anaesthetic agents were frequently employed, the anaesthetist would be embarrassed by the presence of salivary and bronchial secretions which could seriously upset the smooth course of the anaesthetic. Increased secretion could lead to laryngeal spasm, bronchospasm, coughing and possibly post-operative atelectasis. Excessive secretion could trigger off vomiting under light anaesthesia. Today, with anaesthetic agents which are less irritating to the upper respiratory tract the antisialogogue effect may be less necessary, but in certain situations is still an advantage. It is usually necessary to prescribe a drying agent pre-operatively if ether, cyclopropane, divinyl ether, or ketamine are to be used. Suxamethonium can produce excessive salivary secretion, particularly in small children and in association with electro-convulsive therapy.

The antisialogogues in present day use are atropine, promethazine, hyoscine and propantheline (Pro-Banthine). On the whole, hyoscyamine, methantheline bromide, hexcylium and oxyphenonium are unsatisfactory either because of side effects, or because of inadequate drying action. Hyoscine can cause very severe distress and difficulty with swallowing, which can be particularly upsetting if operation is delayed. It should be remembered that it can cause delirium in the aged and is an antanalgesic.

Doses: for doses of these drugs with the exception of atropine see above.

Atropine. Atropine has for many years been a constituent of standard routine premedication, but recently doubt has been cast on the justification for its routine use. It is argued that it upsets the autonomic balance; a low dose may cause excessive vagotonia, and a high dose produce vagal blockade, with sympathetic tone predominating. In 1922 Levy condemned the routine use of atropine before chloroform anaesthesia because it tended to increase ventricular irritability. Given intravenously during anaesthesia under diethyl ether, cyclopropane, or chloroform it can provoke ventricular extrasystoles; it can upset cardiovascular homeostasis by causing hypotension when the head is tilted up and feet down; it can provoke pulmonary oedema in patients with mitral stenosis and it is also thought by some to be dangerous when given to patients suffering with glaucoma.

Burton (1962) when studying the effects of dry gases on the respiratory mucous membrane, showed that atropine decreased the rate of production and movement of mucus and it is also known to alter the nature of bronchial secretions by causing them to become more viscous. Many workers have noted the antisialogogue effect of atropine and recently it has been suggested that, as modern techniques are unlikely to provoke secretions, its routine use for this purpose be abandoned. Though having undoubted anti-emetic properties, it may cause relaxation of the cardiac sphincter. It is ineffective as an agent to counteract respiratory depression, and indeed its use may be positively harmful in this situation. In addition it is ineffective for the treatment of laryngeal spasm.

Mongols have been reported as having fatal idiosyncrasies following the administration of atropine, though the evidence for this is somewhat tenuous. Other anaphylactic idiosyncrasies have also been reported. Atropine causes the mechanism which controls the temperature of the body to be disturbed, tending to lead to a rise in the metabolic rate and a reduction of sweating. It should be avoided in children who are pyrexial, as there is a very real danger of provoking convulsions and it has been implicated as a cause of hypoxaemia, though recent studies have suggested that the findings are not due to atropine.

Intravenous injection: the average adult will tolerate intravenous injections of 0.6–1.2 mg atropine and very much larger doses in nerve gas poisoning.

Subcutaneous injection: peak effect occurs about one hour after injection.

Premedication by mouth: in order to avoid the administration of atropine by injection, some authorities recommend administration by mouth in a dose of 0.6 mg.

The writers are in favour of the routine administration of atropine but should its general use be discontinued it *must* be administered in the following circumstances:

where suxamethonium is to be used, particularly in repeated doses in small children
as a premedication prior to electro-convulsive therapy
prior to the reversal of non-depolarizing block by neostigmine
in some cases of bradycardia (e.g. in relation to halothane anaesthesia)
addition its use should be considered in ocular surgery in an attempt to obtund the oculo-cardiac reflex.

2 *Apparatus*

Since the introduction of general anaesthesia in the mid-19th century there has been a steady development of anaesthetic apparatus. Essentially, such equipment has been designed to ensure that adequate and precise concentrations and volumes of gases and vapours can be delivered to the patient. All these items of equipment carry with them problems of physics which must be properly understood if the anaesthetist is fully to appreciate their clinical use.

The face mask

The ideal mask should be designed to fit the contours of the face and ensure that 'apparatus dead space', inevitable whenever a mask is used, is kept to a minimum. Of special interest are the masks which are efficient even in the edentulous patient and the disposable masks. Transparent masks are also available, and may help in the early observation of regurgitation of stomach contents.

The expiratory port

Ideally, all the expired gases should be voided from the breathing circuit, thereby preventing rebreathing; there should be neither loss from the circuit during inspiration, nor adulteration by air leaking into it and the expiratory port should be as near to the patient as possible in order to prevent rebreathing of gases. The characteristics of an ideal Heidbrink expiratory valve should be such that, when in the inverted position, it will open at a pressure of 0.5–1.0 cm water, this requirement being determined by the characteristics of the reservoir bag. This pressure should be exceeded as little as possible in the upright position and for flows up to 30–40 litres per minute. It is desirable for the valve to open and vent large flows for a small pressure drop. A modified angle piece and expiratory valve has been designed to obviate the dead space of the normal angle piece and to provide a lightweight valve (Vale, 1959).

Recently attention has been focused on the potential hazards of contamination of the theatre atmosphere by anaesthetics. Several items of equipment have been devised to conduct these exhaled gases away from the theatre, or to absorb them by passing them over activated charcoal.

Resistance to air flow

The importance of unrestricted movement of gases through anaesthetic equipment and the patient's air passages cannot be over estimated. Of particular significance is the resistance offered to airflow through endotracheal tubes and their connectors. Straight connections offer the least resistance, and curved tubes considerably less than ones bent at a right angle: the radius of any bend should be 6–7 times that of the length of the connector. The resistance of a tube depends on the following factors:

volume of gas flow per unit time
viscosity and density of the gas
diameter and length of the tubing
the nature of the flow – varying or continuous, turbulent or laminar

Although patients under general anaesthetic have some ability to compensate for increased resistance to airflow, this should not be relied upon. Further, no external pressure on the chest wall and upper abdomen should be tolerated during normal anaesthesia, for the latter in particular may cause grave reduction in ventilation.

Anaesthetic circuits

Non-rebreathing circuits. These circuits, which employ uni-directional valves, ensure the inhalation of gas mixtures of unvarying composition and permit rapid washout of unwanted gas from the lungs (i.e. nitrogen): at the same time, rapid 'wash-in' occurs and therefore there is minimal impairment of uptake of the anaesthetic agent and induction of anaesthesia. The composition of the inspired gas is that which is displayed on the flowmeters and vaporizers. These circuits have the added attraction that they are simple and by carefully observing that the reservoir bag neither overfills nor empties whilst adjusting the flowmeters, the precise minute volume of the patient is known. They have the disadvantage that: they allow the inspiration of non-humidified gases; they tend to be noisy; the valves occasionally stick. A pressure limiting bag has been designed to overcome this difficulty when using the Ruben valve (Waters, 1967); the circuits are extremely wasteful of gases. The function of these valves has been admirably reviewed by Sykes (1959), Steen and Chen (1963), and Askrog *et al.* (1966).

Some of these valves can also be used during manually controlled ventilation. Here they are to be preferred to other circuits where carbon dioxide absorption is not employed as, ideally, loss from the circuit should occur during expiration and not inspiration. Certain valves have, however, been devised to allow spill during controlled ventilation and a miniature valve system has also been devised for automatic ventilation (see page 33). A comprehensive list and details of individual valves is published elsewhere (Mushin *et al.*, 1969). Bullough (1955) has used the circle absorber as a semi-closed circuit, with the soda lime turned off, the expiratory valve at the face open, a flow rate of fresh gases of 81 min^{-1}, and a clamp across the expiratory hosing near the face piece. With the Marrett apparatus the expiratory hosing is simply removed from the machine, the stopper inserted, and the hose reconnected.

Circuits with a fresh gas flow, which if great enough will flush out the expired gas before the ensuing inspiration (See Fig. 1) (Sykes, 1968)

The Magill attachment Mapleson A classification. In an ideal semi-closed system, such as Magill's, a total minute volume of fresh gases, equal to

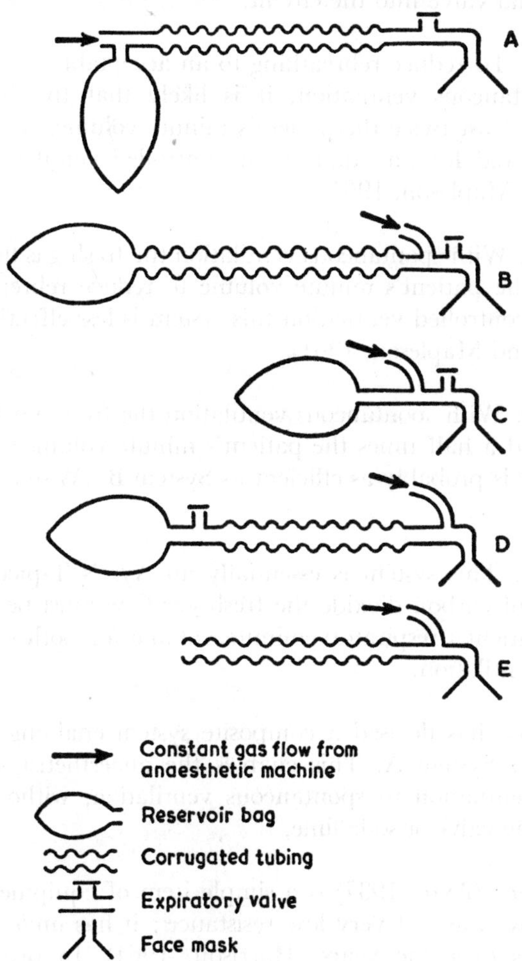

Fig. 1.1 Mapleson (1954) classification of anaesthetic circuits (courtesy of British Journal of Anaesthesia)

the patient's minute volume, will eliminate the rebreathing of expired gases containing carbon dioxide; it will also ensure delivery to the patient of a gas mixture containing oxygen in a concentration equal to that in the fresh gases entering the reservoir bag from the machine. However, Kain *et al.* (1967); Norman *et al.* (1968) have suggested that under certain circumstances carbon dioxide accumulation may not occur, even when the fresh gas flow is less than the minute volume. (The minimum fresh gas flow to prevent rebreathing may be as low as 70% of the patient's minute volume.) The Magill circuit should not be employed routinely for controlled ventilation, as rebreathing can only partially be prevented by very high gas flow, or, completely, by incorporating a uni-directional valve into the circuit.

Mapleson B. To reduce rebreathing to an acceptable level in this circuit, during spontaneous ventilation, it is likely that the fresh gas supply should be at least twice the patient's minute volume. A similar fresh gas flow is required for an adult when controlled ventilation is employed (Waters and Mapleson, 1961).

Mapleson C. With spontaneous ventilation the fresh gas flow should be at least twice the patient's minute volume to reduce rebreathing to a safe level. With controlled ventilation this system is less effective than System B. (Waters and Mapleson, 1961).

Mapleson D. With spontaneous ventilation the fresh gas flow must be at least two and a half times the patient's minute volume: with controlled ventilation it is probably as efficient as System B. (Waters and Mapleson, 1961).

Mapleson E. This system is essentially an Ayre's T-piece. For efficient elimination of carbon dioxide the fresh gas flow must be at least 2 to 2½ times the patient's respiratory minute volume for both spontaneous and controlled ventilation.

Waters (1961) has devised a composite system enabling a change from System D to System A. This enables the anaesthetist to change from controlled ventilation to spontaneous ventilation, without the use of a non-breathing valve or soda lime.

Ayre's T-piece (Ayre, 1937) is a simple item of equipment which offers the great advantage of very low resistance: it has undergone numerous modifications over the years (Harrison, 1964). In order to eliminate rebreathing with spontaneous ventilation, flows in excess of 2 to 2½ times the minute volume are necessary. With such a flow-rate, the volume of the reservoir tube should be at least $\frac{1}{3}$ of the tidal volume, and the diameter at least 1 cm in the neonate to 3–4 cm in the adult. With controlled ventilation volumes up to three times the minute volume, or more, may be necessary to prevent rebreathing, depending on the respiratory pattern and the rate of ventilation. The lung can be ventilated by a variety of methods; the end of the expiratory limb can be occluded with a finger, a bag can be attached (Rees, 1950), or a ventilator employed (Keuskamp, 1963). If a bag is used it should be separated from the patient by a tube with an internal volume which exceeds the patient's tidal volume, otherwise re-inhalation from the bag may occur (Sykes, 1968). The Ayre's T-piece has also been modified to reduce turbulence and resultant increase in resistance to breathing at the point of entry of the fresh gases (Deen, 1963). With a fresh gas flow of 120 ml/lb body weight/min (260 ml/kg body weight/min), and with a minimum flow of 3 l/min, carbon dioxide elimination from Ayre's T-piece system is satisfactory in children (Nightingale *et al.*, 1965). Where the Jackson Rees modification is employed the matter of carbon dioxide elimination is more complex.

It should be noted that the Mapleson A System has a marked advantage over the other semi-closed systems from the point of view of economy of gases. System E has a marked advantage over the others from the point of view of resistance to breathing. All the other systems involve the use of expiratory valves which impose an appreciable resistance to expiration, particularly when a large gas flow is used, as they will need to do in systems B, C and D.

Bullough (1952) has devised a system which employs the twin tubing of a circle system. The inspiratory limb is plugged into the reservoir bag on a continuous flow machine. The expiratory limb lies open to the atmosphere and the patient is connected up in the normal manner. In order to encourage adequate carbon dioxide elimination a flow of at least 8 l/min must be maintained; indeed, the reservoir bag must be distended before the onset of each inspiration.

Lee (1964) has described a combined T-piece and non-rebreathing valve, which utilizes both whilst eliminating the disadvantages.

Circuits which employ the use of absorbents for the elimination of carbon dioxide

These circuits are generally of the closed variety, and have certain disadvantages. A 'closed-circuit' originally meant just what it says, i.e. no gases are voided to the atmosphere, but are continuously re-cycled, the carbon dioxide being absorbed by soda lime, and only sufficient oxygen being added to replenish that used in metabolism. A small amount of anaesthetic gas or vapour is also added, to compensate for that lost from the brain by redistribution, loss from the skin and operation wound and in leaks from apparatus. In practice these losses are difficult to balance exactly, so that a slight surplus of oxygen and gases is used, with a compensatory valve 'blow-off'. In theory, therefore, there should be great economy of gases, retention of heat and moisture and minimal contamination of the theatre atmosphere by anaesthetic agents. It is estimated that a non-rebreathing system may result in the loss of 28 mg of water from the respiratory tract to every litre of dry inspired gas.

There is, however, the disadvantage that the elimination of carbon dioxide is not always efficient. Heavy and cumbersome equipment is often necessary, and although elimination of carbon dioxide occurs, rebreathing of other exhaled gases take place, thus leading to dilution of the fresh gas mixture; this results in prolonged uptake of anaesthetic agents with slow induction. The inspired concentration is thus not the same as that of the fresh inflow of gases and may be appreciably lower.

Carbon dioxide absorption is generally carried out by allowing granules of the absorbent to come into contact with the exhaled gas. The reaction is an exothermic one – 13 700 calories are produced for every mole (18 grams) of water formed. The absorbent commonly used is soda lime which is made up of 95% calcium hydroxide and 5% sodium hydroxide with the addition of silicates to prevent powdering. The size of the granules is of importance (the mesh size should be 4–8) because efficiency depends on the surface area of absorbent presenting to the reacting gas. Resistance to airflow, and the dead space between the granules are also dependent on their size. The moisture content is also of importance. Mixtures of barium and calcium hydroxide have been used. 'Baralyme', which is composed of 80% calcium hydroxide and 20% barium hydroxide, has an absorptive efficiency parallel to that of soda lime. Soda lime is often impregnated with dyes which change colour when the hydroxides are neutralized and converted to carbonates. It has been found however, that the physiological end point (i.e. the point when hypercarbia becomes intolerable to most patients), does not coincide with the chemical end point (i.e. the point at which the colour change occurs). Chemical indicators therefore, are on the whole unreliable, except where two canisters are connected in series; the only reliable way of determining whether the soda lime is exhausted is to monitor the carbon dioxide content of the circuit, but, despite simple colorimetric devices, this is not always practicable. The exothermic reaction is as follows:

$$Co_2 + 2NaOH \rightarrow H_2O + Na_2CO_3 + Heat$$
$$Na_2CO_3 + Ca(OH)_2 \rightarrow 2NaOH + CaCO_3$$

Small quantities of CO_2 are absorbed thus:

$$CO_2 + Ca(OH)_2 \rightarrow H_2O + CaCO_3 + \text{Heat}$$

Note that 1 gram of soda lime absorbs approximately 88 ml of carbon dioxide and a temperature of up to 60°C can be developed within the canisters. The surface of the soda lime rapidly becomes exhausted; there are pores, however, which penetrate into the interior and allow carbon dioxide to diffuse inwards. Even in apparent exhaustion there is still a nucleus of unused hydroxide ions in the centre, but 'resting' the soda lime allows fresh hydroxide ions to diffuse out and carbonate ions to diffuse even deeper. After a suitable interval the soda lime can be used again: at first the efficiency will be high, but this will rapidly fall away. Many types of equipment have been developed which incorporate carbon dioxide absorption in the closed circuit. These depend on providing adequate basal oxygen (approximately 300 ml/min) and maintaining an appropriate concentration of anaesthetic to produce the required level of anaesthesia.

The 'to and fro' canister. Waters (1926) noted the optimal size for a 'to and fro' canister stating that it should be 8 × 13 cm for the adult patient. The space between the granules should be approximately equal to the patient's tidal volume. In a to and fro canister the granules nearest the patient are rendered useless first; as this occurs the size of the dead space increases. Furthermore, if the canister is not tightly packed, (and particularly if it is also positioned horizontally), the gases tend to flow along the uppermost side of the canister and therefore carbon dioxide elimination becomes deficient. Compression of the granules by an ordinary pot-scourer can remedy this. It should be stressed that with the 'to and fro' system the anaesthetic gases are only in static contact with the soda lime for a very short period of the respiratory cycle (expiratory pause) and therefore the system is not as efficient as a true circle absorber. The efficiency can be improved, however, by permitting a high inflow of gases with a resultant leak from the circuit. The resistance of the to and fro circuit amounts to no more than 2–3 cm of water during normal quiet spontaneous ventilation.

Absorbers associated with a circle closed circuit apparatus. Not all these absorbers employ uni-directional flow through the soda lime. With uni-directional flow the expired gas is in static contact with the soda lime for the duration of inspiration; as a result, absorption is more efficient. With the to and fro circle system dead space is also likely to increase with duration of closed circuit anaesthesia. With a uni-directional system and a total gas flow of 7 l/min efficiency is at its optimum. However, this is an uneconomical way of using the equipment. As with the to and fro apparatus, normal, quiet breathing rarely produces a pressure exceeding

2–3 cm of water. The very real danger associated with the administration of trichloroethylene in relation to closed circuit anaesthesia and absorption of carbon dioxide with soda lime must be recognised. Nerve palsies, attributed to oxidation products formed by the interaction of soda lime with trichloroethylene, have occurred. Though the formation of these toxic substances can be greatly reduced by using high quality soda lime and restricting the heat and moisture content, it is to be strongly advised that trichloroethylene is never used in the presence of soda lime. Furthermore, great care should be taken when contemplating closed circuit anasthesia in obstetric cases to make sure that the mother has not had trichloroethylene and air administered during labour: in these cases trichloroethylene is excreted in the breath in sufficient quantities to react with soda lime, for some hours after inhalation has ceased.

It should be stressed that the employment of a carbon dioxide absorber in a closed circuit does not confer immunity from hypercapnia. Unless the patient's alveolar ventilation is normal, severe hypercapnia may go unrecognized because of the high oxygen concentrations in the circuit.

Flowmeters

The presentation to the patient of accurate concentrations of anaesthetic gases is clearly of importance both from the point of view of safety and for the maintainance of a stable anaesthetic state. The flow rate of gases to the patient may be metered in several ways.

Variable orifice flowmeters. With the variable orifice the pressure drop is constant despite the flowrate. These include the Coxeter Bobbin flowmeter, the Rotameter, the Heidbrink meter, and the Connell meter.

Fixed orifice flowmeters. Here the gas flows through a fixed orifice and the pressure drop across the orifice is taken as a measure of the flowmeter. These include pressure gauge meters, water depression meters and water sight meters.

All flowmeters are influenced by the viscosity and density of the gases flowing through them. Because the density of a gas is related to the atmospheric pressure, the performance of such flowmeters is significantly affected in hyperbaric conditions, and at high altitudes. The bobbin may tend to stick to the wall of certain flowmeters because of deposits in the glass tube or static electricity; this may be overcome by exposing the bobbin to a gamma radioactive source which ionizes the flowmeter, or using conducting materials or sprays. Static electricity may cause a flowmeter inaccuracy of 35%. It is possible to calibrate a rotameter over a range of 10 times, i.e. the lowest accurate reading will be one-tenth of a full scale measurement – c.f. nitrous oxide: maximum reading 10 l/min, minimum 1 l/min (Epstein and Hunter, 1968).

Reducing valves

Reducing valves are used by anaesthetists for three main reasons:

(1) Adjustment of the flowrate tap is made more easy.

(2) Once the flow of gas has been set for any particular level, frequent re-adjustment of the flowmeter controls are obviated.

(3) The pressure within the tubing on the patient's side of the reducing valve is limited and the transmission of an excessively high pressure thereby minimized.

It should be noted that reduction to 60 lbf/in^2 (4.15 $\times$ 10^{5}N/m^2 : 4.2 kp/cm^2) is found on some of the recent models of anaesthetic apparatus. The standard British equipment reduces pressure with the carbon dioxide cylinder 740 lbf/in^2 (5.1 $\times$ 10^{6}N/m^2 : 52.0 kp/cm^2); the nitrous oxide cylinder 700 lbf/in^2 (4.8 $\times$ 10^{6}N/m^2 : 49.2 kp/cm^2) and the oxygen cylinder approximately 1950 lbf/in^2 (1.4 $\times$ 10^7 N/m^2 : 137.1 kp/cm^2) to 4, 5, 10, 12 or 60 lbf/in^2, depending on the type of machine employed.

Pipe lines

It is more economical and convenient to have a central store of gases, usually in the liquid state, and a pipe line conveying them to the various outlet points as required. Although the ultimate responsibility for the correct working of the installation must remain with the engineer, the anaesthetist may wish to satisfy himself as to the nature of the gas which emerges from each outlet. Sophisticated equipment will be required for this purpose. A paramagnetic analyser (Beckman or Servomex) is at the moment available for the specific analysis of oxygen concentration. During the commissioning of a piped gas system it is advisable for any anaesthetist who may be concerned, to seek the guidance of his employing authority before involving himself. (The legal implications of medical practitioners concerning themselves in the commissioning of pipe lines has not at the time of writing been clearly defined.)

The supply of pre-mixed 50% nitrous oxide and 50% oxygen (Entonox) by a pipeline from a bank of modern 5000 litre cylinders fitted with internal tubes discharging concurrently is a safe and practical undertaking.

Intermittent flow machines

Intermittent gas flow machines at one time had widespread popularity because of the fact that conservation of gases was achieved. They not only found a place in dental and obstetric anaesthetic and analgesic practice, but also in general surgical anaesthesia. Much attention has recently been focused on the inaccuracies of these machines, particularly older models. The BOC Walton Mark V, the Cyprane AE and the McKesson Anaesthesor or Simplor are the ones with which anaesthetists are most familiar. The Walton Mark V and the Cyprane AE would appear to be the more reliable (Nainby-Luxmore, 1967). Recent developments have favoured continuous rather than intermittent flow for dental out patient anaesthesia.

Ideally, intermittent flow machines should have a safety device which automatically cuts off the nitrous oxide, should the oxygen supply fail. (The BOC Walton Mark V and the AE Gas-Oxygen (optional extra) machines incorporate such a device). An automatic air inspiratory valve and a nitrous oxide failure warning are also desirable features. There should be a built-in relief valve set to prevent pressures in excess of 50 cm water reaching the patient. The machine must be accurate in the concentrations it delivers even when working with tidal volumes in excess of one litre, and in the range of 7.5–20 l/min of minute volume.

Vaporizers

Certain of the inhalational agents used for general anaesthesia exist in part as a liquid at room temperature and pressure. In order to induce and maintain general anaesthesia, well defined concentrations of vapours or gases are required in the inspired mixture. Inaccurate concentrations of agents presented to the patient may well prove lethal, particularly if potent drugs such as chloroform or halothane are to be employed. Reference to Table 2.1 will give some guide to the concentrations required for general anaesthesia.

Table 2.1 *Concentration of inhalational agents for general anaesthesia*

Agent	*Induction*	*Maintenance*
chloroform	up to 4%	0·5–1·5%
diethyl ether	up to 20%	3·5%
halothane	up to 3·5% (approx)	0·5–2·5%
trichloroethylene	0·5–2·0%	0·35–0·5%*
methoxyflurane	up to 1·5%	0·5% or less*

* analgesia

These figures are only approximations but give a rough guide as to the individual specifications of the vaporizers. Other factors must of course be considered; such as the physical status of the patient, the alveolar ventilation, cardiac output, and the presence or absence of shunting of blood past the lungs. Increased alveolar ventilation will increase the speed of induction of anaesthesia, decreased alveolar ventilation, or increased 'shunting' may lead to a prolongation of induction. The anaesthetist should bear these factors in mind when inducing anaesthesia in subjects where these factors are likely to be disturbed (e.g. hypovolaemia with associated low cardiac output).

The degree of ease with which the concentrations listed above can be achieved at room temperature with simple equipment is dependent upon the saturated vapour pressure at room temperature of each agent (Table 2.2).

Table 2.2 *Saturated vapour pressures of inhalational agents at room temperature*

Agent	*Boiling point* (°C)	*Saturated vapour pressure at* 20°C (mmHg)	*Saturated vapour concentration at* 20°C (v/v)
chloroform	61·2	160	20
diethyl ether	34·6	460	60
halothane	50·2	240	32
trichloroethylene	87·1	60	8
methoxyflurane	105	30	4 (at 25°C)

Air saturated with chloroform at room temperature contains 20% chloroform, a percentage very much higher than the 4% maximum that it is justified to use for induction purposes. With halothane, which has a saturated vapour pressure of approximately one third of an atmosphere, it is also necessary to dilute the saturated vapour with gas approximately eight to thirty times. On the other hand, methoxyflurane has an extremely low volatility and therefore the concentration necessary for induction purposes is not readily achieved unless a highly efficient vaporizer is employed: the low volatility together with the high blood solubility of methoxyflurane leads to a prolonged induction. The vaporizer must therefore not only be highly efficient, but must also deliver accurate concentration of agents under conditions of widely varying flow and temperature. As liquid evaporates the temperature tends to fall with consequent reduction in the concentration of the vapour. The standard Boyle bottle was used for as a vaporizer and suffered the severe disadvantage of temperature fall, although attempts were often made to maintain the temperature by placing warm water in a container placed around the bottle. Temperature compensation in its simplest form is seen in the Oxford vaporizer which relies upon the latent heat of crystallization of calcium chloride. More recently, vaporizers have contained sophisticated temperature compensating devices, such as the bimetallic strip or bellows. In order to overcome the effects of altitude, the bellows are now no longer filled with air, but liquid with a high coefficient of expansion, such as alcohol.

The Gardiner vaporizer. This is a versatile temperature compensated vaporizer which can be used for a variety of anaesthetic agents.

The EMO vaporizer. In its basic form, the Epstein Macintosh Oxford (EMO) vaporizer requires no medical gases; it is easily portable and robust. Automatic compensation for changes of temperature ensures that the vapour concentration that reaches the patient remains constant. Resistance to breathing is less than 12 cm of water at a constant flow rate of 40 litres per minute. The EMO vaporizer delivers consistently accurate pre-determined concentration of vapour under a wide range of conditions of flow, depth and rate of respiration, and ambient temperature; together with an inflating bellows it can be used for controlled ventilation using muscle relaxants. There is the danger of high concentrations being achieved if the inflating device is not placed between the vaporizer and the patient. The vaporizing chamber is surrounded by a jacket which, when filled with water at room temperature, serves as a buffer against extreme changes in ambient temperature. Concentrations of ether in air of up to 20% can be achieved. An EMO has also been developed for the use with halothane, which, because of the fact that it attacks a large variety of metals, needs to be constructed of special material. The vaporizer, which may be used for the azeotropic mixture of halothane and ether, is calibrated to deliver 0–2.6% of 1.3% azeotropic mixture. EMO vaporizers can also be supplied for trichloroethylene, chloroform, and methoxyflurane.

The Bryce-Smith induction unit. This unit is for use with a draw-over inhaler such as the EMO and overcomes the respiratory difficulties of ether induction. It is free of controls and is operative immediately it is charged. Approximately 3 ml of halothane are poured into the well surmounting the unit; the wick container is removed, inverted and allowed to stand in the liquid halothane for the few seconds necessary for complete absorption; then the wick container is replaced and the induction unit connected to the outlet port of the EMO inhaler. The mask is lowered on to the patient's face and as there are no on/off controls the patient will be breathing halothane/air and unconsciousness reached in 30 seconds. The EMO lever is now set at 2% and progressively advanced until 15–20% ether is reached in $3\frac{1}{2}$–4 minutes. Ether increases should be by increments of 2%, each increase being accompanied by a pause of 4 to 5 breaths without coughing or breath-holding. By the time 15–20% ether is attained the halothane will be exhausted.

The Oxford miniature vaporizer (OMV) is designed primarily for halothane, but other volatile anaesthetics may also be used. It is designed for short period use, its capacity being small in order to minimize wastage of the residual liquid.

Drager Vapor. The Vapor vaporizer operates on a wide range of gas flows of 0.3 to 12 l/min, precision being controlled by two valves of special design – a by-pass valve and a concentration valve. The output concentration of halothane can be accurately set at between 0.3% and 5% v/v and constant vaporization temperature is achieved by the use of an accurately dimensioned copper block surrounding the vaporization chamber. The high thermal conductivity of the copper supplies the latent heat necessary for the vaporization process, and keeps the liquid halothane temperature constant for long periods whether the gas flow is steady or intermittent. The vaporizer incorporates a unique alternating pressure compensator which accurately maintains the 'set calibration' of the vaporizer: the effects of pressure fluctuations are completely obviated. The Vapor can be supplied for use with ether giving concentrations of 2% to 20% v/v.

Halothane PDV and Penthrane PDV. The PDV (Penlon-draw-over-vaporizer), is an accurate, temperature compensated vaporizer, which, like the OMV, is surrounded by a water jacket, to compensate against extreme temperature changes. It can be used for draw-over purposes, or with a continuous flow of gases.

Abingdon vaporizers are thermo-compensated, with good flow rate characteristics: types are available for use with ether, halothane and methoxyflurane.

Drip feed. Hart (1958) has devised a simple drip feed for halothane, based on the principle that 1 ml of liquid halothane produces 227 ml of vapour at 20°C. If a gas flow of 10 litres is applied with a drip rate of 60 drops/minute (1 ml liquid equals 120 drops), 1% halothane will result.

In order to increase further the efficiency of vaporizers, copper sinks and wicks have been employed, not only to provide a reserve of heat, but also to increase the surface area of the liquid exposed to the carrier gas. In practice, modern calibrated vaporizers consist of a reservoir of saturated vapour and a control for varying the concentrations.

The copper kettle allows a precise and fine control of concentrations and moderate thermostability, with a reserve of heat provided by the use of a copper table top. It relies upon the metering of a variable but separate flow of carrier gas, allowing it to pass through a sintered bronze disc placed within a copper container. The carrier gas bubbles through the liquid anaesthetic and is subsequently mixed with known volumes of diluent gas. This vaporizer can be used for chloroform, ether, halothane, but has the serious disadvantage that the concentration cannot be read directly, as a calculation has to be made in terms of the relative flow of gases from the vaporizer and diluent. This can, however, be determined by the use of a table, which incorporates a knowledge of the vapour pressure of the anaesthetic in use, the temperature of the vaporizing oxygen and the flow rate of the diluent. In practice, it is easier to handle than at first appears, because the final concentration is always modified according to the patient's requirements. The Halox is an English version of this principle. The copper kettle can be classified as a 'by-pass' vaporizer, whereas the PDV, Fluotec III, Pentec, Halothane 4, 2 or 10, Trilene 1.5, Ether 20, Penthrane 1.5, Cyprane and Gardiner vaporizers are 'divergent flow' vaporizers. With these vaporizers the main flow of gases by-passes the vaporizing chamber when the dial is turned to the off position. When the dial is opened a varying proportion of fresh gas flow can be diverted through the vaporizing chamber. The Fluotec Mark III and Pentec Mark II vaporizers are independent of flow rate, temperature variation, duration of use and pressure fluctuations due to the use of ventilators or assisted ventilation. Excess thymol residues no longer cause the controls to seize (see below).

The Goldman Vaporizer is not temperature compensated and thus will suffer a fall in concentration as the temperature of the liquid falls. Wicks of blotting paper placed in the container can greatly improve the performance of the vaporizer. In order to overcome some of these disadvantages, Goldman has introduced a new vaporizer which is essentially a pressurized version of the Vapor or Halox vaporizer. Vaporization occurs within a gas pressure of 60 lb/in^2 (4.15 $\times$ 10 N/m^2). As a result there is little change in vol.% of halothane with change in temperature, rates of flow, and altitude. Concentrations of 3.0% v/v halothane can be obtained with rates of gas flow up to 5 1/min.

The effects of back pressure upon the performance of vaporizers. The effect of intermittent positive pressure on the output of a vaporizer in a closed circuit system (the vaporizer being outside the circle), is to produce a higher concentration from a Fluotec vaporizer than would be expected from the vaporizer setting. A valve has been devised for the use of Fluotec Mark II vaporizer to overcome the pressure fluctuation transmitted to the vaporizer. (The Fluotec Mark III has such a mechanism incorporated within it.) On the other hand (Cole, 1966) it is found that with the Manley and Barnet ventilators, the concentration output of the Fluotec Mark II is less than that expected from the dial setting. This apparent difference is thought to be due to the lower mean pressures, the intermittent application of pressure, and the low flowrates, employed when using the closed circuit. The build-up in anaesthetic concentration when a circle system with carbon dioxide absorption is employed depends upon many factors, amongst which the position of the vaporizer (in or outside the circle) is of major importance.

Deposits of thymol in halothane vaporizers. Thymol, which is added as a stabilizer in 0.01% concentration in halothane, being of low volatility, tends to accumulate in vaporizers if they are not periodically emptied, crystallizing on the thermocompensating device and interfering with the correct working of the vaporizer. It is of the greatest importance that the vaporizers are serviced at least once per year, and allowed to run low once per week, the residues being discarded.

Humidification

Endotracheal intubation by-passes the warming and humidifying mechanisms of the upper respiratory tract; consequently inhalation of dry gases from cylinders, or even from the atmosphere, will lead to drying and crusting of secretions within the tracheobronchial tree. The exposure of the respiratory mucosa to the dry gases delivered by most anaesthetic machines may cause severe changes such as hyperaemia, excess mucus, and diminished ciliary action. 28 mg of water may be lost from the respiratory tract for every litre of dry inspired gas, and clearly closed circuit equipment should be employed, or some form of humidification used for any case where dry gases are inspired for any length of time. When the gases are properly humidified (50–75% relative humidity at body temperature), and by-pass the nasal passages by endotracheal intubation, no adverse effects occur except in the region of the inflated cuff, where ciliary action is stopped. The simplest method of providing moisture, to prevent inspiration and crusting in the tracheo-bronchial tree, is to moisten the tubing and reservoir bag of the system. Equipment which ensures near saturation of inspired air at body temperature prevents drying of mucous membrane and loosens and liquefies previously thickened or dried mucus.

Of particular value in the management of tracheostomies is a blower humidifier (East-Radcliffe) which will produce a relative humidity in excess of 90% at 32°C under normal environmental conditions. Hot water humidifiers are also available to be used in conjunction with ventilators (e.g. Cape-Waine). The elevation of the water bath temperature to 50°C will not only ensure a high humidity in the inspired gas, but it will also exert a bacteriostic effect.

A condenser-humidifier can substantially increase the water content of inspired gas, although it cannot return any more water that the subject expires: they have, however, the advantage that little condensation occurs in valves or meters.

Herzog and Norlander (1964) have described their clinical experience with ultrasonic humidification. Using an ultrasonic aerosol generator they have been able to produce particle sizes from 0.8–1.0 μm, making superhumidification possible, with a water content in the inspired gas of 240 g/m^2 as contrasted with the saturated amount of 44 g/m^2 at 37°C. Great caution is necessary because of the danger of the introduction or large quantities of water into the lungs.

It cannot be overstressed that full sterilization of such equipment is essential between all cases. The possibility that *Ps. pyocyaneus* acquired from the air might multiply in a vapour condenser humidifier must be considered. It would seem that there is little danger from aerially acquired *Ps. pyocyaneus,* if the condenser humidifier is changed every three hours.

Portable apparatus

From time to time the anaesthetist may be called upon to administer a general anaesthetic in situations where adequate equipment is not readily available. In its simplest form the equipment should consist of a chloroform bottle with dropper and a Schimmelbusch mask. However, many of these situations arise in relation to emergency work and ideally oxygen should be procurable. Certainly, a means of applying suction to clear debris from the respiratory tract is essential, and, failing a supply of oxygen, some means of inflating the lungs artificially. A laryngoscope and a selection of endotracheal tubes are essential items and many portable items have been devised (Boulton, 1966), Stephens (1965), Merrifield *et al.* (1967). The Haloxair allows for the administration of halothane and air, with enrichment with oxygen if required: controlled ventilation, with or without the addition of oxygen, can also be carried out. Another similar item of equipment, the Porta Blease has been evaluated by Merrifield *et al.* (1967).

In its simplest form, a vaporizer may take the form of the Flagg can – a modification of this can be made with a simple glass jar (Boulton, 1966). Trichloroethylene, in particular, can be employed using the Flagg can, and because of its relatively high boiling point, stability in the concentration of trichloroethylene vapour can be readily achieved. In addition, because of its cheapness and non-inflamability it has attractions for use in the emergency situation. The CON apparatus employs a single dose non-explosive mixture of cyclopropane, oxygen and nitrogen, and enables, on one charge of the apparatus from 'sparklets', a duration of anaesthesia of approximately 4 minutes. More sophisticated apparatus can include vaporizers which are temperature compensated. The EMO inhaler, being a draw-over inhaler with facilities for artificial ventilation, is particularly suitable for this type of work. The OMV or Bryce-Smith induction unit facilitates the induction of ether anaesthesia by means of halothane. Care should, however, be taken when employing controlled ventilation to see that the bellows, e.g. the Ambu Bag or Oxford Bellows, lie between the patient and the vaporizer in order to avoid giving high concentrations of vapour to the patient.

Artificial ventilation. In emergency situations this can be readily performed by mouth to mouth ventilation provided that general anaesthesia is not required. Such a method of ventilation can be greatly facilitated by using a special airway such as the Brook, or applying the mouth to a face mask. During anaesthesia manual ventilation using an Ambu Bag, Cardiff or Oxford Bellows, or mechanical ventilation using a portable ventilator, may be necessary.

Vellore ventilator. This machine made by Penlon is useful for ward work but rather inconvenient for theatre use. Power is obtained from compressed air at 1–2 lb/in^2 derived from a cylinder or compressor; it has variable speed and is volume cycled with a variable inspiratory/expiratory ratio.

East-Radcliffe M2 or B2 ventilator. This machine is suitable for both ward and theatre work. A time-cycled constant pressure generator, it has a variable inspiratory/expiratory ratio, is driven by either mains (a.c.) or battery motor and has a single speed. When used with an inflating valve (East magnetic valve supplied), it can be used with a draw-over vaporizer.

Cape Minor ventilator can be used for ward or theatre work. It has a built-in single speed ac motor (15 rev/min) and, being a time cycled flow generator, the inspiratory/expiratory time increases with tidal volume. It uses an inflating valve and can be employed as a minute volume divider with draw-over vaporizers.

Miniature ventilators

Several small portable ventilators have been designed for use during the administration of anaesthesia, to supply automatic, intermittent, positive pressure, ventilation to apnoeic patients.

The Carden Microvent has these characteristics: variable volume 50 to 1000 ml; variable inflation pressure; full control of inspiratory/expiratory ratio; very small dead space; allows spontaneous ventilation (Carden, 1969).

The Cohen Minivent (Cohen, 1966) can be used with any nitrous oxide and oxygen machine having flow meters and reservoir bag. Its method of action is such that a positive pressure is permitted to build up in the reservoir bag, and this pressure is intermittenly released to the patient's lungs during inflation.

The screwing of a knurled control knob outwards will increase the ratio of ventilation. The minute volume being delivered to the patient may be read directly from the flow meters of the anaesthetic machine.

The East Freeman Automatic-Vent operates by using the resilience of the normal reservoir bag on the anaesthetic machine and the volume to be delivered is set directly on the flow meters. By adjusting a magnetic ring the rate of ventilation can be altered.

The Mitchell-East Magnetic-Poi. The operation of this valve (Mitchell and Epstein, 1966) is controlled by two magnets set in opposition, and is actuated by the pressure built up in the reservoir bag.

Lung ventilators

The indications for the use of automatic ventilators include the following:

- controlled ventilation during anaesthesia
- prolonged respiratory control in complete or severe respiratory insufficiency, arising spontaneously or induced by treatment
- prolonged (assisted) ventilation with patient triggering in partial respiratory insufficiency
- ventilation in respiratory insufficiency of the newborn
- ventilatory assistance during the transportation of patients with respiratory insufficiency

The majority of ventilators available to the anaesthetist operate by applying an intermittent pressure, in excess of atmospheric pressure, to the tracheo-bronchial tree. A sub-atmospheric pressure is occasionally applied during the expiratory phase of ventilation, and under these circumstances the 'expiratory reserve volume' (ERV) may be encroached upon.

The design and performance of ventilators have been considered by many workers. On the whole, classifications have been unsatisfactory, for any attempt to classify them according to whether they are time-cycled, pressure-cycled, or volume-cycled overlooks the importance of the ability of the machine to compensate for changes in compliance, or leaks from the apparatus. An important group of ventilators consists of machines in which the minute volume is one of the most assigned parameters. Such machines are termed 'minute volume dividers'. Regardless of the manipulation of the other controls, these machines deliver the assigned minute volume. Usually it is determined by the output of gas from an anaesthetic machine or the output from the air compressor. Minute volume dividers cannot compensate for leaks in the circuit.

In choosing a pulmonary ventilator, the anaesthetist must first decide what he requires the ventilator to do. The machine should be capable of delivering tidal volumes in the range of 200–1000 ml for adults, and down to as little as 30 ml for small children. The expired volume should be capable of being measured. The upper range of rate of ventilation should be about 40 cycles per minute in the case of the neonate : and the lower, 10–15 cycles per minute in the case of the adult. The inspiratory phase should consist of a period of inspiratory flow followed by as brief an inspiratory pause as possible. The duration of the inspiratory phase should be capable of variation between 0.5 s and 3.0 s, but it should be as short as possible in order to reduce the mean intrathoracic pressure. However, a relatively long inspiratory time (1.0–1.5 s) permits better distribution of gas and better mixing. The inspiratory flow rate should be such that high instantaneous or peak flow rates are achieved, so allowing the inflation of the lungs to take place during a short inspiratory phase. Peak flow rates of 100 l/min are ideal, but peak rates of 80 l/min are adequate. The expiratory phase consists of a period during which the lung is exhausted of gases: expiration should commence immediately after the required tidal volume has entered the lungs. Under normal circumstances an inspiration/expiration ratio of $\frac{1}{2}$–$\frac{1}{3}$ will be satisfactory. The amount of resistance to expiration should not normally exceed 2 cm water at a flow rate of 0.5 l/s, under certain circumstances (e.g. respiratory distress syndrome), or else the mean intrathoracic pressure will be raised. If a sub-atmospheric phase is provided this should be controllable, with pressure down to minus 10 cm water. A sudden application of negative pressure will decrease lung compliance and increase dead space. Large sub-atmospheric pressures are believed to produce narrowing of the bronchi and increased expiratory resistance. Furthermore, increased venous admixture may also arise from collapse of smaller airways. Opinion is divided as to whether indeed there is any advantage in employing a negative phase at all. Patient-triggered inspiration is sometimes called for, particularly during the difficult phase of 'weaning' patients off the ventilator. The trigger mechanism must be variable in its sensitivity and capable of over-riding control so as to allow automatic ventilation should the patient fail to trigger the machine. Should this occur it is essential that the normal time-cycling device should operate.

All machines should be so designed that accidental high pressure build-up cannot occur. If they rely on an extraneous source of power, there should be the facility to ventilate the patient by hand should the supply fail. If the machines are to be used for theatre work, particular attention should be paid to insulation and isolation of any electrical circuits, so that they can be guaranteed free from the risk of explosion. They should be as simple as possible, small and light in weight, and easy to sterilize. Light-weight portable ventilators suitable for anaesthesia and supportive therapy have been devised for use in emergency and difficult circumstances (see page 33).

The majority of patients compensate surprisingly well for the rise in the mean intrathoracic pressure during IPPV (intermittent positive pressure ventilation). They respond by an increase of peripheral venous blood pressure which restores the driving pressure for venous flow, so that the cardiac output returns to previous values. This venoconstrictive reaction requires a responsive sympathetic nervous system which may be absent following an epidural anaesthetic, or the administration of a ganglion blocking agent or a cervical cord transection, and in patients suffering a reduction of blood volume.

New ventilators are continuously being introduced and modifications made to existing ones. For details of their characteristics and working mechanism reference should be made to the standard work by Mushin *et al.* (1969) and to manufacturers' specifications.

Sterilization of equipment

The anaesthetist should develop the habit of keeping his anaesthetic machine clean and uncontaminated by used endotracheal tubes, airways, suction catheters, and dirty syringes. All equipment which has been used on a patient should be segregated from the clean and disposed of by the theatre attendant or nurse. Some anaesthetists will keep the top shelf of their anaesthetic machines clear for 'clean' and employ the bottom shelf for 'dirty'.

Certain items of equipment will require to be cleaned and sterilized between cases. Masks, tubes, laryngoscopes, and other equipment coming into contact with the patient's skin or mucous membrane, should be sterilized after use and stored under clean, if not sterile conditions and handled with as much attention to asepsis as possible. Equipment such as airways, endotracheal tubes, and other equipment used within the patient's respiratory tract should be autoclaved; Y-pieces, angle-pieces and endotracheal mounts should be boiled or autoclaved after use; corrugated tubing, reservoir bags and Water's canisters should be autoclaved daily and circle absorbers sterilized at regular intervals. With a known infective case the circle absorber is best avoided and the Water's canister used in preference. Masks are prone to damage by autoclaving or boiling, and are often treated either by thorough washing with soap and water followed by immersion in a bowl of water at 60°–70°C for two minutes or, following washing, immersed in 0.1% chlorhexidine or 2% aqueous activated dialdehyde solution (Cidex) for half an hour. Although autoclaving markedly shortens the life of endotracheal tubes and airways, it is suggested that endotracheal tubes should be sterilized by autoclaving between cases, and discarded after approximately six uses. Numerous pathogenic organisms have been cultured from anaesthetic machines though *Pseudomonas pyocyaneus* has never been detected from within a soda lime canister. Anaesthetic machines should be sprayed down with 1% chlorhexidine in alcohol and all cylinders washed down with Lysol prior to being brought into the theatre. Expensive endotracheal tubes and blockers may be sterilized by ethylene oxide.

Ethylene oxide in the non-explosive mixture of 10% in 90% carbon dioxide (preferably under pressure) may be used for the sterilization of bulky equipment that cannot be exposed to autoclaving or high pressure steam without deterioration. Heart-lung machines can be handled in this way, but it is difficult to control the variables associated with ethylene oxide sterilization: it has good penetrating powers, but it is extremely toxic and has to be handled with very great care as it may cause pulmonary oedema. Where possible it is better to employ pre-sterilized disposable equipment for perfusion work. Ethylene oxide/carbon dioxide mixture has been used for the sterilization of ventilators. Using a large Terylene bag proofed with Neoprene the machine is allowed to cycle for up to 24 hours, either with the machine within the bag or by ventilating in and out of the bag: indicator devices are sometimes used to control the sterilization. A non-explosive mixture of ethylene oxide and freon has also been used for the sterilization of anaesthetic equipment, but as ethylene oxide is highly soluble in rubber and plastic materials the machines should be thoroughly ventilated with air before use. Humidified ethylene oxide under pressure is more effective for sterilization. Plastic should be aerated for at least 48 hours, and rubber 72 hours, before coming into contact with a patient. However, until ventilators can be developed which permit the separation of the patient's breathing circuit, this method of sterilization is only available for those of the smaller ventilators which can be effectively sterilized by placing them in the chamber of the sterilizing apparatus. It would appear unwise to vent the gas into the hospital vacuum system.

Formaldehyde. Another method which has been employed for the sterilization of ventilators is the use of formaldehyde. This may be used either by 'boiling' formalin solution in the humidifier whilst cycling the machine (Sykes, 1964) or combining low pressure steam with formaldehyde in an autoclave chamber (Whitby, 1970).

Nebulized alcohol or hydrogen peroxide. Nebulized alcohol in nitrogen and hydrogen peroxide have recently been introduced for the sterilization of ventilators and humidifiers. Particular size is of importance and nebulization may be achieved either by using an ultrasonic nebulizer (such as the MNE, DeVilbiss, or Monaghan apparatus) or a gas driven nebulizer (Harlow) (Robinson, 1970).

Sterilization of local anaesthetic agents. It is essential to sterilize the outside of containers for local anaesthetic agents which are employed for spinal subarachnoid or epidural work. On no account should the ampoules be placed in a sterilizing solution such as carbolic acid, as there is a very real danger of sterilizing solution entering the ampoule should there be a flaw in the glass. It has been shown that formalin vapour is effective for the sterilization of the outside of ampoules after one hour's exposure but slight traces can be found within the ampoule if cracked.

To avoid contamination of solutions, autoclaving is the only reliable way to ensure sterilization. Autoclaving at 19 lb/in^2 (1.3 kp/cm^2) pressure at 260°–270°C for three hours does not reduce the potency of amethocaine, procaine, or nupercaine crystals, and chlorprocaine, mepivacaine, lignocaine, or hexycaine solutions. Repeated autoclaving of 1.5% and 2% lignocaine containing 1 :200 000–1 :50 000 adrenaline does not alter the potency or pH.

Ventilators. In order to overcome the disadvantage of sterilization with ethylene or formalin, heated or siliconized filters have been devised to sterilize the inspired and expired air during intermittent positive pressure ventilation. The dry filters will remove pathogenic organisms from the inspired air to a diameter of 0.5 μm, with an efficiency of 99.9%, thus ensuring complete sterility from airborne bacteria. In order to prevent contamination of the surrounding atmosphere a filter must also be supplied to the expiratory port. Unless the filter is heated or treated with silicone, condensation of water vapour on the expiratory side will reduce its efficiency.

Disposable items. Many of the materials used by anaesthetists today have been sterilized by being subjected to gamma irradiation, and are not suitable for re-sterilization after use. Care must be taken that the packages have not been damaged, or sterility would then be suspect.

'British Standards'. The British Standards Institution publishes among its British Standards a number which are directly concerned with apparatus for anaesthesia. The review of these by E. K. Hillard will still provide a useful account of them (Hillard, 1968).

3 *Management of Anaesthesia*

Prior to the commencement of the operating list, the anaesthetist must allow ample time to select and meticulously check all apparatus and drugs. It must never be assumed that the anaesthetic machine and such items of equipment as the laryngoscope are serviceable, and the responsibility as to their reliability rests with the anaesthetist and no one else.

Anaesthesia should not be induced until the anaesthetist has satisfied himself that the patient is the one that he has seen on his pre-operative visit for this operation, that consent for the operation and anaesthesia is signed (see page 435) and the premedication has been administered.

Intravenous induction agents

Thiopentone (Pentothal, Intraval). This should be freshly prepared by dissolving the powder in distilled water; the 2.5% rather than the 5% solution should be used as it is less likely to produce severe damage to tisues in the event of extravenous injections. An induction dose of 4–8 mg/kg, in the fit adult is usually employed, but the dose must be gauged on the response of the subject to the initial 2–4 ml. Increase in depth and frequency of ventilation is found with the first few breaths during the induction of anaesthesia with thiopentone, especially when a respiratory depressant has been used in the pre-medication. This increase in amplitude is usually followed by a decrease. The initial respiratory effect is thought to be due to the passage of the alkaline bolus of thiopentone through the carotid chemoreceptors. It must be remembered that thiopentone is a potent myocardial depressant and vasodilator and great care must be excercised when using it in cardio-vascular disease or oligaemic states. Increased sensitivity to thiopentone in dystrophia myotonica has been reported and it should be avoided in cases of porphyria.

Thiopentone anaphylaxis. Several cases have been reported of anaphylaxis occurring in relation to the injection of thiopentone. There are several salient features about these cases: they have occurred in subjects who have received multiple general anaesthetics; often there is a history of adverse reactions to oral barbiturates; the clinical picture is characterized by peripheral circulatory failure, respiratory distress, prolonged unconsciousness, and sometimes skin manifestations. However, there is usually a rapid return to normal, and treatment should be directed towards respiratory and circulatory support along the conventional lines.

Methohexitone (Brietal). The solution is prepared by mixing the powder in distilled water and can be kept for a few days in refrigerated conditions. A 1% solution is usually employed but 2% has been used : in view of the narrow safety margin and the increased risk of thrombophlebitis the 5% solution cannot be recommended. In 1% solution it is said to be less irritant to the tissues than 2.5% thiopentone but methohexitone should be avoided in subjects with an epileptic diathesis and known porphyria. The average induction dose for the fit adult varies from 1 mg–1.5 mg/kg. Ventilation is often transiently depressed during induction, the degree of depression being a function of the rate of injection. This agent is often employed for outpatient anaesthesia, but it is doubtful whether it should be used for the maintenance of anaesthesia.

Propanidid (Epontol). This is available as a 5% solution. The adult dose varies from 5–7 mg/kg and in children the dose is 7–8 mg/kg but in the frail or elderly patient the dose should be reduced to 4–5 mg/kg, the solution being diluted to half-strength with normal saline. Induction is associated with hyperpnoea, which may be followed by a period of apnoea. Though a useful induction agent for outpatient and day cases in particular, propanidid is unsuitable as the sole agent for the maintenance of anaesthesia. The period of narcotic activity is extremely short, but because of its rapid clearance from the body it does not potentiate the action of alcohol and therefore can be recommended as an agent of choice in patients who are alcohol dependent. It does potentiate the action of suxamethonium, prolonging the action slightly. Sudden and unexpected cardio-vascular collapse has been reported, which can give rise to great concern.

Hydroxydione (Viadril, Pressuren). This substance is a synthetic steroid, a white crystalline solid, freely soluble in water, and with potent narcotic action. In doses normally employed, it can cause deep sleep in from three to twenty minutes according to the rate of injection. It is given intravenously in doses of 0.5–1.0 g according to the age and condition of the patient; a rapid injection of 5–10% hydroxydione in procaine (0.25–0.5%) lessens the incidence of venous complications. Analgesia is poor and the agent usually requires supplementing with analgesics or general anaesthetic agents. Depression of ventilation is minimal, but with excessive dosage can occur. The laryngeal reflex is depressed and there is often an appreciable fall in blood pressure. However, the main disadvantage is the slow onset of action and slow recovery rate. This agent is no longer freely available.

Chlormethiazole (Heminevrin). This substance when given intravenously in a 0.8% solution, quickly induces a sleep which is initially rather deep, and may be accompanied by muscle relaxation, disappearance of reflexes and marked meiosis: after 5–10 minutes this passees into a condition remarkably like physiological sleep. The patient can be awakened whenever required, and neither analgesia nor anaesthesia are present if moderate doses are given, but there is amnesia even after violent reactions to painful stimuli. It may have a place in obstetrics and in the treatment of status epilepticus.

Gamma-hydroxy-butyric acid (Gamma-OH). This is a derivative of gamma-amino-butyric acid, found in the central nervous system. Gamma-OH when given intravenously in a dose of 70 mg/kg, produces unconsciousness in 10–15 minutes, the time being less if a heavy premedication has been given: its duration of effect is about one to one and a half hours. Although pharyngeal and laryngeal reflexes are usually present, analgesia and unconsciousness permit a satisfactory state for procedures such as cardiac catheterization. Because clonic movements of the limbs sometimes complicate induction, thiopentone can be given to cover the first 5–10 minutes whilst the action of the drug is becoming established. Untoward psychic disturbances have been reported in the post-operative period though these are not nearly so severe as with 'Sernyl' (phencylidine: CI 395). Gamma-OH produces a state of dissociation from the surroundings, with analgesia, but if the incidence of hallucinations and other post-operative psychotic effects, proves to be high, its potentiality may not be achieved.

Ketamine (Ketalar). This is a drug related to phencylidine and has many of the acceptable properties of that drug without, apparently, the severe side effects. 1.0–2.0 mg/kg, may be given intravenously and produces analgesia and unconsciousness within one minute that lasts for 5–10 minutes, or it may be given intramuscularly in a dose of 6.5–13.0 mg/kg. There is usually some slight ventilatory depression, and occasionally mild hypertension associated with tachycardia. Unfortunately, like Gamma-OH and phencylidine, dreams have been reported, though perhaps not so severe as with phencylidine; but it is claimed that the tendency to such dreams is significantly reduced by attention to premedication and allowing the patient to recover from the effects of the drug without being disturbed. The drug would appear to be useful in plastic surgery and possibly for children. Ketamine should be avoided in the hypertensive patient.

Althesin. This steroid anaesthetic agent, a mixture of two pregnanediones, appears to have the merits of hydroxydione and the barbiturates without their disadvantages. When injected intravenously it produces immediate induction of anaesthesia of short duration, which is characterized by a rise in respiratory rate and pulse rate, with a slight fall in systolic and diastolic pressure. It has a high therapeutic ratio and is free from vascular irritation effects, even when injected intra-arterially in the experimental animal. Because of its short duration of action althesin may prove to be of value in outpatient anaesthesia, and in alcohol dependent patients. Unfortunately, like propanidid a number of cases of cardio-vascular collapse associated with skin flushing have been reported. The dose for intravenous administration is 0.05 ml to 0.075 ml/kg given slowly.

Complications of intravenous anaesthesia

Arterial complications. The anaesthetist should take every step to avoid intra-arterial injection by carefuly palpating the selected vessel prior to injection and by choosing a site where arteries are least likely to be present. The medial aspect of the antecubital fossa should never be used. One or more of the three important arteries of the antecubital fossa are in a superficial situation in about 18% of the population and consequently such a vessel is involved in about one quarter of inadvertent arterial injections. The radial artery is most often found in an aberrant site, usually running under the bicipital aponeurosis and taking a superficial position in the forearm: the ulnar artery is likely to be superficial for a shorter distance. Both often appear as satellite arteries of antecubital veins, and observation of parallel vessels in the fossa should arouse suspicion of a superficial artery. *The anaesthetist should always inject a small test dose of the drug, asking the patient whether pain is experienced at the site of the injection and/or down the arm.* (The typical pain of the intra-arterial injection radiates distally from the injection site to the fingers). The solutions used should be those which have the least likelihood of causing damage and the concentration of the thiopentone solution should never exceed 2.5% (5% propanidid is thought to be less likely to cause serious damage if injected intra-arterially). With intra-arterial injection in the antecubital fossa, the resultant thrombosis is likely to cause extensive gangrene, since collateral vessels are often inadequate in the distal part of the arm. The anaesthetist should be equally cautious when using the back of the hand for an intravenous injection, as intra-arterial injection has been reported. Should intra-arterial injection occur, the needle should be left in the artery and 2% procaine solution injected: anti-coagulant therapy should be considered and an intra-arterial injection of tolazoline (Priscol) 5 ml of 1% solution given. As the likely underlying phenomenon is the deposition of crystals in the smaller vessels, there might be some case for flushing the vessels with a dextran solution.

Sympathetic blockade of the upper limb may be undertaken and the whole body should be warmed, leaving the affected part exposed to the atmosphere.

Venous complications. Thrombophlebitis may arise at the site of injection of intravenous drugs. Hydroxydione, in particular, predisposes to a high incidence of thrombophlebitis and attempts to reduce this complication have been made by running the solution into a saline drip. The incidence of venous complications has been studied under comparable conditions in 700 cases following equipotent doses of 5% thiopentone, 2% methohexitone, and 3.5% and 5% propanidid, using two sizes of disposable needle (Hewitt *et al.*, 1966). There was no difference between the effects of thiopentone and methohexitone, but propanidid in 5% solution, while acceptable for clinical use, had significantly more sequelae. This viscous solution was more easily injected through the larger of the two needles, but there was a higher incidence of local ecchymoses. Thiopentone, chlorpromazine, diazepam, propanidid, and pethidine can all give rise to thrombophlebitis. If a vein of the dorsum of the hand is chosen for injection, the most practical way of reducing haematomata is to elevate the hand above the level of the heart and apply firm pressure with a pad for at least four minutes. An analysis of cases referred to one particular medical defence organization because of sequelae from injection of thiopentone, revealed three cases of gangrene, five cases of damage to nerve and muscle, and ten cases of local tissue necrosis over a seven year period.

Extravascular injections of most induction agents can cause degrees of necrosis of tissue and should be carefully guarded against: because of its position in the antecubital fossa, the median nerve is particularly vulnerable here.

Technique of intravenous injection

Choice of vessel. The medial aspect of the antecubital fossa should be treated with the greatest of respect for intravenous injection, however prominent the vessels may be. First of all, the site and course of the brachial artery should be determined; a tourniquet should be applied to the limb proximal to the site of the injection; the vein should be encouraged to distend by gently squeezing the fist, 'flicking' the vessel with the finger, and by applying local warmth. Having determined the site for injection, the tourniquet should be momentarily released and the vessel palpated for possible pulsation. Should pulsation of the vessel be absent, the tourniquet should be reapplied and puncture of the skin made at a point approximately 0.5–1.0 cm away from the proposed point of puncture of the vein, holding the barrel of the loaded syringe in one hand,

and with the thumb of the other hand, tensing the skin and placing the vein in a taut position. The needle should then be advanced in the subcutaneous tissues until the vein is punctured, and further advanced along the vein until its tip is 0.5–1.0 cm from the point of entry into the vein. As soon as venepuncture is accomplished the thumb of the left-hand (in a right-handed person) is firmly applied to the point where the shaft of the needle joins the syringe, the fingers of the hand being under the limb, thus securely anchoring the needle in situ. The plunger should be gently withdrawn, using the free hand, the entry of blood into the syringe noted and the tourniquet released, with the hand other than the one holding the syringe. An injection of 1–2 ml of solution is then made, whilst at the same time observing the site of injection for possible extravenous deposition. Having asked the patient whether he feels any discomfort, a further 2 ml of solution is quickly followed and the reaction of the patient's ventilation noted – this will give an indication of the circulation time. A further quantity is then injected, according to the degree of depression of ventilation and the degree of unconsciousness of the patient : care in the choice of the total dose and the rate of administration is necessary to prevent apnoea. At the completion of the injection the needle should be withdrawn, at the same time applying firm pressure at the puncture site, for four minutes at least, with the puncture site elevated above the level of the heart.

Inhalational agents

The ideal general anaesthetic agent should :

- produce unconsciousness with its associated analgesia and amnesia
- be readily acceptable to the patient
- produce muscular relaxation when required
- be easily reversible
- *should not* impair bodily functions i.e.,
  - the normal acid-base balance should not be upset
  - adequate tissue perfusion, particularly of the brain, liver and kidneys should be maintained
  - oxygen requirements of the body must be satisfied
  - the agent should not produce damage to the organs, such as the liver
  - the patient should not suffer from side effects, such as vomiting

Principle properties of inhalational agents

In considering the suitability of an inhalational anaesthetic agent for the production of the general anaesthetic state, the following main physical and pharmacological properties should be compared :

- flammability

cardiovascular effects
respiratory effects
blood/gas solubility ratio – this has a direct bearing on the rapidity of induction and recovery
potency – the concept of minimum alveolar concentration (MAC) (see page 51) applies

Commonly used inhalational anaesthetic agents

Halothane: boiling point 50.2 °C. This is non-explosive and non-flammable; the blood/gas solubility coefficient in 2.3 and hence induction of and recovery from anaesthesia tend to be quick. The oil/gas coefficient is 224. The MAC is 0.77 and halothane lacks analgesic properties. Ventilation is depressed with increasing anaesthetic depth and tachypnoea may occur. Depression of the blood pressure and bradycardia are associated with the use of halothane. Sympathetic ganglionic blockade is of no consequence in halothane anaesthesia as the predominant cause of fall in blood pressure as this cardiovascular effect is due to myocardial depression. There is no failure of ventricular filling but failure of ventricular emptying. Although there is increased baroreceptor discharge and increased activity in sympathetic post-ganglionic nerves during halothane anaesthesia, particularly with hypotension, the predominant effect is on the effector cell. Halothane does not in itself cause a significant reduction in vascular resistance. In the absence of hypercapnia, ventricular extrasystoles as a result of halothane administration are extremely uncommon. Adrenaline should not be administered to a subject breathing halothane. However, some authorities are prepared to permit such administration if the patient has received β-adrenergic blocking agents. Skeletal muscle is relaxed, and uterine contractility is depressed with increasing concentrations of halothane. Like most anaesthetic agents it crosses the placenta. There is some evidence to suggest that halothane, when given repeatedly, especially over a short interval, may produce an adverse effect on the liver.

Trichloroethylene: boiling point 87.1 °C. This is non-explosive and non-flammable in concentrations used in clinical practice; the blood/gas solubility coefficient is 9.15 and the oil/gas 960. Induction and recovery tend to be slow. The derived MAC is approximately 0.16 and thus trichloroethylene has good analgesic properties. Tachypnoea is common. Dysrhythmias may occur and adrenaline should not be administered to subject breathing trichloroethylene. Blood pressure is not significantly affected. In concentrations up to 0.5% there is minimal effect on uterine contractions, and relaxation of skeletal muscle is poor. Trichloroethylene rapidly crosses the placenta. There is no evidence of liver damage associated with its use.

Diethyl ether: boiling point 34.6°C. This is both flammable and explosive if used in conjunction with oxygen or nitrous oxide. In air, however, it is flammable only. The blood/gas solubility is 12.1 and hence both induction and recovery tend to be prolonged. The oil/gas solubility is 65 and the MAC is 1.9. Diethyl ether is irritant to the respiratory tract, increasing both salivary and bronchial secretions. It is a broncho-dilator, causing rather less respiratory depression than equipotent alveolar concentrations of halothane or methoxyflurane. Like all general anaesthetic agents, it is a myocardial depressant with increasing dose, but, because of increased sympathetic activity, the direct action on the heart is masked. Adrenaline may be administered during ether anaesthesia. Skeletal muscle is relaxed with increasing concentrations of ether, and a similar effect is seen with uterine contractility. It crosses the placenta readily. Ether causes mobilization of liver glycogen producing a rise in blood sugar. Post operative vomiting often occurs.

Cyclopropane (this gas is stored under pressure, and the liquid form has a boiling point of −33°C). It is flammable and explosive in both air and oxygen, but this danger can be reduced by adding diluents. The blood/gas solubility coefficient is 0.46 and hence induction and recovery tend to be rapid. The oil/gas solubility is 11.8 and the MAC 9.2%. Cyclopropane tends to cause increased salivation. Depression of ventilation occurs with increase in depth of anaesthesia. Likewise, myocardial depression tends to occur with increasing dose. Dysrhythmias are associated with carbon dioxide retention during the use of cyclopropane, and adrenaline should not be used. The effect on uterine contractility varies with depth, and it crosses the placenta. Skeletal muscle is progressively relaxed. Post-operative vomiting is often associated with its use. Employing a closed circuit apparatus 50% cyclopropane is used for induction and 5–10% for maintenance.

Methoxyflurane (boiling point 104.6°C). In concentrations above 4% methoxyflurane may ignite at vapour temperature in excess of 75°C. This situation does not occur in normal clinical practice. The blood/gas solubility coefficient is 13.0 and hence induction of and recovery from anaesthesia tend to be slow. The effect on induction is further accentuated by the very low volatility. The oil/gas solubility is 970 and the MAC 0.16%. Methoxyflurane has good analgesic properties. Reduction in ventilation occurs with increasing depth of anaesthesia and when associated with carbon dioxide retention may provoke extrasystoles. Methoxyflurane is a rather more potent myocardial depressant than other agents, though it seems likely that adrenaline may be used during the course of anaesthesia. Skeletal muscle is progressively relaxed only after prolonged anaesthesia, but there appears to be little effect on uterine contractility. It crosses the placenta. Nausea and vomiting during recovery are about as common as after the use of halothane. There is some evidence of nephrotoxicity occurring after the use of methoxyflurane.

Nitrous oxide. This gas is stored as a liquid under pressure, and is not flammable or explosive but supports combustion. The blood/gas coefficient of 0.41 leads to rapid induction and recovery. The oil/gas solubility coefficient is 1.4. The administration of 70% to 75% N_2O to man decreases by two-thirds the alveolar concentration of halothane necessary to prevent movement in response to a surgical incision. It is a very good analgesic but has no significant relaxing effect on skeletal or uterine muscle. Evidence as to the effect on blood pressure by nitrous oxide is conflicting, but in any case the effect is of no clinical importance. It readily crosses the placenta. Nausea and vomiting are not common when oxygenation has been adequate. Adrenaline may be used in its presence. Prolonged use over several days, e.g. for patients on a ventilator, may lead to bone marrow depression.

Azeotropes

The azeotropic mixture of two or more liquids is one which boils at a constant temperature and has a fixed composition. Fluorine compounds, in particular, readily form azeotropic mixtures.

The formation of an azeotropic mixture between diethyl ether and halothane has the objectives of reducing the flammability of ether, overcoming the vagotonic effects of halothane and enhancing induction with ether. This mixture of 31.7% diethyl ether and 68.3% halothane (v/v) remains constant and has a boiling point of 52.7°C and the lower limit of flammability is 7.25% in oxygen (v/v): this concentration is greater than that likely to be required for surgical anaesthesia. 68.7% halothane (v/v) and 31.3% methyl *n*-propyl ether (v/v) has also been employed; this mixture cannot be ignited in concentrations of less than 7.6% (v/v) in oxygen.

Methods of administration of general anaesthesia

The use of air as a vehicle to carry anaesthetic vapours

The open method employing the Schimmelbusch mask has been used for many years. It can be used for the administration of diethyl ether, divinyl ether, chloroform, ethyl chloride, halothane and fluroxene, although the administration of halothane in this way is extremely expensive and has little to recommend it. Using halothane, the drop rate on to a Schimmelbusch mask should commence at a rate of 20–50 drops/min reducing for maintenance to 5–20 drops/min. Unfortunately, hypoxaemia may occur when air is used and oxygen therefore needs to be given. Agents with a low vapour pressure at room temperature, such as methoxyflurane, are not suitable for use with an open mask. It is recommended that the administration of chloroform employing a Schimmelbusch mask should be carried out with no more than four layers of gauze. Chloroform, at the rate of one drop every three seconds, increasing slowly to a rate of 30 drops per minute, should be allowed to fall on to the lower quadrants of the mask. When surgical anaesthesia supervenes, the rate should be slowed to maintain the appropriate level of anaesthesia. Prolonged administration of chloroform, other than in an emergency situation, should not be allowed.

The use of air has obvious attractions in the armed services from the point of view of supply and transport of anaesthetic equipment and cylinders. There are, however, certain disadvantages, amongst them being the danger of hypoxaemia. Unless there is gross alveolar hypoventilation, desaturation can often be corrected by allowing a gentle flow of oxygen to enter under the mask; this will also reduce the amount of rebreathing.

Air may be employed in draw-over equipment, in which case the patient's own tidal volume is used to volatilize the liquid anaesthetic. An alternative method of blowing air over the liquid is now obsolete (Junker's Inhaler). The Epstein McIntosh Oxford Inhaler (EMO) is a temperature compensated vaporizer, which allows the concentration of anaesthetic vapour to be predetermined and, although primarily designed for ether, it can be used for other anaesthetic liquids. It can be used for controlled ventilation, in which case bellows are used, the resulting vapour being passed to the patient by intermittent positive pressure ventilation: *care should be taken to ensure that the bellows lie between the vaporizer and the patient.*

The equipment is portable and enables anaesthesia to be conducted with safety without further apparatus though oxygen can be added to the mixtures if required. After induction with thiopentone, concentrations of diethyl ether will be required of the order of 15%: this concentration should be reduced to approximately 7% for maintenance with spontaneous ventilation. Where controlled ventilation is employed smaller concentrations of the order of 2–5% with muscle relaxants will be required.

Halothane may be used as an induction agent. Using the Halothane Induction Unit interposed between the EMO inhaler and the Oxford inflation bellows, induction with thiopentone is followed by placing the mask over the face, and using the induction unit, 2% ether is turned on, increasing to 4%, and finally to 15%. The Halothane Induction Unit is designed to facilitate induction of ether anaesthesia and 3 ml of halothane vaporized over a period of 4 minutes is sufficient to enable a patient to breathe concentrations of 15–20% ether. The Goldman vaporizer is satisfactory for this purpose, but the Rowbotham vaporizer has too high a resistance: the Maggio-Vogelsanger Basel (MVB) vaporizer limits the volume to 5 ml. Trichloroethylene can be employed instead of halothane to facilitate induction with ether. The Fluoxair equipment has a temperature compensated vaporizer and inflating bellows, enabling halothane and air to be administered with or without added oxygen.

When using air as a vehicle, despite adequate alveolar ventilation, there may be a disproportionate fall in arterial oxygen tension during spontaneous ventilation, which suggests that venous admixture occurs. This venous admixture presumably arises because some parts of the lung have decreased ventilation/perfusion ratios. A fall in cardiac output could be a further contributory factor towards arterial hypoxaemia. It is likely therefore that when air is employed as the vehicle for carrying anaesthetic vapour, some degree of hypoxaemia may occur. The body oxygen store can be increased by the addition of oxygen, and therefore reduce the degree of hypoxaemia which may arise from momentary obstruction.

Trichloroethylene/air or methoxyflurane/air is used for obstetric pain relief. In addition, trichloroethylene/air (0.5% or less) has been used in conjunction with muscle relaxants for general anaesthesia using a specially calibrated EMO inhaler: such a technique may well have a place in emergency situations.

The use of air hyperventilation and muscle relaxants

Hyperventilation with air for operations upon the abdomen has been employed. Following premedication with hyoscine 0.6 mg and papaveretum 10 mg, anaesthesia can be induced with D-tubocurarine 30–40 mg, followed immediately by thiopentone 300–400 mg. Following intubation anaesthesia is maintained by hyperventilating the patient with air using tidal volumes between 600–900 ml with minute volumes of 35–40 l: further doses of curare are given as required. Because of the risk of recollection of the operative procedure, it is our opinion that this is not a justifiable technique to employ in normal clinical practice; the technique may, however, have a place in the extreme emergency situation. Its success will depend on the degree of narcosis achieved with premedication, the raising of the pain threshold with hyperventilation, and the reduction of afferent impulses, particularly proprioceptive, produced by the lissive effect of curare on the muscle spindles.

The use of oxygen to volatilize liquid anaesthetic agents

The use of halothane and oxygen alone in a closed circuit has been advocated by a number of anaesthetists. This method clearly has economic advantages and reduces the contamination of the theatre atmosphere with vapour. Some anaesthetists advocate the use of closed circuit halothane and oxygen, allowing the patients to breathe spontaneously, claiming that good relaxation occurs. Simple circuits have been suggested for this particular use. Bodman *et al.* (1967) employ a cheap circuit for the use with halothane and oxygen during spontaneous ventilation, using such a Water's canister, a Goldman vaporizer and a form of undirectional valve. The very real danger of using such a circuit for controlled ventilation cannot be over-stressed, as build-up of excessively high concentrations of halothane may quickly lead to overdosage. For spontaneous ventilation using Bodman's circuit, the Goldman vaporizer should be set at position 2 and then reduced to position 1 : position 3 should never be used.

The use of the Rowbotham vaporizer within the closed circuit has been described. During spontaneous ventilation, with the vaporizer placed on the inspiratory side of a circle absorber, a fresh gas flow of 2 litres of nitrous oxide and 1 litre of oxygen, and the lever at 3/4 setting, a concentration of 2.25% can be achieved. The theoretical objection to this method is that there is some resistance to breathing because of this vaporizer. The use of the Goldman vaporizer in a circle system has been reported and a Goldman drip-feed may also be employed. Others have used the intermittent injection of halothane into a closed circuit : 1 ml of liquid halothane produces 226 ml of vapour at 20°C and 760 mmHg.

If spontaneous ventilation occurs with the vaporizer within the circuit (VIC), then the amount of agent vaporized will depend on the tidal volumes resultant upon the depth of anaesthesia. Depression of ventilation will tend to cause a lightening of anaesthesia because less anaesthetic is taken up by the lungs : this will be followed by an increase in depth of ventilation with increased uptake and a recurrence of some degree of further respiratory depression. If patients are permitted to breathe spontaneously whilst breathing halothane and oxygen, carbon dioxide retention occurs and the resulting high levels of carbon dioxide, within the body, may lead to cardiac dysrhythmias. As very high levels of carbon dioxide tension have been reported using spontaneous ventilation with VIC it would seem unwise to employ VIC as a routine. Although closed circuit halothane and oxygen and controlled ventilation with the vaporizer inside the circuit (VIC) has great potential dangers, it is sometimes employed; Bodman *et al.* (1967) have taken the precaution of monitoring the halothane concentration continuously within the circuit. However, we believe that controlled ventilation with VIC is not a technique to be employed by the inexperienced and should not be undertaken lightly.

Some workers employ the vaporizer outside the circuit (VOC), particularly when controlled ventilation is used. With low flow rates (i.e. 200–300 ml/min of fresh gas), vaporization with VOC is often inadequate and therefore high flow rates with consequent loss of gas are necessary. Thus, with VOC, the amount of halothane being added to the anaesthetic circuit is dependent upon the flow of fresh gases entering the circuit. A highly efficient vaporizer is therefore particularly desirable if low flow rates are employed: a vaporizer which will deliver 10% halothane under these conditions has, in fact, been developed.

Circulatory collapse and cardiac arrest following the administration of nitrous oxide to patients under anaesthesia with halothane/oxygen have been reported. Care should therefore be taken when terminating anaesthesia after a prolonged period of halothane/oxygen.

Maintenance of general anaesthesia

The concept of 'depth' is so firmly established in the anaesthetist's vocabulary that it seems justifiable to use it in establishing a general principle: *that anaesthesia should be controlled at a depth appropriate to the surgical procedure.* The Minimal Alveolar Concentration (MAC) is that concentration of anaesthetic agent, at alveolar level, that adequately prevents reflex response to a standard stimulus. 'Light' anaesthesia implies a low concentration, because if the stimulus is of low intensity there will be no reflex movement whereas if the intensity is greater there may be some reflex movement. 'Deep' anaesthesia is associated with higher concentrations at alveolar level and a lack of reflex response to stimuli at high intensity (i.e. stretching of the anal sphincter or dilatation of the cervix).

Light general anaesthesia with spontaneous ventilation is usually acceptable for surgery of the arms and legs and the surface of the body. General anaesthesia associated with spontaneous ventilation, with the possible exception of 'light ether', is inevitably associated with alveolar hypoventilation and carbon dioxide retention. Such retention of carbon dioxide, particularly in the presence of cyclopropane and halothane, may be harmful. Operations of a prolonged nature, and those requiring 'deeper' anaesthesia associated with muscular relaxation, must always be intubated and artificially ventilated. The combination of analgesia, drug-induced hypnosis, and controlled relaxation (the so-called balanced anaesthesia), is possibly least harmful to the patient and allows the preservation of compensatory cardiovascular reflexes. This triad can be best achieved by adequate pre-operative sedation, induction with thiopentone or methohexitone, and maintenance of controlled ventilation with nitrous oxide/oxygen with or without an agent such as halothane, plus relaxation with neuromuscular blocking agents. The associated use of hyperventilation has its protagonists, but recent studies suggests that this technique may not be as innocuous as was previously believed, particularly if halothane is used. If associated with nitrous oxide/oxygen alone, the hyperventilation technique may also carry the risk of awareness during the operation. Care must be taken to avoid overdosage with inhalational agents during controlled ventilation. As an alternative to using an inhalational agent such as halothane, to ensure a balanced condition, general anaesthesia may be maintained by careful administration of analgesic agents that may also produce central respiratory depression. By careful adjustment of dosage a state of affairs is achieved where there is neither a complete respiratory depression nor a complete peripheral neuromuscular blockade. In divided doses such agents as phenoperidine (up to 2 mg), pethidine (up to 100 mg), levorphanol (Dromoran) (up to 2.0 mg), dipipanone (up to 25 mg) or fentanyl (up to 0.6 mg) may be used, but it is essential to maintain adequate alveolar ventilation. Their effects may be reversed at the termination of anaesthesia by nalorphine, naloxone or similar drugs. However, levallorphan or nalorphine can themselves produce ventilatory depression if given in excess.

When muscular relaxation is required, the writers are in favour of controlled ventilation, employing 0.5–1% halothane in nitrous oxide and oxygen in the proportion of 2 to 1, the relaxation being achieved by the administration of a neuromuscular blocking agent such as gallamine triethiodide or pancuronium bromide. It should be noted that D-tubocurarine carries the disadvantage of hypotension when associated with halothane. Signs of lightness such as movement of limbs, tears, swallowing attemped respiration, twitching of facial muscles, or sweating may be treated by increasing the halothane by a further 0.5–1.0% or by administering a further dose of relaxant. Special note should be taken of the risk of using halothane in obstetric cases.

Control of depth of anaesthesia

For many years anaesthetists have been accustomed to thinking of the degree of depth of anaesthesia in terms of the classical description of the 'stages' and 'planes' as described by Guedel in relation to diethyl ether. With the introduction of neuromuscular blocking agents, the use of hyperventilation, and the employment of other inhalational agents such as halothane, these clear stages of anaesthesia have become less well defined. It has been felt for some time that patients react beneficially to trauma more effectively if anaesthesia is not too deep, so that compensatory, autonomic reflexes are unimpaired. On the other hand, a patient who is too light may react adversely to strong surgical stimuli. A balance is therefore necessary and the anaesthetist today must ensure that the patient is unconscious but not too deeply narcotized, and that, when relaxation is required, neuromuscular blocking agents are given rather than increased quantities of inhalational anaesthetic agents.

Anaesthesia may be induced by using an agent such as thiopentone or methohexitone. Following induction, the patient should be immediately presented with the inhalational agent in sufficient concentration to continue smooth deepening of anaesthesia. Should intubation be required, but spontaneous ventilation be desired, a short acting neuromuscular blocking agent (such as suxamethonium) may be employed: alternatively anaesthesia may be deepened by using up to 3.5% halothane for a short while. Anaesthesia is maintained by agents such as halothane, methoxyflurane, or trichloroethylene, using oxygen or nitrous oxide/oxygen as vehicle gases. Accumulated experience has shown the concentration of agents necessary to ensure unconsciousness; 80% nitrous oxide barely produces unconsciousness unless other intravenous or inhalational agents are employed: on the other hand, halothane 0.5% to 1%, will generally maintain unconsciousness once anaesthesia has been induced. If intravenous induction is contraindicated, induction and intubation can be carried out by using rapidly increasing concentrations of halothane (up to 3.5%) with nitrous oxide and oxygen until the appropriate level of anaesthesia is reached.

Provided that it is possible to maintain a patent airway by positioning the head and jaws it is wiser not to insert an artificial airway too early as, if the patient is too light, swallowing, vomiting and excessive laryngeal irritation may be provoked. When breathing is regular and automatic, an oro-pharyngeal airway may be inserted if felt necessary, the mask fastened and the operation commenced. If halothane is being employed, the concentration is turned down to a maintenance dose of 0.5% to 1.5%, and this may be further decreased if ventilation is depressed, or increased if the patient moves his limbs, sweats or swallows. Where relaxation is required, neuromuscular blockade combined with controlled ventilation is indicated. The anaesthetist should aim at maintaining anaesthesia with little depression of blood pressure and little or no deviation of the pulse rate from basal. The patient should, as far as possible have a warm periphery, a dry skin, and a good colour. The onset of surgical anaesthesia, apart from the lack of response to surgical stimuli, is characterized by regular automatic ventilation. Signs of lightening of anaesthesia are the accumulation of tears, eye movements and slowing or acceleration of the heart rate, depending on the degree of surgical stimulus. Excessive parasympathetic stimulation may be accompanied by a slow pulse, pallor and hypotension, which may sometimes be alleviated by the administration of 0.6 mg atropine intravenously. Sweating usually signifies too light anaesthesia. When using halothane during controlled ventilation with muscle relaxants, the halothane should be discontinued approximately ten minutes before reversal of neuromuscular blockade with neostigmine.

Non-depolarizing neuromuscular block

D-Tubocurarine, gallamine triethiodide (Flaxedil), alcuronium (Alloferin) and pancuronium (Pavulon), are neuromuscular blocking agents which produce their effect by competing with acetylcholine for the receptors at the neuromuscular endplate. In normal doses in the normal individual, these agents are readily reversible by the administration of neostigmine. Patients suffering from myasthenia gravis, the myasthenic syndrome, electrolyte and acid-base disturbances, have an increased susceptibility to these agents. The ganglion blocking agents hexamethonium, trimetaphan, and phenactropinium can produce a complete neuromuscular block of a non-depolarizing type.

D-*tubocurarine.* This is normally administered intravenously, though the intramuscular route is sometimes employed for long term therapeutic neuromuscular blockade. In the normal fit adult male a dose of 30 mg is usually an effective paralytic dose and allows good conditions for orotracheal intubation. Some authorities administer a test dose of 5 mg intravenously in order to allow detection of patients sensitive to the agent: two to three minutes should normally be allowed for the agent to commence its effect. The duration of action lasts approximately 30 minutes and potentiation of its effects will occur with most of the inhalational general anaesthetic agents. Varying degrees of histamine release are sometimes associated with its administration, and it is probably best avoided in patients with a history of bronchospasm and patients with a phaechromocytoma. It may be used in subjects with renal disease, but patients with liver disorder sometimes demonstrate a resistance. Hyperventilation and hypothermia reduce its effect, and hypotension sometimes occurs following the intravenous injection of D-tubocurarine, possibly due to its histamine-releasing effects.

Gallamine triethiodide (Flaxedil) is similar in its action to D-tubocurarine, though of somewhat shorter duration. A dose of 120 mg is approximately as effective as a dose of 30 mg of D-tubocurarine. Tachycardia is associated with its use, and the combination of gallamine with halothane is not hypotensive in its effect, the vagotonic effects of halothane being countered by gallamine. The duration of action is prolonged with hyperventilation and antagonized by respiratory or metabolic acidosis. Gallamine crosses the placenta freely and probably should not be used in obstetric work. It is eliminated from the body almost entirely by the kidneys, and should never be employed in the presence of renal disease.

Alcuronium (Alloferin) is derived from an alkaloid of calabash curare, toxiferine. It is shorter acting in equipotent dosage than D-tubocurarine, more readily reversible, and does not cause marked tachycardia nor serious hypotension. It is about twice as potent as D-tubocurarine: doses from 5–25 mg may be given to the adult depending on the clinical conditions required. In view of the fact that histamine release is less likely than with D-tubocurarine, alcuronium may be safer in cases with a history of asthma.

Pancuronium bromide (Pavulon) is a potent neuromuscular blocking agent: an amino-steroid with a powerful non-depolarizing action, it is free from hormonal action. Pancuronium has more rapid onset of action than other non-depolarizing agents, with a duration of effect similar to D-tubocurarine. There is a lack of histamine release and associated bronchospasm; no ganglion blockade; no occurrence of hypotension and the pulse rate is not altered. In the adult, 4–6 mg is usually given as an initial dose and this may be followed by increments of up to 2 mg. Because it is a rapidly acting agent it fulfils the need for a non-depolarizing neuromuscular blocking agent for intubation purposes. Although there is no evidence that its use is contraindicated in either liver or renal disease, it should be administered cautiously in both.

Reversal of non-depolarizing agents

As a general principle, the administration of muscle relaxants should be avoided during the last 20 m of an operation. Any case receiving non-depolarizing blocking agents should receive adequate dosage of neostigmine at the termination of anaesthesia. In order to counteract the slowing effect of neostigmine upon the heart it is customary to block its effect by the prior administration of atropine.

Cases of cardiac arrest have been reported after the administration of atropine and neostigmine at the termination of anaesthesia. Small doses of atropine given intravenously have been shown to cause bradycardia; this effect, coupled with the slowing associated with the muscarinic effect of neostigmine, has been thought to lead to cardiac arrest in certain cases. Serious cardiac irregularities may follow the therapeutic dose of atropine, if carbon dioxide retention is present. It has been suggested that the heart is protected from the effects of neostigmine if a respiratory alkalosis is producd by artificial ventilation, therefore it has been advised that atropine and neostigmine should be given before spontaneous ventilation is allowed to return. The effect of atropine on the heart rate has been the subject of much investigation, and is largely dependent on the relationship between the existing heart rate and the intrinsic heart rate. If the heart rate is already at or above the intrinsic rate (approximately 100 beats/min in man) atropine will cause no significant change. If there is a pre-existing bradycardia of vagal origin, injection of atropine may cause marked increase of heart rate, but never to more than the intrinsic rate.

The following appears to be the most acceptable routine to follow for the reversal of neuromuscular blockade:

(1) Atropine should not be administered in the presence of carbon dioxide retention, i.e. spontaneous ventilation should not be permitted before the administration of atropine and neostigmine.

(2) Atropine in a dose of 1.2 mg intravenously should be given if the pulse rate is below 80/min: if the rate is above 80/min, 0.6 mg

should be given intravenously. This is followed by 2.5 mg neostigmine after two minutes and up to a total of 5.0 mg may be given in further divided doses. If the subjects have had 0.6 mg of atropine it may be advisable to repeat this if doses over 2.5 mg neostigmine are given.

(3) Spontaneous ventilation will usually take place once the neuromuscular block has been reversed, provided central depression does not exist. Certain stimuli might be required to trigger off spontaneous ventilation, e.g. administration of carbon dioxide 5–10% for one minute, carinal stimulation by means of a narrow bore catheter passed down the endotracheal tube, and deflation of the cuff of the endotracheal tube. Nikethamide 2–5 ml intravenously is sometimes of benefit, particularly with the respiratory cripple. Although pyridostigmine is said to be longer acting than neostigmine (5 mg pyridostigmine being equivalent to 2.5 mg neostigmine) it has been found to be unreliable in its action.

Depolarizing neuro-muscular block

Decamethonium (C10 Eulissin), suxamethonium (Scoline, Anectine), and suxethonium (Brevedil E), are neuromuscular blocking agents which produce their effect by depolarizing the motor end-plate. Their duration of action is dependent upon the rapidity with which they are hydrolysed or otherwise eliminated.

Decamethonium in an initial dose of 5 mg in the fit adult male, it will produce its maximum effect in 3–4 minutes, and has a duration of action of approximately 20 minutes. Decamethonium causes significantly less histamine release than D-tubocurarine and has little effect upon the cardiovascular system. A total dose of 10 mg should not be exceeded for fear of dual block. Pentamethonium has been employed to counter the neuromuscular blocking effect of decamethonium iodide, but on the whole is unsatisfactory, as pentamethonium has a marked hypotensive action through its effect in blocking sympathetic ganglia. Decamethonium is employed as a test for myasthenia gravis, but is now little used in anaesthesia, and is not readily available. Phase I block (depolarizing) is antagonized by hexafluorenium and potentiated by edrophonium and Phase II block (non-depolarizing) potentiated by hexafluorenium, and antagonized by edrophonium.

Suxamethonium and Suxethonium produce their effect in a similar manner to decamethonium, but, because they are normally more rapidly hydrolysed, their duration of action is short, lasting only about four minutes. There is no significant difference in action between the two drugs, nor difference in the incidence of muscle pains after their administration. The dose of suxamethonium varies from 25 to 100 mg in a single paralytic dose, but a dose exceeding 50 mg is rarely required for intubation in the adult. More may be administered intermittently, or continuously as a 0.1% drip to maintain neuromuscular blockade, though Phase II block progressively increases with increasing dose.

Potentiation of the neuromuscular blocking action of suxamethonium. Certain agents are known to potentiate the effects of suxamethonium. Hexafluorenium (Mylaxen) produces an extension of suxamethonium block by inhibition of plasma cholinesterase: it should not be given if operative procedures are expected to last less than one hour, or in patients with extensive hepatic disease or with low plasma cholinesterase. Propanidid is said to extend the course of action of suxamethonium. Tetrahydroaminacrine (Tacrine, Romotol) possesses both anti-cholinesterase and neuromuscular blocking effects and may be employed to reduce the dose and increase the effect of suxamethonium. Tacrine does not potentiate the neuromuscular blocking action of suxamethonium at the neuromuscular junction, but works primarily by depressing the plasma cholinesterase. Atropine should always be given to counter the powerful muscarinic effects as the combination of Tacrine and suxamethonium can give rise to alarming bradycardia and salivation. 15 mg Tacrine is followed by 30 mg suxamethonium. It is claimed that suxamethonium after-pains are reduced to insignificant proportions and the time scale of the intermittent technique is extended, thus reducing the risk of dual block. However, it is likely that dual block still occurs even with relatively small doses of suxamethonium combined with Tacrine. The respiratory stimulant effect of Tacrine, although usually present, is inconstant in its action and in addition, the drug has undesirable side effects which include nausea and abdominal cramps. Because of the 'analeptic' properties of Tacrine its use is suggested for Caesarean section, forceps, and poor risk cases. It has a mild cardio-inhibitor action in the anaesthestized patients, but in those premedicated with atropine, the intensity of effect is slight, unlike that of neostigmine. It is unsatisfactory as an antidote to non-depolarizing blockers.

Procaine amide and quinidine have also been shown to potentiate the neuromuscular blocking effects of suxamethonium. Diazepam has been found to increase the duration of neuromuscular block produced by gallamine and to reduce that produced by succinylcholine, although this has not been generally confirmed. In certain other clinical situations, caution should be exercised when using suxamethonium, e.g. ecothiopate iodide eye drops in ophthalmology, some anti-cancer agents such as cyclophosphamide, and aprotinin (Trasylol), all cause potentiation of effect.

Ideally all cases receiving neuromuscular blocking agents should be intubated and ventilated artificially.

Suxamethonium after-pains. The use of suxamethonium as a short-acting relaxant is often followed by severe and incapacitating muscle pains, the severity of which can outweigh the undoubted advantages of the agent. There is a lower incidence in elderly males, young children, and patients of great muscular fitness. There is apparently no correlation between the intensity of fasciculation and subsequent pain nor does the administration of suxamethonium intramuscularly decrease the incidence of pain. There would appear to be no difference in incidence if the bromide rather than the chloride is given. The prior administration of gallamine (20–40 mg) has been used to lessen the frequency of pain but at least two minutes must be given to allow the gallamine to act: 3 mg of D-tubocurarine has also been found to produce the same effect. This practice is not to be encouraged. Early ambulation increases the incidence of after-pain and therefore suxamethonium has serious limitations when used for outpatient anaesthesia. Attenion has been focused upon the extension of the effect of suxamethonium by tetrahydroaminacrine and it has been noted that the incidence of muscle pains is significantly reduced after this combination of agents. Intravenous lignocaine has also been given in an attempt to reduce the incidence of muscle pains.

Neuromuscular blocking effects of antibiotics

The first reported case of respiratory insufficiency associated with antibiotics occurred in relation to the use of neomycin in a patient undergoing anaesthesia. Since that time there have been numerous reports of difficulties arising with the use of neomycin, streptomycin, dihydrostreptomycin, kanamycin, bacitracin, polymyxin B and other antibiotics in patients receiving general anaesthesia. There have also been several reports of neuromuscular paralysis in patients who have received no general anaesthetic agents, and in others who had received a general anaesthetic which did not include neuromuscular blocking agents in the technique. Most of the cases have arisen where excessive doses have been given either into the pleural or peritoneal cavities, or intramuscularly. However, at least four cases have been reported of respiratory insufficiency arising as a result of oral neomycin, which, under normal conditions, is not absorbed by the intestinal tract. It may be that orally administered neomycin can be absorbed in appreciable quantity from damaged intestinal mucosa or in cases of large bowel obstruction. It has also been shown that large doses of streptomycin injected into dogs produce not only neuromuscular blockade but also marked hypotension. The administration of neostigmine in patients receiving streptomycin produces a slow and incomplete recovery, but calcium chloride alone, or after neostigmine, causes a quick and complete recovery of blood pressure.

The treatment of this condition should include immediate IPPV and steps to avoid vasomotor collapse. Calcium should be given intravenously in a slow injection of 10 ml of 10% calcium chloride. It should be noted that the neuromuscular blocking effect of some antibiotics is not so readily reversible.

Hyperventilation

The protagonists of the employment of hyperventilation during anaesthesia have claimed that the potentially harmful effects of respiratory acidosis are avoided, indeed, that respiratory alkalosis is a useful adjunct of light anaesthesia, because cerebral function is depressed, analgesia is enhanced, and the total dose of curare reduced. The heart is also said to be protected against the potentially dangerous effects of neostigmine.

The technique implies an alveolar ventilation in excess of that required to maintain adequate elimination of carbon dioxide. It is a useful adjunct to the thiopentone/nitrous oxide/oxygen/relaxant technique. It has also been used in the treatment of crush injury of the chest, and the management of general anaesthesia for patients suffering from chronic respiratory disease.

For many years it has been argued that hyperventilation increases the arterial oxygen tension. However, hyperventilation under general anaesthesia may significantly reduce the cardiac output, and the reason for this is thought to be related to the reduction in arterial carbon dioxide tension. Such a reduction in cardiac output lowers the amount of oxygen available to the tissues; for a given oxygen consumption the mixed venous oxygen content falls, and the venous admixture of this blood through normal shunts leads to arterial hypoxaemia.

The raised pain threshold associated with hyperventilation is probably not due to cerebral hypoxia, though recent work suggests that, when hyperventilation has been employed during general anaesthesia, prolonged effects can arise and are carried through into the post-operative period. The cause of the raised pain threshold has been thought to be a decrease in discharge from the reticular activating system, associated with a lowering of the carbon dioxide tension: indeed, it should be remembered that if hyperventilation is momentarily allowed to cease the patient might become conscious. It has also been claimed that hyperventilation prolongs the action of relaxants, and this is certainly true where gallamine is concerned. However, recent work suggests that the action of curare is antagonized. Afferent neural blockade, by employing local conduction anaesthesia, enhances the effectiveness of hyperventilation anaesthesia.

There is no doubt that hyperventilation anaesthesia is a useful adjunct to the thiopentone/nitrous oxide/oxygen/relaxant technique, but a satisfactory result is dependent upon good pre-anaesthetic medication and adequate neuromuscular blockade. Although recent work has suggested that there may be harmful effects from its use, the present evidence requires further support before the method can be finally evaluated. A report (Sullivan and Patterson, 1968), suggests that prolonged hypoventilation in the post-operative period may result from hyperventilation during anaesthesia.

Post-operative apnoea

The causes of post-operative apnoea are many and various. One particular group of patients consists of those that can be described as being moribund. These patients very often have severe disturbances of electrolytes, with associated metabolic acidosis, poor peripheral blood flow, and other complicating factors. Relative or absolute overdosage with general anaesthetic agents may cause apnoea, particularly in such patients, because of their increased susceptibility to anaesthetic agents as a whole. Underventilation may give rise to carbon dioxide retention, hypoxaemia and metabolic acidosis, all of which alter the response of the patient to neuromuscular blocking agents and delay recovery. In particular, a low plasma pH is known to potentiate the action of D-tubocurarine. Overventilation may give rise to apnoea due to excessive carbon dioxide elimination. Reflex inhibition of ventilation may occur as a result of afferent stimulation, such as may arise from painful stimuli, or the presence of an endotracheal tube. Lack of afferent stimuli may also lead to apnoea (gentle stimulation of the carina with a suction catheter, or even the command to breathe to the conscious apnoeic subject, may re-establish breathing). Poor peripheral blood flow, arising from oligaemic states or any other cause, may lead to incomplete removal of neuromuscular blocking agent from the region of the motor end-plate. As a result of the altered response of muscles to the hypothermic state prolonged relaxant action may occur. Metabolic acidosis may cause 'neostigmine-fast' curarization, particularly in debilitated patients who have sustained a prolonged loss of fluids and electrolytes; although spontaneous ventilation usually returns in these patients at the end of the operation, it is inadequate and sometimes associated with 'tracheal tug'. The relaxant action is not reversed completely by neostigmine, the patient remains unconscious or semi-conscious and there is generally evidence of cardiovascular impairment. This condition is often improved by the administration of sodium bicarbonate solution and, where facilities for blood gas analysis exist, the amount of bicarbonate to be given should be titrated against the patient's base deficit. Potassium deficency is known to produce a susceptibility to D-tubocurarine, so the cautious administration of potassium to these patients can be of value.

Depolarizing blockers: apnoea may arise in association with the use of suxamethonium. Absence of plasma cholinesterase, reduced quantities, or the presence of an atypical cholinesterase may lead to prolongation of the action of suxamethonium. Reduced quantities of plasma cholinesterase are found in association with gross liver disease, chronic anaemia, massive blood transfusion, burns, malignant states such as bronchial neoplasm, malnutrition, heart failure and acute infections. Exposure to organo-phosphorus compounds and certain drugs also lead to low levels of plasma cholinesterase : ecothiopate iodide, used as eye drops in the ophthalmic treatment of glaucoma, and strabismus in small children, reduces the plasma cholinesterase, giving rise to signs of cholinergic intoxication when the level falls to 20–30% of its initial value. Therapeutic radiation, dialysis, and chemotherapy with anti-cancer agents such as AB-132 and cyclo-phosphamide are further causes of reduction in cholinesterase activities. Prolongation of the action of suxamethonium in association with low levels of normal plasma cholinesterase generally gives rise to apnoea lasting no more than one hour. However, the low levels are sometimes associated with an atypical cholinesterase and the apnoea may be prolonged for several hours: such a condition occurs in about 1 in 3000 of the population and is genetically determined. In such patients abnormal enzymes are present, which are more resistant to a variety of inhibitors, such as dibucaine, and differ from the normal enzymes in being less active in hydrolysing suxamethonium. Trimetaphan, a potent inhibitor of pseudocholinesterase, prolongs the duration of apnoea and care should therefore be taken when using suxamethonium in cases receiving deliberate hypotension with trimetaphan. Hexamethonium, phenactropinium, hexafluorenium, procaine and quinidine also extend the duration of effect of suxamethonium and tetrahydroaminacrine (Romotol, Tacrine) has a similar action. Repeated doses of 20 mg suxamethonium can give rise to dual block when a total dose of 200 mg is reached in the adult. If an infusion technique is used dual block may not occur until higher dosage has been reached. Suxamethonium is therefore an unsuitable agent to employ if relaxation is required for more than 20 minutes. Dual block also arises in association with a low and/or abnormal plasma cholinesterase. Succinylmonocholine (a breakdown product of suxamethonium) produces a depolarizing myoneural blocking action, slower in onset, less complete, and longer lasting than succinyldicholine (suxamethonium) but with a marked cumulative effect. This may only be of significance if large doses of suxamethonium have been used.

Non-depolarizing blockers. Sensitivity to these agents in the Myasthenic state is well recognized. Prolonged paralysis may occur after the use of gallamine in patients with kidney failure.

Diagnosis and treatment of apnoea

It has been pointed out that there are three main causes for post-operative ventilatory inadequacy or apnoea. These are: depression of the respiratory centre; mechanical defects of the respiratory system; and peripheral causes related to the use of muscle relaxants.

The only satisfactory way of distinguishing a peripheral cause, from the other two groups, is by the use of a peripheral nerve stimulator. There are a number of these stimulators available and several have been described. Application of the appropriate electrical stimulus to the ulnar nerve at the elbow joint just behind the medial epicondyle will, under normal circumstances, provoke a response in the muscles of the hypothenar eminence. Therefore, in a case of apnoea, if there is marked activity in this muscle group when the nerve is stimulated, it can be concluded that the respiratory muscles have at least partly recovered from the effects of the muscle relaxant. The return of activity in the stimulated group does not necessarily mean, however, that muscles of other groups are equally free from neuromuscular block. Where there is adequate response to nerve stimulus, apnoea must be of central, or mechanical origin. (The only exception to this rule is found in certain severe cases of myasthenia gravis, where the respiratory muscles rather than the upper limb muscles are involved in the disease). The mechanical movement of the muscles of the hand consequent upon electrical stimulation of the ulnar nerve is characteristic.

Depolarizing block: there is no improvement in the response after a prolonged burst of tetanic stimulation and no post-tetanic facilitation.

Non-depolarizing block: fade is seen in response to electrical stimulation and, following a prolonged burst of tetanus, there is a temporary marked improvement. Such a response is likely to be improved by the giving of anticholinesterase drugs. Intravenous edrophonium 10 mg should be given first, and if the response improves, neostigmine administration should be considered. Several authorities have advocated the routine use of a nerve stimulator, as not only will it enable the anaesthetist to become familiar with its use in case of emergency, but it can also guide the anaesthetist in accurate titration of the dose of neostigmine required to reverse paralysis.

Treatment of apnoea: whilst attempts are being made to determine the cause of the ventilatory inadequacy, the patient should be artificially ventilated. More than 30% oxygen should be administered, but the patient should be kept unconscious by delivering 50%–60% nitrous oxide. Conversation should be kept to the minimum, and at no time should the patient's problem be discussed in his presence, in case he is returning to consciousness. Where facilities allow, arterial blood should be taken for estimation of carbon dioxide tension; if suxamethonium has been employed, a heparinized sample of blood should be taken for subsequent cholinesterase estimation; for which rapid tests have been devised. If relaxants have been given, edrophonium 10 mg intravenously may be administered. It should be remembered that subjects apnoeic due to deficiencies of cholinesterase pass through a stage of dual blockade where edrophonium may be of value. If central depression is thought to be the cause of the patient's ventilatory inadequacy, then the appropriate antidote may be given.

If any doubt exists as to the cause of the trouble, the administration of drugs must be avoided so as not to complicate the picture. Treatment should be directed towards sustaining the patient's respiratory and cardiovascular systems, waiting until any drugs which may be causing the difficulties can be detoxicated and/or excreted. Where it is thought that the apnoea is due to cholinesterase deficiency consideration should be given to the administration of plasma. The cholinesterase content of fresh frozen plasma stored at 20°C has a short life of about 21 days, and contains on average 120 μg/ml cholinesterase as against 30 μg/ml in whole blood. The rapid infusion of 400–800 ml of double strength plasma or triple-strength plasma has been suggested, but great care should be taken in doing this, on account of the deleterious effects of the high potassium content of the plasma on cardiac action. However, there is no doubt that plasma is better than the whole blood recommended by some.

Myasthenic syndrome

The myasthenic state is not only associated with myasthenia gravis, but also with bronchial carcinoma, amyotrophic sclerosis, certain of the collagen diseases, polymyositis, dermatomyositis, systemic lupus erythematosis and polyarteritis nodosa. Neostigmine has proved beneficial in myasthenia associated with these disorders. Myasthenia is also associated with the use of certain antibiotics.

Bronchial carcinoma

The myasthenic syndrome is sometimes associated with bronchial carcinoma. The weakness and fatiguability, which mainly affect the proximal muscles, respond poorly to neostigmine, in contrast with its action in myasthenia gravis. The muscular weakness often precedes the discovery of the carcinoma, but an electromyograph will help in the differential diagnosis. Abnormally small action potentials which decrease in size, are recorded at slow rates of supramaximal nerve stimulation and marked growth of potentials occurs on tetanic stimulation; whereas in myasthenia gravis, fade of successive potentials is shown. In bronchial carcinoma the ocular and bulbar muscles are frequently involved in the myasthenic process and a short-lived increase in strength on exertion is sometimes observed. There is a particular susceptibility to the non-depolarizing relaxants, the neuromuscular block not being readily reversed with neostigmine. Muscle relaxants should be avoided, although when profound relaxation is required, small doses of suxamethonium may be justifiable.

Low cholinesterase activity is sometimes present in association with bronchial carcinoma without apparent liver involvement, and should suxamethonium be used, prolonged response accompanied by paralysis of the respiratory muscles may occur, though this will seldom last longer than one hour.

Amyotrophic lateral sclerosis

Amyotrophic lateral sclerosis (motor neurone disease) is an adult disease of the motor system, which begins insidiously and progresses to a fatal termination uually within three years. A defect in neuromuscular transmission similar to that observed in myasthenia gravis is often found in these patients, and therefore neuromuscular blocking agents, particularly the non-depolarizing agents, should be avoided.

Syringomyelia

Patients suffering from syringomyelia react in a way similar to the myasthenic syndrome. Neuromuscular blocking agents as a whole are best avoided.

Poliomyelitis

The wasted muscles of patients recovering from poliomyelitis are sensitive to non-depolarizing blocking agents.

Collagen diseases

Polymyositis, dermatomysitis, systemic lupus erythematosis and polyarteritis nodosa are often associated with excessive muscle weakness and increased response to neostigmine. Neuromuscular blocking agents are again best avoided in these states. Low serum cholinesterase has been reported in relation to polyarteritis and it is assumed that this is due to liver involvement.

Familial periodic paralysis

This is a rare disorder associated with low levels of serum potassium leading to muscular weakness. Non-depolarizing relaxants can provoke difficulties which may be corrected by the cautious administration of potassium.

Myasthenia gravis

The incidence of this condition is about 1 in 40 000 patients. The classical case of myasthenia gravis presents with bilateral ptosis, chin supported on one hand and saliva drooling from the corner of the mouth. Usually, however, the presenting sign is solitary, and in 25% of cases it is ocular, diplopia and ptosis being the commonest signs; generalized muscular weakness is next. Spontaneous remissions frequently occur and these may vary in length from a few days to several years. When myasthenia is localized to the extrinsic eye muscles for two or three years, further involvement is unlikely.

The anaesthetist may not be confronted with such a clear-cut clinical picture and mild cases, in particular, may create difficulties for him, especially if he employs muscle relaxants. Where there is doubt as to the nature of the condition, diagnostic tests can be employed.

Neostigmine test

Atropine 1.2 mg and neostigmine 2.5 mg can be administered intravenously. An improvement in muscle tone and power will give an indication that the subject is a possible myasthenic. If it is preferred that the action of the anti-cholinesterase be short-lived, edrophonium 10 mg instead of neostigmine should be given with the atropine.

Use of muscle relaxants

Curare. Approximately 84% of myasthenic patients exhibit sensitivity to 0.016 mg/kg of D-tubocurarine chloride.

Suxamethonium. Myasthenia gravis of a very mild nature will show increased resistance to this agent: patients with clinical weakness have the tendency to develop dual block.

Decamethonium. This test has been devised by Churchill-Davidson and Richardson (1953). There are three distinct stages.

The stage of resistance: the patients show clinical weakness and yet, whereas normal subjects will develop complete paralysis with a dose of 3.0 mg of decamethonium, patients suffering from myasthenia gravis who are in this stage show a complete resistance to this dose. The dose of decamethonium is given cautiously in divided doses of 1.0 mg at a time, until a total of 2.5–3.0 mg has been given.

The stage of dual block: the administration of 3.0 mg produces paralysis which is partially reversible by administering edrophonium.

The stage of myopathy: the sensitivity of the patient to decamethonium will vary according to the degree of involvement of the muscle fibres in the myopathic state which has arisen because of disuse of the fibres.

The response of the muscles of the hypothenar eminence of the hand to stimulation of the ulnar nerve at the elbow can be recorded electromyographically during the course of decamethonium administration and will greatly assist in the establishment of a diagnosis. *All these tests involve the risk of paralysing the patient and means of artificially ventilating the lungs must be readily available.*

Treatment of myasthenia gravis. Tumours of the thymus are present in about 15% of myasthenic patients and with careful radiological techniques, if a tumour is present, it can usually be seen. A survey of 294 patients who have been operated upon for removal of the thymus (Keynes, 1966) compared with 110 patients who had not been operated upon, showed that fewer females died of myasthenia if the thymus had been removed than would have been expected had they been treated with drugs alone. Thymectomy was also shown to greatly increase the number of women who had improved ten years after the onset of the illness. The best results are obtained in patients with a younger than average age of onset, with a short pre-operative duration of the disease and who are younger at the age of operation. The prognosis is poor if a thymoma is present pre-operatively, though pre-operative radiotherapy may be beneficial. The indications for operation in the absence of thymoma are found in two groups: patients under 50 years of age, with a history of less than two years, in whom symptoms are not adequately controlled by drugs; and a smaller group, irrespective of age of onset, with symptoms for 5 years or less who are severely handicapped, despite energetic medical treatment.

Provided that the operation is not carried out as an emergency in a crisis, the results employing these criteria are found to be entirely satisfactory in 70% of cases.

Pre-operative management

Many of these patients are severely debilitated and, because of muscle weakness, have difficulty in voiding accumulated secretions within the lung. Every attempt should be made to improve the condition of the lung by physiotherapy, postural drainage, antibiotics, mucolytics and antispasmodics.

Drugs. Neostigmine is often administered to these patients and is given orally as 15 mg tablets, in doses up to 45 mg four hourly, occasionally in greater quantity. Pyridostigmine causes less gastric irritation, and has a longer duration of action than neostigmine: 60 mg of pyridostigmine is equivalent to 15 mg neostigmine. Ambenonium chloride is somewhat similar in its action to neostigmine, 6 mg of ambenonium being equivalent to 15 mg neostigmine. The dose of these drugs should be so regulated as to be the minimum quantity compatible with maximum effect. Excessive salivation and colic can occur, particularly when the dose of anti-cholinesterase is increased, but atropine is of value in countering these side effects, and rest in hospital may allow a reduction in the total dose of anti-cholinesterase administered. ACTH may be employed in addition to the above.

Preparation for operation

Premedication. If possible, the oral route for neostigmine administration should be employed. Anti-sialogogues are usually unnecessary, particularly if cyclopropane and ether are avoided : anti-cholinesterase drugs enhance the action of the opiates and similar drugs, and the inclusion of these latter drugs in the premedication is also best avoided. If sedation is required this can be best achieved by the administration of phenothiazines.

Anaesthesia for patients with myasthenia gravis

General principles. There is no contraindication to the use of intravenous induction agents provided small amounts are given slowly. Unnecessary intubation should be avoided, as this may increase the tracheitis often present in some of these cases. *Patients with myasthenia gravis should only be given neuromuscular blocking agents if ventilation is to be supported, not only during the operation, but also as a deliberate regime in the post-operative period.* This is because the need for such an agent is rarely necessary in the presence of the poor muscle tone, and might seriously complicate what could otherwise be a relatively straight forward anaesthetic procedure (see above). If controlled ventilation is required this can be achieved by using inhalational agents combined with hyperventilation. Spontaneous ventilation is adequate for many surgical procedures in the well-controlled patients provided that tidal volume is carefully monitored. Trichloroethylene is often a very suitable agent when spontaneous ventilation is employed.

Anaesthesia for thymectomy: these patients should be intubated as controlled ventilation is invariably employed.

As it is usual to deliberately ventilate them in the post-operative period until adequate muscle power returns, there is no contraindication to the continuous use of neuromuscular blocking agents of the non-depolarizing group.

Post-operative care. In all cases of surgery upon patients with myasthenia gravis the need for careful respiratory care must be emphasized. It is essential to prevent pulmonary complications by encouraging the voiding of secretions, by humidification of inspired gases, suction, and active physiotherapy. The medication must be continuously readjusted with the object of achieving optimal muscle power. Full facilities for the support of ventilation must always be readily available.

Hypothermia

The term hypothermia is generally used when the body temperature falls below 35°C. The associated depression of metabolism by hypothermia is the primary physiological basis for the clinical use of this technique. The fall in oxygen uptake is said to be exponential with the fall in core temperature: however, the fall in oxygen consumption of the brain is linear down to 27–25°C in animals, though this relationship is not so consistent in man. During hypothermia the blood flow to the brain is reduced to balance the fall in oxygen consumption. In general the oxygen requirement is reduced in the following manner:

65–70% at 32°C
50–55% at 30°C
40% at 28°C
20–25% at 20°C
10% at 10°C

This reduction in the oxygen requirements of the body will enable the blood supply to certain organs to be temporarily suspended, thus permitting the surgeon to operate unhindered by the presence of blood.

The safe periods of circulatory arrest may vary in accordance with the age, the cardiopulmonary status, the depth of hypothermia of the patient and the anaesthesia used. Based upon clinical, biochemical and EEG criteria, arrest of flow in the brain may be reasonably safe within the following limits:

°C	37	30	28	25	20	10
Minutes	3	6	8–10	12–15	20	40

Deliberate hypothermia has been employed to facilitate intracranial operations, and operations upon the heart and great vessels. The production of the hypothermic state can be achieved by surface, veno-venous, or veno-arterial cooling.

Surface cooling

This technique is largely employed in situations where the surgical diagnosis is definite before cooling commences: unnecessary cooling is thus avoided. The technique is seldom employed today for intracardiac operations, but is sometimes used for operations upon the abdominal aorta, where the blood supply to the kidneys may be temporarily interrupted, and in intracranial operations.

Technique. Many techniques have been evolved for the production of the hypothermic state by surface cooling, but, whatever technique is employed, careful monitoring of the patient's vital functions is of paramount importance. The success of the procedure will be influenced by the amount of shivering and cutaneous vasoconstriction that occurs and also the degree of metabolic acidosis that results.

Preparation. This should include a careful assessment of the patient's cardiovascular function, with particular attention to the presence of myocardial disease. An electrocardiographic study should be carried out.

Premedication. There are many views regarding this matter. Where surface cooling is used, it is important to ensure adequate cutaneous vasodilatation, and with this in mind many anaesthetists incorporate in the premedication chlorpromazine and/or promethazine. The presence of chlorpromazine in particular will reduce the likelihood of shivering. However, associated with this deliberate attempt to produce cutaneous vasodilation is the associated risk of hypotension at an early stage of the cooling.

General anaesthesia. General anaesthesia with controlled ventilation must be used. The addition of diethyl ether or halothane to the mixture of nitrous oxide and oxygen will further promote cutaneous vasodilatation, though it should be borne in mind that the myocardial depressant effects of halothane are more marked during hypothermia. Carbon dioxide inhalation enhances cutaneous vasodilatation, maintains cardiac output and heart rate, and prevents the extreme hypocapnia that may occur during hypothermia (Broome and Sellick, 1965). Neuromuscular blocking agents will not only facilitate controlled ventilation but also prevent shivering: however, the altered response to these agents of reduction of body temperature must be borne in mind. D-Tubocurarine decreases in sensitivity with reduction in temperature whereas suxamethonium has the reverse effect. Care should, therefore, be taken to avoid giving additional neuromuscular blocking agents towards the end of operation, because of the possible increase in neuromuscular blocking effect associated with rewarming of the patient. Lack of appreciation of this effect may create difficulties with ventilation in the post-operative period.

Technique of cooling. The object of this technique is to cool the blood circulating through the skin and thus, by the process of circulation, lead to a reduction of body temperature. Using the skin as a heat exchanger in this way leads to a relatively slow reduction in body temperature: this method of cooling is also associated with a slower temperature drop of the core than the shell (the superficial tissues). During cooling, the heart temperature is an index of the core temperature, and the oesophageal temperature has proved to be a reliable guide to this, much more so than the rectal, which can be most misleading. The pharyngeal temperature or temperature of the external auditory meatus is fairly closely related to the temperature of the brain. (The use of the external auditory meatus for this purpose carries the real risk of injury which can be reduced by inserting the probe whilst the patient is conscious.)

After the cessation of surface cooling a further fall in temperature is often experienced. This fall varies in degree and is dependent on the amount of vasodilatation and subcutaneous fat of the subject, the rate of cooling, and other factors such as shell/core gradient. Great care must be exhibited in timing the termination of active cooling to avoid running in to the zone of temperature where cardiac dysrhythmias and cardiac arrest occur. A similar after-swing may be experienced in association with active rewarming.

Many methods are available for the production of surface cooling. They vary from the use of wind tunnels, and the application of ice bags, to the placing of the subjects in a bath of cold water, and the use of 'circulating' blankets. The ease with which the technique can be applied differs with each method. Particular care must be taken to avoid placing ice in direct contact with the skin, or ice bags in one position for a prolonged period of time, as necrosis of the underlying tissues may follow. To facilitate the application of cooling liquids to the surface of the body special cooling solutions may be employed. Cold Cetavalon added to water tends to cling to the skin surface and not to run off like pure water.

Another danger of surface cooling is that cardiac arrest can occur if accurate and careful observation of the patient's temperature is not insisted upon. The advantages of this technique are its simplicity and safety. It is rarely employed today for intra-thoracic operations, as the cardiac surgeons in particular usually prefer to confirm the diagnosis with direct observation of the heart, before embarking upon the hypothermic technique.

Veno-venous and veno-arterial cooling

These techniques are sometimes combined with cardio-pulmonary by-pass. Instead of using the skin as a heat exchanger, efficient systems for heat exchange are incorporated within the perfusion apparatus. The advantage of veno-venous cooling is that it avoids arterial canulation, but has the disadvantage that, should the heart fail, there is no means readily available for supporting the circulation other than by cardiac massage. The Drew Technique which uses the patient's own lungs to oxygenate the blood, allows for more profound degrees of cooling; the volume of blood necessary to 'prime' the system is also smaller than with mechanical oxygenators. However, the Drew Technique requires thoracotomy for the insertion of cannulae. Other pump-oxygenators have the facility of cooling the blood, and at the same time of supporting the circulation when it fails to be effective. Both systems require heparinization of the patient prior to the insertion of cannulae.

Monitoring the hypothermic patient

It is essential to have an accurate and continuous record of the temperature of the patient. The oesophageal temperature should be obtained from a sensing device placed immediately behind the heart. The temperature of the pharynx or external auditory meatus will give a guide to the temperature of the blood circulating to the brain. This may be 1–2°C higher than the oesophageal temperature. Care should be taken to ensure that the patient's temperature does not fall below 28°–29°C following the after-drop; depending on the rate of cooling, the active cooling should cease in good time to prevent this occurrence. The blood pressure, also, should be monitored throughout, either from an indwelling arterial catheter or indirectly, by use of a sphygmomanometer. The blood pressure will tend to fall as the cardiac output becomes reduced: at 32°C the cardiac output is reduced to 75% of normal, and at 28°C to 54% of normal. In addition the electrocardiograph should be monitored throughout. Patients usually exhibit no abnormality in the ECG until the temperature falls below 32°C, but below this level the first abnormality appears in the form of an increased PR interval, the QRS complex widens and the QT interval becomes prolonged. The first dysrhythmia to occur is normally atrial fibrillation, which is frequently noted below 28°C. ST changes associated with elevation appear below 26°C: provided that the heart is well oxygenated, and not manipulated, it will not fibrillate above 28°C unless it is already diseased or poisoned by drugs, but below 28°C the incidence of ventricular fibrillation increases rapidly. Rapid cooling of the circulation using direct cooling, may force cold blood into the coronary circulation long before the body core temperature is reduced; the perfusion of the heart by this cold blood may well provoke ventricular fibrillation and leave vital organs of the body exposed to an inadequate blood supply.

Dysrhythmias. The successful use of propranolol in the reversion to normal rhythm in a case undergoing moderate hypothermia which developed a cardia dysrhythmia has been reported. Great care should be exercised, however, in the use of β-adrenergic blockers in this situation, particularly if metabolic acidosis is present, as severe cardiovascular depression may occur. Certainly not more than 0.5 mg of propanolol should be used.

Acid-base balance. Poor peripheral blood flow, associated with vasoconstriction and superadded shivering, will contribute to the development of a metabolic acidosis. Such a metabolic acidosis is not an inevitable accompaniment of hypothermia *per se* and, though usually a reflection of the period and degree of anaerobic metabolism, it is more an index of the ability of the liver to remove and cope with such metabolites. The most common cause of metabolic acidosis during hypothermia is the infusion of ACD blood.

Electro-anaesthesia

The history of electrical anaesthesia began some eighty years ago. Recent research has perfected techniques for use in animals, but much more investigation is required before the technique can be satisfactorily employed in human beings.

Hypnosis

Hypnosis, by highly selected and trained practitioners, is occasionally employed to produce conditions for surgical anaesthesia, but the impossibility of forecasting suitable subjects makes the general use of hypnosis impracticable. Probably not more than 25% of all cases could be operated on under hypnosis and not more than 15% for major surgical operations.

The technique of acupuncture, widely used in China, has recently been the subject of interest in the Western World. (For further reading: Mann, F., 1973. *Acupuncture: Cure of many diseases,* Pan Books, London.)

Posture

The patient is positioned upon the operating table in such a way as to facilitate the operative procedure, bearing in mind that he may be held immobile for prolonged periods. Damage to tissues, joints and nerves may result and certain positions may, in addition, embarrass ventilation and blood flow. Careless positioning may also increase the hazard of diathermy burns.

The Trendelenberg position

This position is often adopted for pelvic operations in order to prevent abdominal contents obtruding into the operative field.

Effect on ventilation. Although the Trendelenberg position has been shown to reduce ventilation by about 14–24% in patients breathing spontaneously under halothane anaesthesia, further work has suggested that no significant changes occur in arterial gas tensions, respiratory minute volumes or rates.

Effect on cerebral blood flow. A 30° head down tilt after haemorrhage causes a reduction of carotid blood flow, suggesting that this traditional manoeuvre is perhaps not beneficial to the patient.

Effect on the nervous system. The use of shoulder rests to prevent the patient slipping off the table is to be strongly condemned. Damage to the brachial plexus may occur, particularly if the arm is placed at right angles to the long axis of the body. The Langton Hewer ribbed mattress obviates the need for shoulder rests.

Intermittent positive pressure ventilation should be adopted for intra-abdominal cases placed in this position, the mandatory use of a cuffed endotracheal tube thus also preventing the aspiration of regurgitated gastric contents.

The lithotomy position

This position is adopted for certain gynaecological and genito-urinary operations. Great care must be taken in raising the legs into position, particularly if disease of the hip joints is present. Both legs should always be raised at the same time, never independently; they should be well padded against the upright support and the lateral popliteal nerve never allowed to press against it.

Prolonged spontaneous ventilation in this position should not be allowed, as pressure on the diaphragm by abdominal contents, particularly in the obese subject, will increase the work of breathing. This position should never be used for the induction of anaesthesia.

The supine position

This posture creates no great difficulties apart from the fact that managing the unconscious subject in this posture increases the likelihood of inhalation of stomach contents, should they be regurgitated or vomited. The *supine hypotensive syndrome* may occur as a result of an abdominal tumour or gravid uterus pressing upon the inferior vena cava and impeding venous return to the heart. The use of a lumbar bridge may produce excessive bleeding in pelvic operations, because of kinking of the inferior vena cava.

The prone position

This posture is adopted for operation upon the back and vertebral column. As the chest movement is restricted, impairment of respiratory movement may occur if the abdomen is not raised off the table by pillows placed under the iliac crests and upper chest and shoulders. Prolonged maintenance of this posture will call for controlled ventilation. Sagging of the vertebral column may arise from placing pillows under the pelvis and give rise to venous oozing, due to impairment of venous return through the vena cava. This venous oozing can seriously embarrass a surgeon operating on the vertebral column and spinal cord, and calls for very careful positioning.

The knee-elbow position

This position is used for certain orthopaedic procedures such as spinal operations and in gynaecology. Great care should be exercised to ensure the stability of the patient and to avoid pressure damage to legs, arms and neck: this can best be achieved by the judicious use of padding and strapping. The patient must be intubated and controlled ventilation used throughout.

The sitting position

Varying degrees of this position are often employed for operations on the head and neck. The brain will be particularly vulnerable when this position is adopted if reduction in blood flow occurs to the upper part of the body. There is often a fall in the arm blood pressure with this position, the intensity and duration of which will depend on whether cardiovascular reflexes have been obtunded by general anaesthesia. It should be remembered that the pressure ten inches above the brachial artery will be approximately 20 mmHg less than at the brachial artery and further, the cerebral arteries may not be able to dilate in the presence of atheroma. Should a fall in cerebral perfusion occur during anaesthesia (particularly in the dental chair) this may pass unnoticed at the time with subsequent dire consequences. The question of inhalation of particulate matter is dealt with on page 342.

The lateral or semi-prone position

The latter is the best position for nursing the unconscious patient.

Patient monitoring

During the course of a general anaesthetic the anaesthetist will not only be concerned with the assessment of the depth of anaesthesia and the maintenance of the appropriate level, but must also satisfy himself that the patient's vital functions are not impaired. In the past the anaesthetist has relied upon sight, hearing, touch, and even olfactory stimuli, to sense various functions and integrate these at his own cortical level. These afferent impulses have been supplemented by the use of sensing devices.

The sphygmomanometer and the electrocardiograph have enabled him to measure to a varying degree the efficiency of the myocardium in response both to the surgical procedure and the general anaesthetic agents.

One major concern has been the flow of adequate amounts of oxygen to the tissues, in particular the flow of oxygen to the brain and, to a lesser degree, to the kidneys, liver and heart. A rough guide of peripheral blood flow has been the colour of blood in the cutaneous tissues and the capacity of the skin to refill after pressure has been exerted upon it. The colour can, however, be an unreliable index of the oxygenation of the blood, because the assessment is subject to many variables such as the amount of haemoglobin present, the visual acuity of the anaesthetist and the type of lighting (the spectral requirements for the artificial illumination have been investigated and are laid down in MRC Memo No 43, 'Spectral requirements of light sources for clinical purposes', 1966 obtainable from Her Majesty's Stationery Office). The presence of blood in the ear lobe and the tip of the nose – conventional sites for observation from the point of view of the anaesthetist – and the ability of tissues blanched under pressure to refill are useful rough guides as to the efficiency of peripheral flow. The presence or absence of a spurting artery in the operation site will further help to form a picture of blood flow to the tissues, but will in no way permit one to quantitate flow. The depth of anaesthesia tends to be assessed purely on clinical grounds, such as the patient's response to a given surgical stimulus, the presence or absence of sweating, lacrimation, and muscle tone.

In order to replace the clinical assessment, a monitoring device must be 100% reliable. Eye-sight, and the use of a finger over a pulse, together with the integration of the cerebral cortex, are undoubtedly features with which present day monitoring devices cannot compete, provided that the attention of the observer does not wander, and fatigue does not supervene. However, if the anaesthetist is aware of the limitations of certain monitoring devices, they can be a most useful supplement to the information he collates from moment to moment regarding the patient. Care must be taken, however, that he does not become 'hypnotized' by the equipment, and disregard such features as change in the patient's colour, pulse and blood pressure.

The anaesthetist is concerned with the transport of adequate amounts of oxygen to the tissues. If the haemoglobin content of the blood is adequate and the haemoglobin is fully saturated, the amount of oxygen being supplied to the tissues is a function of the cardiac output and its distribution. A knowledge of the blood pressure will give an index of the effect of cardiac output upon the arterial side of the vascular tree, but it will not necessarily give a measure of the adequacy of flow of oxygenated haemoglobin to the tissues. Similarly, the monitoring of the central venous pressure will not only give an index of the tone within the venous system, but also the ability of the myocardium to deal with the blood being returned to the right side of the heart. The pulse pressure may be measured directly or displayed employing the signal resulting from a sensing device in contact with the pulp of the finger: such a sensing device may be a photo-electric system or carbon microphone, and the signal so obtained will be a function of the degree of peripheral vasoconstriction, amongst other factors. The blood pressure thus obtained generally under-reads when compared with that obtained from the palpation of the brachial artery. A study of the pulse rate and rhythm, and in particular any changes therein, may give some indication of the response of the heart to the surgery, the anaesthetic agents, and the depth of anaesthesia. The presence of dysrhythmias may be related to the anaesthetic agent and to other features, such as the presence of hypercapnia and hypoxia, and lead the anaesthetist to take the appropriate action.

The electrocardiograph may be continuously displayed on an oscilloscope and/or on a paper record. Such recording is desirable during the course of hypothermic procedures and major cardiac surgery, but also has some application during routine general anaesthesia. However, the electrocardiograph may, at times, be misleading as the normal ECG complex has been observed during complete cardiac standstill: indeed, it is of more value to know what blood flow is being delivered from the heart. Although it is now technically possible to quantitate blood flow this is not practicable in the majority of cases, as either a major vessel has to be exposed to enable an electro-magnetic flowmeter to be placed in position, or canulation of an artery is necessary in order to monitor the passage of tracer during cardiac output studies. However, developments in impedence plethysmography and the application of the Doppler phenomenon have enabled some measure of blood flow to be made without the disadvantage of vessel exposure. A study of the electroencephalograph may enable the anaesthetist to detect not only variations in the level of anaesthesia, but also the presence or absence of cerebral oxygen deprivation. The routine application of continuous EEG monitoring, however, is of doubtful applicability because of its sophistication and vagaries. *It must be remembered that a silent EEG pattern does not necessarily indicate brain death.*

The anaesthetist must know the efficiency of alveolar ventilation. The monitoring of alveolar or arterial carbon dioxide tension is of particular value but again methods are not readily available for routine patient monitoring. Similarly monitoring of the arterial blood for arterial oxygen saturation and/or tension is not at the moment practicable and the use of the ear oximeter is, on the whole, unreliable. However, the measurement of the expired volume will give some measure of alveolar ventilation. It may be monitored by a variety of means, such as the Wright anemometer, the Drager meter, the dry gas meter or the spirometer. The ventilatory activity can be achieved by use of impedence plethysmography, a strain gauge placed around the chest, or by a temperature sensing device with a fast response time placed within the lumen of the conducting air passages.

The monitoring of temperature is an essential requisite of hypothermic techniques and paediatric anaesthesia. The transducer may be a thermistor, a thermocouple, or a simple high and low reading mercury thermometer: the pharynx, nasal passages, oesophagus, rectum, muscle, skin or external auditory meatus may be used as sites for measurement.

The electromyograph, recorded in response to stimulation of a nerve with an electrical current, is a useful guide to the degree of recovery from neuromuscular blockade. There is a possibility that the continuous measurement of skin resistance to the passage of an electric current may give a guide to the depth of anaesthesia in relation to the intensity of the surgical stimulus. Variations in blood flow and the degree of moisture on the skin surface cause variations in the electrical resistance.

Awareness during anaesthesia

With the introduction of neuromuscular blocking agents and the present tendency to maintain general anaesthesia on a light plane, there have been disturbing reports in the literature of patients recalling episodes that occurred during the course of a surgical operation.

Provided that the patient is hyperventilated, 70% nitrous oxide in oxygen should alone be sufficient to maintain unawareness, particularly if there has been an ample premedication. Passive hyperventilation with air has been shown to produce a state of indifference to the environment, at the same time raising the pain threshold. Hyperventilation, therefore, forms an integral part of some anaesthetic techniques. A possible explanation for the phenomenon is that hypocapnia produced by alveolar hyperventilation damps down the reticular activating system within the central nervous system: care should thus be taken that a state of awareness does not develop as the result of a pause in manual hyperventilation.

Certain other factors may influence the patient's conscious appreciation of pain: thiopentone, pentobarbitone, and certain phenothiazines (e.g. promethazine), have an antanalgesic action, i.e. they reduce the threshold to pain. Halothane has poor analgesic properties which makes itself particularly apparent in the immediate post-operative period. Anaesthetic mixtures may also become weakened by leakage into the system. Where premedication is relied upon as part of the anaesthetic technique, dosage and timing must be correct.

Quantities of induction agents should likewise be adequate, bearing in mind the present tendency to use solutions of low concentration. There is a danger that if a relaxant drug is given prior to the injection of thiopentone, the intravenous needle may become displaced before the narcotic can be administered. The practice of giving 100% oxygen to an obstetric patient immediately prior to the delivery of the baby should be carried out with particular care if anaesthesia has been maintained with nitrous oxide/oxygen only. Procedures such as bronchoscopy may outlast the effect of a single dose of drug such as thiopentone, and this operation in particular is usually carried out under relaxants without any inhalational supplements.

It must be remembered that the sense of hearing is the last to go and the first to return when associated with anaesthesia, and conversations are readily recalled when consciousness returns. The view is held by some that adequate paralysis and its consequent lack of proprioception encourages the unconscious state.

In conclusion the anaesthetist must not be unduly influenced by the fact that a very small proportion of patients have recalled certain episodes during an operation, nor allow this to bias his choice of anaesthetic to the extent of endangering the patient's safety.

Post-operative amnesia

Older patients tend to have more post-operative amnesia than young. The use of hyoscine in the pre-anaesthetic medication leads to a significant prolongation of post-operative amnesia. If post-operative drugs are administered during the amnesic period it is significantly prolonged. Diazepam is being employed to produce sedation for conservative dentistry. When used intravenously for this work this agent carries a high incidence of anterograde amnesia.

Care of the post-operative unconscious patient

The ideal method of nursing these cases is in the lateral semi-prone position – the so-called post-tonsillectomy position. The patient is rolled onto his side, with the pelvis and thorax at an angle of about 45° with the horizontal. A pillow is placed beneath the chest, and the upper arm is placed over this, as though hugging it. The lower arm is either in front of or behind the trunk, depending on the girth of the patient – it is difficult to place it behind in the obese. Both legs are bent at the knee, the upper more than the lower, as this prevents pressure between the thighs, though some workers claim that if the lower is more flexed, the patient is more stable. The head may be on a very flat pillow, or rest directly on the mattress.

Post-operative trolleys should have facilities for lowering or raising the head and legs. The attendant must stand at the head of the trolley or bed, with her hand cupped under the patient's jaw to maintain an airway, and to enable her to feel each respiration on the palm of her hand. It should be stressed to all such attendants that respirations must be felt or quietly heard, and that absolutely no reliance should be placed on the movement of chest or abdomen, which can take place even when the respiratory passage is completely obstructed. The pulse should be regularly palpated, and the colour observed. A source of oxygen and means of artificial ventilation must be ready to hand, together with facilities for suction, a mouth gag, swabs, airways, and a laryngoscope. The patient should not leave the precincts of the theatre and proximity of the anaesthetist until the return of consciousness and the vital reflexes.

Owing to the small size of the pharynx and glottis, all children are particularly at risk and must be nursed as above, but many adults are nursed prone. This is because they are expected to be unconscious for only a few minutes, and the recovery trolley may be very narrow. If this is done, the head must not be on a pillow, but be turned well to the side, and a pillow should be under the contralateral shoulder. All other provisos must still apply.

Diathermy

Most diathermy units of British manufacture have outputs of the order of 250–300 W. At the point of application of the active electrodes, as the area of contact is small, the current density is high : heat is generated at this point, with the desired effect of section, desiccation, or coagulation of tissue and vessels. (The current is transmitted as a frequency of 3–10 MHz.) The plate or patient electrode, used with surgical diathermy equipment, is required to provide a return path for diathermy currents which enter the body at the 'active' diathermy electrode. The plate electrode must have good contact with the body, and be of sufficient area to provide a low impedence path for the diathermy current and to reduce the current density in the underlying tissues to as low a value as possible, in order to keep to a minimum unwanted heat generation from the passage of the current. Since the maximum power output of most surgical diathermy units is seldom used, the comparatively large plate electrode (30 in^2, 187 cm^2) advised in the Report of the Working Party on Anaesthetic Explosions (1956) provides for a fair margin of error in the reduction of contact area, due to imperfect application. Smaller plate electrodes have been used with infants. When electrodes of a reduced size are used, it is even more important to see that contact between the electrode and the body is good : the use of two plate electrodes connected in a parallel is recommended where practicable, so that the total area of contact is kept as large as possible. To overcome the problem associated with the use of diathermy apparatus in small children, large sheets of aluminium foil may be employed.

Saline-soaked pads may be used for covering the plate electrode; these pads have the advantage that intimate contact with the skin is obtained by a solution of good electrical conductivity and the pad itself tends to reduce the effect of slight irregularities in the surface of the electrode. Recent work has shown that normal physiological saline (0.9% w/v) is as satisfactory as stronger solutions and has the advantage of not irritating sensitive skin (Dobbie, 1969). The use of wet saline pads particularly in small infants may lead to hypothermia. The drying of these pads during the course of a long operation leads to imperfect conduction of the electric current; under such circumstances current may flow to earth through any alternative contact that is offered (e.g. metal of operating table that may be touching the skin), resulting in a burn at such point of contact. It is likely that smooth, flat, metal pads, requiring no covers or even electrode jelly will be more extensively accepted. Great care should always be taken to ensure that, when positioning the patient prior to operation, he is not in contact with any metallic or conducting parts of the operating table. Burns can also arise if the earth electrode is imperfectly connected to the diathermy apparatus, so the plate electrode should always be tested for efficient continuity prior to application to the patient, by using the contact point provided on the machine, unless a warning device is incorporated in the machine. The electrode should be flattened periodically and discarded when cracked or hardened. If contact cream is used, it should be removed from the pad afterwards to prevent a dry film forming and impairing conductivity. Areas where bone is directly subcutaneous should be avoided. Provided that the earth path through the indifferent electrode is adequately secured by the above measures there would appear to be no danger to the patient from the diathermy when electrical monitoring equipment is used e.g. ECG (Dobbie, 1969), provided the latter is protected from diathermy current frequencies by an adequate impedence.

Explosions

New work has recently revised attitudes regarding safety precautions in the operating theatre during the use of flammable anaesthetic agents such as diethyl ether, divinyl ether (Vinesthene), cyclopropane and ethyl chloride. Diathermy or cautery should not, of course, be used on a patient receiving such a flammable or explosive anaesthetic. But it is possible that in the past the so called 'zone of risk' that surrounds a patient receiving one of these agents has been exaggerated and the previously advised 4 ft 6 in (135 cm) can possibly be reduced to a radius of 25 cm around any part of the anaesthetic circuit.

The following precautions would still appear advisable. Theatre clothing should be of cotton, and no woollen blankets nor man-made fibres should be used on patients or by staff. However, this does not apply to close-fitting stockings nor underclothes, as they soon have a film of conducting moisture forming on them. All footwear must be anti-static. The theatre and its equipment: floors should be of anti-static material, as should all wheeled apparatus in the theatre, all rubber mattresses, and tubing on anaesthetic or suction machines.

Suction apparatus must be spark-proof so that explosive gases do not come into contact with sparks. The relative humidity of a theatre should be about 60% : this, also, is to eliminate the formation of static electrical charges that might cause a spark. No open flame, or radiator that can become hotter than 60°C, should be allowed in the theatre. Endoscopic instruments and headlamps should be run off an 'intrinsically safe circuit' – i.e. one of 4–6 V, as such a circuit is unlikely to generate a spark in case of sudden disconnection. Transformers, and not resistances, should be used to reduce mains voltages. All foot switches should be gas tight.

Further reading

Recommendations of the Association of Anaesthetists of Great Britain and Ireland (1971) 'Explosion hazards'. *Anaesthesia, 26* : 155.

4 *The Extremes of Age*

Paediatrics

The extremes of age present particular problems to the anaesthetist. Table 4.1 lists the commoner physiological data in children. The young, by virtue of their immaturity, cannot be treated as smaller versions of the adult, for each system of the body is in the process of developing its own inherent stability in response to the environment in which the new human finds himself. Not only is the central nervous system laying down the pattern which will be adopted in the mature individual, but other systems of the body are also undergoing profound changes. It is, therefore, to be expected that such an immature being will react to anaesthesia and surgical trauma in a different way from the adult. Three phases may be differentiated in this development from a neonate to a mature individual. The two systems predominantly affected by this change are the respiratory and cardiovascular. The first phase concerns the commencement of spontaneous ventilation, and is associated with a number of circulatory alterations which are associated with expansion of the lungs; this is followed by the phase of consolidation, in which the internal control of respiration and the re-adjustment within the circulatory system are stabilized. The final phase concerns the transition from the neonatal pattern to that of the child, and this is followed by a relatively smooth development to the adult pattern. Apart from predominantly cardiovascular and respiratory changes (see Table 4.1), there are other changes which, in many ways, are equally important. The development of the central nervous system is associated with the development of the higher centres and appreciation of the environment. As development proceeds, heat regulation becomes more stable and metabolism adopts the adult pattern.

Heat regulation

The instability of the heat regulating mechanism in children is often demonstrated by the marked variations in temperature accompanying relatively trivial episodes such as 'teething'. In the early months of life the general tendency is for infants to lose heat, and this presents a very

Table 4.1 *Paediatric physiological values*

Value	*Age* *Newborn*	*Later*
Metabolic rate cal/h/m² body surface area	approx. 60 in infancy	approx. 40 school age to adolescence approx. 30–35 adult
Oxygen consumption ml/kg/min	6	3·5–4·0
Respiratory rate /min	average 40 (range 20–50)	falls to 12–16 at 15 years
Tidal volume ml (= 3 × dead space) – see below	approx. 17 at birth	increasing to approx. 360 at 15 years
Alveolar ventilation ml/min	approx. 380 at 1 week	increasing to approx. 3 litres at 15 years
Dead space 2·2 × wt. (kg)	ml	*age*
	6	1 week
	22	1 year
	32	3 years
	40	5 years
	58	8 years
	140	15 years
Cardiac output	l/min	*age* (years)
	1·9	1
	2·7	3
	3·2	5
	4·4	8
	5·7	12
	at birth	*later*
Blood volume ml/kg	84·7 neonate	decreasing to 65 by 2 years
Pulse rate /min	90–180 (average 125)	
Blood pressure mmHg	75–85 systolic 40–50 diastolic	95 systolic at approx. 14 days
Haemoglobin %	may exceed 150	falling to as low as 75 in some patients at 3 months: then rises slowly to normal values

Electrolytes and water (baby's weight 3–5 kg):
2·4 kg water; 66 g total nitrogen; 243 Na^+ mEq; 160 Cl^- mEq; 28·2 Ca^{++} mEq.

real problem in young infants undergoing surgery and anaesthesia. Monitoring of temperature is mandatory in all neonates. The thermometer must be capable of recording temperatures as low as 28°C. Every attempt must be made to prevent heat loss, from the time the baby is first seen. If the temperature is low the operation should be postponed to allow the temperature to rise. Under anaesthesia, with an immature temperature control further depressed by the anaesthetic agent, there are many factors tending to lower the temperature. Of these, the open wound both radiating heat and allowing evaporation is the most important and least amenable to control. In addition, the use of dry anaesthetic gases encourages tracheal heat loss, and cold blood and infusion liquid may cause problems.

To combat losses, the theatre temperatures should be high (24°C–29°C) and the baby exposed for as little time as possible. If intravenous infusions have to be employed, the baby, apart from the arm or leg, should be wrapped in warmed gauze or a silvered rescue blanket. The baby should be on an electric or hot water blanket. Heating blankets should be suitably controlled to prevent excessive temperatures with the risk of burns. Two thermostats are recommended. A water blanket connected to a pump unit with a thermostat delivering water at normal body temperature, is probably more satisfactory as the temperature can be more accurately controlled; it is useful for warming blood either by putting the bottle in the unit or for warming a coil.

It should be remembered that a high temperature gradient cannot be allowed between the heating blanket and the baby. This creates a practical limit on heat transfer. It is therefore easier to maintain the temperature than to raise it. As the child matures, the danger of hyperpyrexia develops. Hyperpyrexia will occur if normal heat loss is prevented by the use of atropine, Mackintosh sheeting, and an excessively warm and humid operating theatre such as may be found in less temperate climates. It must be borne in mind that small children have a higher metabolic rate than adults, and any factor that further increases this rate, such as pyrexial illness, hyperpnoea, dehydration, and drugs such as atropine, will create an imbalance between heat production and heat loss.

'Ether convulsions', attributed not only to ether but atropine, Mackintosh sheeting, pyrexial illness and dehydration, very rarely occur. A true convulsion occurring under anaesthesia must be treated very seriously and the possibility of malignant hyperpyrexia borne in mind. The routine monitoring of temperature in all patients is the only way to diagnose this complication at a stage early enough to permit effective treatment.

Malignant hyperpyrexia. Recently a new syndrome has been reported in the literature (Relton *et al.*, 1968). This consists of a sudden and inexplicable rise in body temperature sometimes associated with muscular rigidity, occurring under general anaesthesia. Many theories as to its origin have been put forward, but there is as yet no general agreement. Although most patients are young, the condition has been reported in adults and may have a familial incidence, which may be associated with a familial incidence of myopathy. However, the patients are more often healthy, and apyrexial at the time of induction. First signs are increased ventilation, tachycardia, sweating and peripheral cyanosis or flushing, sometimes associated with muscular rigidity. The body temperature may rise to 42°C or more and cause death. When associated with suxamethonium, imperfect relaxation is often present. It is possible that the muscular spasm is due to some agent acting directly on muscle fibres, as it is not relieved by the administration of D-tubocurarine. Treatment must be instituted immediately. Artificial ventilation with 100% oxygen should be given and vigorous surface cooling initiated. If a water blanket is available the heater should be switched off and ice poured into the tank. Low blood pressure is best treated with a 5% dextrose infusion to which 2 mg isoprenaline is added, and sodium bicarbonate should be given for metabolic acidosis. Procaine, up to 40 mg/kg i.v. is suggested as being a specific treatment. A non-depolarizing relaxant may occasionally help to reduce heat production from muscular activity and make artificial ventilation easier.

Body temperature should be monitored as a routine in all young patients undergoing general anaesthesia.

Response to drugs

It need hardly be said that the child, by virtue of its small size, will detoxicate and eliminate drugs at a rate in proportion to the body size and metabolic rate. The response of the child to a particular drug will vary according to the type used. Drugs which act by reducing metabolism, will, on the whole, require to be given in rather larger doses relative to body size than in the adult, on account of the higher metabolic rate. Adjustment of dosage to body weight rather than age is particularly important with all drugs. Local anaesthetic agents should always be calculated on the basis of weight. Children tolerate atropine well, and half the adult dose may be employed from the age of 2 years to 10 years.

Oxygenation

The body oxygen stores of the small child are relatively small in comparison to the oxygen consumption. Therefore, should respiratory obstruction or depression occur, desaturation of arterial blood arises more rapidly than in the adult. To guard against this it is important to pre-oxygenate a child to ensure nitrogen washout before attempting any endotracheal manoeuvre, and this applies equally to extubation as to intubation. An increased oxygen store in the alveoli permits a longer safe apnoeic time.

Starvation

Deliberate and unnecessary restriction of fluid and carbohydrate intake in infants leads very rapidly to metabolic acidosis and ketosis. Whilst recognizing the fact that oral intake in the immediate pre-operative period may hazard the patient if vomiting or regurgitation should occur, clearly some degree of continued hydration must be allowed up to the four hours preceding operation. Oral feeding should recommence as early as possible in the post-operative period. If oral intake cannot be ensured, parenteral therapy must be instituted. Here guidance by an experienced paediatrician is invaluable.

Blood loss

Blood loss should be measured as accurately as possible during surgery, particularly in neonates. One simple and inexpensive method is that of swab washing. This permits the use of wet swabs which tend to make swab weighing less accurate. The use of suction is to be discouraged as significant volumes of blood can remain unseen in the tubing. The estimated blood volume can be calculated from the weight (see page 83). A loss of 10% of this value is the upper limit of loss that can be tolerated without replacement in a healthy child e.g. in a neonate of 3.2 kg the estimated blood volume is 256 ml. A loss of 25 ml would be the upper limit to be allowed before considering replacement. In deciding when to replace, the continuing loss into the tissues after surgery should be taken into account. In considering transfusion it is important to realize that the neonatal haemoglobin may be about 16 g per 100 ml; 'whole blood for transfusion' has a haemoglobin of 11 g. In operations such as meningo-myelocoele repair and the removal of sacro-coccygeal teratomata, the blood loss may be from 50%–100% of the blood volume. In these cases the blood must be given as fast as the loss occurs. 1 ml of 10% calcium gluconate should be given for each 100 ml of blood. Efforts should be made to acquire blood not more than one week old for these operations.

Water and electrolytes

In a baby depleted of electrolytes and water pre-operatively, every effort should be made to restore an adequate blood volume before operation commences. Blood electrolyte estimations are of relatively little value and should not entirely be relied upon as a guide. The presence of peripheral refill of cutaneous tissue after pressure is often a valuable sign of adequate blood volume. Where there is evidence of a depleted blood volume, blood is best given. The use of the umbilical vein for replacement is not recommended because of the risk of bowel ischaemia, and infection. In the post-operative period the neonate should be given breast milk rather than cow's milk as soon as possible. With a gastric operation, feeding should take place via a tube placed in the duodenum. This subject is considered in more detail on page 160.

Premedication

Like the problem of intubation in children, this has been the subject of much discussion. Some feel strongly that children should be oblivious to their surroundings prior to induction of anaesthesia, so that psychic trauma is kept to the minimum. Certainly, an inhalational induction with a frightened child may produce fear of anaesthesia for the rest of his life. On the other hand, many children soon become adapted to hospital life, and an intravenous induction without previous sedation is advocated by others. Certain anaesthetists believe that the mother should be present at induction. Whatever method is adopted, clearly a kind, gentle but firm approach to the patient is necessary. Children's anaesthesia always seems to be difficult to organize, as operating lists often have to be changed due to emergencies, such as the appearance overnight of a rash or diarrhoea, or unexpected findings in an earlier operation. The ordering of premedication should take this into account. Premedication ideally will produce long acting tranquillity rather than short acting sedation. There is also little point of giving an injection in the ward only to avoid the memory of one in the anaesthetic room. A few minutes spent with a child at a pre-anaesthesia visit can obviate the need for any premedication.

Sedation by oral route

Very many syrups and elixirs – and supositories – have been prepared in order to make the sedative agent more acceptable to the child. A syrup or elixir may prove the ideal vehicle for the sedative agent chosen. Occasionally the agent may be prescribed in the form of a tablet, or capsule, in which case it may be necessary to assist the child in swallowing the substance, by means of a small sweet drink, or by disguising the agent with jam or honey. Sedatives administered in this way are unreliable in the onset of action and may well be vomited (see Table 4.2).

D

Table 4.2 *Oral sedatives*

Drug	*Dose*	*Comment*
chloral hydrate	20 mg/lb (44 mg/kg)	Very unpleasant taste and difficult to disguise Useful for a procedure under local anaesthesia
barbiturates		
phenobarbitone*	0·4mg/lb (0·8 mg/kg)	Max. dose 30 mg at 5 years
butobarbitone*	40 mg/stone (6 mg/kg)	Bitter taste of barbiturates is difficult to disguise Some available as an elixir Many are antanalgesics and may lead to post-operative restlessness
pentobarbitone*	40 mg/stone (6 mg/kg)	
quinalbarbitone*	40 mg/stone (6 mg/kg)	
phenothiazines		
pecazine (Pacatal, Mephazine)*	28 mg/stone (4·4 mg/kg)	
trimeprazine tartrate*	14–28 mg/stone (2·0–4·0 mg/kg)	Vallergan Forte syrup contains 6 mg/ml trimeprazine tartrate
promethazine	1·1–2·2 mg/kg	
methylpentynol (Oblivon)*	250 mg/stone (39 mg/kg)	
diazepam*	0·1 mg/lb (0·22 mg/kg)	
glutethamide (Doriden)	125 mg orally at 6 months increasing to 250 mg at 6 years	Give one hour preoperatively

Sedation by injection

Opiates. Morphine or papaveretum in combination with hyoscine or atropine are drugs well suited for the premedication of children over 15.9 kg (35 lb), or about 5 years of age :

morphine*:	0.1 mg/lb (0.3 mg/kg)
papaveretum*:	0.29 mg/lb (0.3 mg/kg)
pethidine*:	0.5–1.0 mg/lb (1.0–3.0 mg/kg)

Methohexitone : an intramuscular dose of 3 mg/lb (6.6 mg/kg) gives a safe, rapid and pleasant induction of sleep.

Great care must be taken to ensure that the airway is maintained and therefore the patient should be treated as though under general anaesthesia.

* These can be given with oral or intramuscular hyoscine: 0·2 mg under 50 lb (23 kg), 0·4 mg over 50 lb.

Diazepam (Valium)* : 0.2 mg/kg i.m. up to 25 kg body weight.

Ketamine : with a dose of 1–4 mg/kg intravenously of this dissociative agent, sleep occurs within a minute, with recovery in 15–20 minutes. When given intramuscularly in a dose of 6.5–13.0 mg/kg sleep occurs in 4–5 minutes, with recovery in about 1 hour.

Neuroleptic agents have been employed for the calming of the particularly difficult child.

Sedation by rectal route

Enema: thiopentone may be administered by the rectal route using either a 5% or 10% solution of thiopentone sodium, or as a paste, or suppository. As a solution, the dose is based on 1 g per 23 kg (or 1 g per 50 lb). Where the solution is employed, the drug should be gently run in with the patient lying in the left lateral position, the catheter gently removed, and the buttocks strapped together.

Suppositories: for children requiring general anaesthesia, those weighing 6–12 kg require a 0.25 g suppository, and those weighing 12–25 kg require a 0.5 g suppository.

The suppositories, which are supplied in 125 mg, 250 mg, and 500 mg sizes are ideally administered 45 minutes prior to induction of anaesthesia. Thiopentone suspension produces a much more profound sedation for a shorter time than the suppositories which are therefore preferable and safer. Quinalbarbitone 32 mg/stone (5 mg/kg) may be given rectally 2–3 hours pre-operatively. Max. dose 200 mg.

Caution : *Where the aim of the pre-medication has been to produce a child who is deeply asleep (e.g. intramuscular methohexitone or rectal thiopentone) the patient must at no time be left unattended, and at all times the airway must be carefully guarded.*

Parasympatholytic agents. It has been the custom in the past to administer as a routine, certain of the parasympatholytic agents, chiefly for their anti-sialogogue effect. In the days when diethyl ether was frequently used for paediatric anaesthesia, it was essential to prevent the secretion of mucus from the upper respiratory tract. As a consequence, atropine or hyoscine are still given routinely in hospitals.

Today, when ether is not likely to be used, atropine or hyoscine may be omitted from the pre-medication. However, if suxamethonium is included in the anaesthetic technique, atropine should be administered beforehand in order to reduce the incidence of severe bradycardia that may be associated with its use. In order to avoid the necessity of an injection in the conscious child, oral atropine has been advocated; it has been claimed that medication by this route is reliable and effective. Extreme caution should be observed when administering atropine to the pyrexial, dehydrated, or toxic child, as there is a very real danger of provoking a hyperpyrexial state which may be accompanied by convulsions. Atropine may also aggravate an existing tachycardia. Dose: atropine 0.02 mg/lb (0.04 mg/kg) reaching a maximum of 0.6 mg at 14 kg. Hyoscine 0.006 mg/lb (0.012 mg/kg) reaching a maximum of 0.4 mg at 32 kg.

Timing of administration will depend on the drug, the route of administration, and the dose. Table 4.3 shows a general scheme.

Table 4.3 *Timing of administration of sedatives*

Route	*Drug*	*Time interval before induction of anaesthesia* (min)
Mouth	chloral	45
	barbiturates* phenothiazines* methylpentynol	90–120
Rectum	thiopentone*	30
	pentobarbitone* quinalbarbitone*	60–90
Injection	atropine	30–40
	opiates pethidine phenothiazines* hyoscine	60–90

* Certain of the barbiturates and phenothiazines are antanalgesics, and may, if used in the premedication, predispose to post-operative restlessness, particularly if the operation is of short duration (e.g. tonsillectomy and adenoidectomy).

Neonates. Pre-anaesthetic medication is generally unnecessary, except for atropine, as the presence of even small amounts of secretion can be troublesome, and bradycardia often occurs when awake intubation is performed.

Children up to 18 months. Pre-anaesthetic medication is generally unnecessary, except for atropine (see above).

Equipment. Particular regard should be paid to the small tidal volumes experienced in neonates and infants. Dead space apparatus should be kept to the minimum and unnecessary resistance to ventilation eliminated. Face masks have been devised for use with small children (Jenkins, 1957), (Rendell-Baker, 1962) and attempts have been made to reduce dead space (Vale, 1958 and 1959), (Voss, 1963). Carbon dioxide absorption has been advocated by some, as it is argued that heat and water loss are thereby minimized. Such apparatus is, however, unnecessarily cumbersome, has an appreciable dead space, and not inconsiderable resistance to the rapid breathing of the children. Others have devised uni-directional valves (Rackow and Salanitre, 1968); there are problems associated with the resistance and dead space of these items of equipment, and some of them do not function satisfactorily and safely with controlled ventilation. A T-piece technique may be employed. Such a technique is particularly valuable in a patient with an endotracheal tube; resistance is minimal, and re-breathing should not occur provided an adequate fresh gas flow is maintained. Controlled ventilation may be employed by intermittently occluding the end of the tube with a finger or an automatic device (Keuskamp, 1963. Alternatively, rapid intermittent pressure on a reservoir bag placed at the end of the tube is satisfactory. An air entrainment device has been produced for use with draw-over vaporizers in children (Farman 1965).

Induction of general anaesthesia

The method of induction is governed by the personal preference of the anaesthetist. Many workers prefer an inhalational method especially with smaller children, and indeed with neonates it is often possible to intubate prior to induction. Other anaesthetists use the intravenous route, claiming that this is less psychologically disturbing especially to the older child. The method used is secondary to the skill and experience of the administrator.

Maintenance of General Anaesthesia. Although there has been a trend towards laryngeal intubation and controlled ventilation using muscle relaxants in children, we feel that the inhalational methods still have a distinct place in paediatric anaesthesia.

The introduction of halothane has displaced the traditional agents, divinyl ether, diethyl ether and Vinesthene Anaesthetic Mixture (VAM). Being non-irritant, supplied from a calibrated vaporizer and being potent in the presence of high concentrations of oxygen, halothane permits intubation without muscle relaxants. Open mask anaesthetics, with their unknown concentrations, both of anaesthetic and oxygen, large mask dead space and general pollution of the atmosphere have little except simplicity to recommend them. The administration of divinyl ether combined with diethyl ether (VAM) on an open mask is satisfactory for operations of short duration, though a trickle of oxygen run through a small tube under the mask is probably advisable. Diethyl ether, divinyl ether, as well as halothane, may also be used with conventional anaesthetic apparatus, though efforts should be made to reduce the dead space and respiratory resistance of the apparatus.

Ethyl chloride should never be employed for general anaesthetic purposes.

We consider that routine laryngeal intubation using neuromuscular blocking agents is not necessary for operations such as circumcisions and repair of inguinal hernia.

Post-operative management

Careful control of acid-base balance, hydration, oxygenation, and temperature is essential. Ventilatory insufficiency should be treated by intermittent positive pressure ventilation through a naso-tracheal tube.

Endotracheal intubation in children

Over the years there has been much controversy over the question of endotracheal intubation in children, particularly the very young. It was argued that the laryngeal mucosa of the infant was very sensitive to even the smallest degree of trauma, and that the slightest laryngeal oedema rapidly gave rise to significant laryngeal obstruction. Much of the disrepute that acrued from intubation arose in the days before neuromuscular blocking agents, when, in some circumstances, relaxation and good visualization of the larynx were difficult to achieve. With the advent of modern relaxant techniques and halothane, good conditions for intubation are the general rule; intubation is far less traumatic to the sensitive tissues and complications are rare. Some authorities recommend relaxant techniques and controlled ventilation for the majority of paediatric anaesthetics irrespective of the duration of the nature of the operation. Such techniques will make intubation mandatory. This procedure would only be recommended in centres with much paediatric work, as routine intubation and ventilation require specialized instruments and equipment not usually found in general surgical theatres.

Laryngoscopy. Because of the anatomical relationships of the larynx in the young, intubation is often not so straightforward as in the adult. There are four main differences in the neonate. The tongue is relatively large, the epiglottis is large and less stiff, the cords slope posteriorly, and the narrowest part of the respiratory tract is at the cricoid ring. For these reasons the ordinary Macintosh laryngoscope is sometimes not suitable and a straight blade laryngoscope is easier to use up to the age of about six months, after which the adult size Macintosh laryngoscope can usually be used. Many laryngoscopes have been devised to facilitate the procedure.

Intubation. In the small child the narrowest part of the air passages into which an endotracheal tube is placed is the immediate subglottic region. The cross-secion of this region roughly corresponds to the cross-section of the external nares. With nasal intubation (see below), if the tube can readily be passed through the nasal air passages, it almost certainly will pass freely into the trachea. The length and diameter of endotracheal tubes for children have been the subject of much study. The traditional method of measuring the length of the tube by assessing the distance between the external nares and the ear lobes is very unreliable. The passage of a tube of incorrect length clearly creates problems; a tube which is too long may pass into the right main bronchus with associated problems. The Magill flexo-metallic tube reduces the chances of passing the tube too far into the tracheo-bronchial tree. Assessment of the length of the orotracheal tube in cm can be determined by dividing the age of the child in years by 2 and adding 12 (Levin, 1958), and another rough guide is shown in Table 4.4 (McIntyre, 1957).

Table 4.4 *Orotracheal tube length and age*

Age (years)	*2*	*3*	*4*	*5*	*6*	*7*	*8*	*9*	*10*	*11*	*12*
Length of tube (cm)	13·25	13·25	13·75	14·25	14·52	14·5	15·25	15·5	15·5	16·25	16·5

The diameter of tubes has also been based on age. For children less than 1 year a tube range of 2.0–4.5 mm is usually satisfactory. For children one year of age and over, put a two in front of the age in years and divide by 4; this will give the largest size tube internal diameter (i.d.) in mm that can be accommodated, and by selecting one size smaller one can be sure that the tube will fit. For children ten years and over add two to the first digit of the age and calculate as above. This is shown in Table 4.5.

Table 4.5 *Orotracheal tube diameter*

Age (years)	neonate	¼–½	½–1	1–2	2–3
Internal diameter of tube (mm)	3	3·5	4	4·5	5

All endotracheal tubes should be carefully prepared for use in a sterile condition and a selection of tubes of sizes roughly in the region of that expected, should be available for immediate use. The largest diameter tube that can be passed with ease should be used. Selective endo-bronchial intubation for thoracic surgery in young children has been tried but no longer employed, because of the small diameters involved.

Tracheostomy versus prolonged naso-tracheal intubation. Where indications have arisen for prolonged by-pass of the upper respiratory tract it has been the custom in the past to perform a tracheostomy. Tracheostomy in children has carried with it a very high morbidity and mortality rate. Despite the theoretical advantage of permitting the ready access to the tracheo-bonchial tree and the resultant ability to apply suction for the removal of secretions, in practice infections have been almost impossible to avoid, despite highly skilled nursing and the provision of intensive therapy units. Crusting of secretions has occurred despite apparently efficient humidification. Even if these hazards can be overcome there is a very real danger of subglottic stenosis. As a result of these potential complications there has been a recent trend towards the naso-tracheal route when intubation is required for prolonged periods of time. Tubes have been designed for this purpose which can be readily anchored to the patient's face without fear of becoming displaced. With efficient humidification pulmonary complications are minimized. Such a procedure may be adopted for periods of seven to ten days with apparently little ill effect. Prior to extubation it is advisable to place the patient on systemic steroids in order to minimize any oedema which may arise at glottic level (their effect can be further supplemented by spraying the cords with hydrocortisone powder, or solution).

Neuromuscular blocking agents

Neonates. The early use of non-depolarizing relaxants in the neonate (less than 28 days old) was abandoned in view of reports of the undue sensitivity of these small, immature children to the drugs. However, there appears to be no obvious sensitivity to the action of D-tubocurarine compared to the adult, when dosage is calculated on the body weight basis stated below, the patient is not deeply anaesthetized, and no hypothermia has been permitted. Provided that small initial doses of D-tubocurarine are used, and reversal with neostigmine is carried out at the termination of anaesthesia, no special hazards exist for infants or children.

It is recommended that initial doses should be 0.25 mg D-tubocurarine in the premature, and 0.5 mg in full-term neonates up to four weeks. After four weeks of age the dose of curare can be given on the basis of 0.5 mg/kg. Divided doses should be given at three minute intervals until paralysis occurs. Increments can be one third to one half of initial dose should muscular activity return. Tubocurarine is best administered in the following manner: 10 mg D-tubocurarine are taken up into a 10 ml or 20 ml syringe and diluted with water. Each ml in the syringe will therefore contain 1.0 mg or 0.5 mg. For reversal atropine 0.6 mg is best diluted in 6 ml and neostigmine 2.5 mg in 10 ml. Residual curarisation is reversed at the end of operation with neostigmine 0.036 mg/lb (0.08 mg/kg) preceded by atropine 0.008 mg/lb (0.018 mg/kg) intravenously, or the dose may be determined thus:

Dose neostigmine = 1/10 × dose curare: Dose atropine = $\frac{1}{4}$ × dose neostigmine.

Potentiating factors such as inhalational agents should be avoided, and the tendency to hypothermia, which is marked when controlled ventilation is used, countered by appropriate means.

For procedures up to 30 minutes duration, intermittent suxamethonium may be used. Doses intravenously (1–2 mg/kg) up to a total not exceeding 15–45 mg may be given. The importance of limiting the total dose is because of the tendency of the neonate to develop dual block with increasing dosage. The incremental dose should be kept as low as 1.0–1.25 mg. In an attempt to reduce the total dose of suxamethonium given, small concentrations of halothane are often added to the inspired mixture. Intramuscular suxamethonium has been recommended in a dose of 1.5 mg/lb (3.3 mg/kg), complete paralysis occurring in about one minute, and spontaneous ventilation returning in about 15–19 minutes when the 10% solution is used. Injection may be given into the tongue, though this practice is not without its dangers. Care should be taken if intramuscular suxamethonium is administered to children – any reduction in muscle blood flow may prolong the effect of the agent. Intramuscular and subcutaneous suxamethonium should be given with caution for intubation as there is a risk that relaxation may be inadequate for intubation but enough to stop respiration.

Infants and children are sometimes said to be more resistant than neonates to both types of neuromuscular blocking agents. An initial injection of 0.65 mg/kg D-tubocurarine in younger children and 0.6 mg/kg in older children is suitable for intubation. Ventilation should be controlled until the action is reversed. Increments should be $\frac{1}{8}$–$\frac{3}{4}$ of the initial dose. The drug should be administered in a solution of 3 mg/ml (i.e. 15 mg D-tubocurarine diluted to 5 ml with water). The dose of D-tubocurarine administered should be reduced if ether or halothane are used. Where a vagolytic effect is required gallamine, in a dose of 1 mg/lb (2.2 mg/kg) may be preferable. Following the administration of gallamine or D-tubocurarine, neostigmine (0.036 mg/lb or 0.08 mg/kg) should always be given, preceded in every case by atropine 0.008 mg/lb (0.018 mg/kg).

D*

Suxamethonium may give rise to bradycardia in children and should always be preceded by atropine or other vagolytic agents. Suxamethonium 0.5 mg/lb (1.1 mg/kg) is recommended for infants and children, and subsequent doses should be $\frac{1}{4}$–$\frac{1}{2}$ of the original.

Alcuronium (Alloferin): in children over the age of one year, this drug is twice as potent as D-tubocurarine in regard to onset of action and duration of clinical relaxation. There is a tendency for the blood pressure to rise following intubation with this drug, but the agent produces less histamine release than curare. The recommended dose is 2 mg/stone (0.32 mg/kg). The reversal with neostigmine is complete.

Pancuronium bromide (Pavulon): this drug has to date received relatively little evaluation in children, but will undoubtedly find a useful role in paediatric anaesthesia. A dose of 0.1 mg/kg is suggested as a paralytic dose.

Controlled ventilation of the lungs

Control of ventilation in children under anaesthesia is easily obtained by neuromuscular blocking agents or by ventilating with halothane. Having intubated the child by using suxamethonium or halothane, some anaesthetists allow the child to breathe halothane spontaneously until positioned on the table. During this time, temperature probe, ECG and stethoscope can be applied and an intravenous infusion set up. With both hands still free the anaesthetic circuit should be checked to ensure that there are no leaks, and the ventilation may then be controlled.

In neonates and small children ventilation can be performed by squeezing a bag on the free limb of an Ayre's T-piece circuit. For this purpose the top should be removed from the neck of the bag. The neck of the bag is regularly occluded just before the bag is squeezed. Alternatively, the end of the tube can be regularly occluded thus causing inspiration, and released during expiration. This latter method avoids any rebreathing but does not allow the anaesthetist to feel any gross changes in compliance. The chest should always be visible so that adequacy of inflation can be observed. A precordial, or oesophageal stethoscope is valuable for listening to breath sounds.

Automatic ventilation of the lungs. Because of the small tidal volumes, rapid respiratory rates, small inspiratory flow rates, and low compliance pressures, automatic ventilators designed for use with adults do not work satisfactorily in small children. The Starling Ideal Pump is, however, well suited for ventilation in children. Other ventilators and modifications of ventilators have been developed (Mushin *et al.*, 1969) but possibly the most suitable is a 'mechanical finger' which can be so placed in an Ayre's T-piece circuit that it intermittently occludes the flow of gases, such as the Amsterdam (Keuskamp, 1963) and the Sheffield ECG (Mushin *et al.*, 1969).

Amongst ventilators more recently marketed is the Bourns Paediatric Respirator. This ventilator, of which there are two models, is specifically designed for small children and infants, and allows volumes to be adjusted from 5 to 50 ml per stroke or 0 to 150 ml per stroke (depending on the model). The maximum pressure is adjustable from 0–60 cm of water and a variable flow control allows rates of inflow from 50–200 ml/s. A breathing frequency from 20–110 breaths per minute can be achieved. A patient triggering device is incorporated, as well as an automatic sigh device. Single direction flow minimizes dead space. The trigger on this machine is particularly sensitive requiring the removal of 0.1 ml from the patient circuit to operate it. The response time is 32 ms which enables the machine to follow very rapid inspiratory efforts. This is particularly valuable in respiratory distress syndrome as it has been found that assisted ventilation raises the PO_2 compared with controlled ventilation.

Using naso-tracheal intubation and Intermittent Positive Pressure Ventilation (IPPV), many workers have been treating the Respiratory Distress Syndrome (RDS) in the newborn, with varying degrees of success. Recently Positive End-Expiratory Pressure (PEEP) has been advocated for the treatment of this condition.

Conditions with special problems for the anaesthetist

Colonic replacement of oesophagus and Duhamel 'pull-through' operation for megacolon. Though both these procedures are carried out at rather different ages, the Duhamel being performed in a more mature child, these formidable operations create problems for the anaesthetist because of the long duration of operation, heat loss, and blood replacement. The patient's body temperature must be continuously monitored and blood loss accurately measured.

Atresia of the oesophagus. Early diagnosis of atresia of the oesophagus is of the greatest importance, so that it can be corrected with the patient in the optimum condition. Maternal hydramnios may alert the paediatrician to the possibility of this problem. The signs are excessive salivation and choking. Confirmation is achieved by the failure to pass a catheter into the stomach. The accumulated secretions in the upper pouch constantly spill into the lungs giving rise to infective sequelae. Three preoperative factors influence survival: associated congenital abnormalities, prematurity, and secondary pulmonary involvement. About 28% of children have associated congenital abnormalities, the most common being found in the gastro-intestinal tract consisting of imperforate anus, omphalocele, duodenal atresia, and Meckel's diverticulum. Cardiovascular abnormalities include ventricular septal defect, coarctation of the aorta and persistent ductus ateriosus. Absence or non-functioning of the kidneys are occasionally found. About 5% of cases have a cleft palate. As the mortality from operation varies between 20%–70% this condition should only be treated where intensive-care facilities exist.

Pre-operative treatment: this should include nursing the patient flat or in a head-down position with no oral feeding. A nasal double-suction catheter (Replogle tube) is inserted and continuous or regular suction of the upper pouch is carried out. Particular attention should be paid to hydration with parenterally administered fluids. Operation should not be delayed for longer than 48 hours. A venous cutdown or venepuncture of a scalp vein using a disposable small vein set should be established prior to the induction of anaesthesia.

Anaesthesia: a premedication of atropine 0.02 mg/kg may be given. If there is pre-operative evidence of excessive accumulation of secretions within the tracheo-bronchial tree, bronchoscopy is best carried out before intubation. Intubation should be carried out with an armoured tube, if possible with the patient conscious. An inhalational induction prior to intubation may be considered in the fitter cases. A thorough tracheo-bronchial toilet should then be performed. The endotracheal tube should be connected to an Ayres T-piece arrangement, modified as desired. Great care must be taken to avoid inflating the gastro-intestinal tract by excessive positive pressure on the airway. Spontaneous ventilation must therefore be used if there is a fistula connecting the trachea to the stomach. The patient should be placed in the left lateral position. The surgeon will attend immediately to any fistula which exists between the tracheo-bronchial tree and gastro-intestinal tract. Once the fistula is closed, controlled ventilation can be instituted. Ether or halothane, or the nitrous oxide/oxygen/relaxant technique may be used for maintenance, depending on the individual preference of the anaesthetist, and whether diathermy is being used. Controlled ventilation can be maintained by intermittent occlusion of the T-piece. Supplementary relaxation can be achieved by using a neuromuscular blocking agent if required. The trachea may become momentarily obstructed during detachment of the oesophageal segment from the trachea. Tracheo-bronchial toilet should be carried out as and when required. During thoracotomy the retractors and packs should be removed and the lungs fully inflated at intervals. All intravenous fluids should be warmed and attention paid to blood balance. Care must be taken to prevent the loss of heat from the body: warming devices should be used. When the oesophageal anastomosis is completed a fine feeding tube is passed from the nose to the stomach. It is well to remember this when sticking down the endotracheal tube and positioning the patient so that the access to the face is possible.

Post-operative measures: chest physiotherapy should be carefully co-ordinated with suction, and regular turning of the patient performed. Oral feeding can be instituted with 4 ml of sterile water hourly. Radiographic examination of the chest should be carried out at regular intervals.

Insertion of Spitz-Holter valve. This operation involves inserting a by-pass between the cerebral right lateral ventricle and the right internal jugular vein. The patients have varying degrees of hydrocephalus, which on account of the large size of the head, may seriously interfere with laryngoscopy and endotracheal intubation. The age varies from 2–3 weeks to 5–6 years, though most of the patients presenting for surgery appear before the end of their first year. Anaesthesia should be induced with nitrous-oxide-halothane, with the patient lying in the supine position, the head turned on one side. The patient should be intubated with an armoured tube but because of the possible difficulty in passing the tube and maintaining an airway in the apnoeic child, neuromuscular blocking agents are best avoided. Maintenance should be facilitated by the use of an Ayre's T-piece, with spontaneous ventilation.

Congenital diaphragmatic hernia. A variety of defects may occur in the diaphragm. Some of these defects may allow abdominal contents to come to lie within the thoracic cavity. The patients will present in most cases with varying degrees of respiratory distress according to the magnitude of the deformity in the diaphragm. These patients travel very poorly and they may require immediate endotracheal intubation as a life-saving measure. On admission a catheter should be passed into the stomach, and constant suction applied. The patients should be nursed in the upright posture, with humidification and oxygen enrichment of the inspired atmosphere. Preparation should include a chest X-ray, haemoglobin determination, crossmatch of blood, and the establishment of an intravenous infusion. The patients are best intubated whilst conscious. Once intubated, ventilation should be controlled and anaesthesia maintained with oxygen and halothane and neuromuscular blockade if required.

Anaesthesia for Fredet-Rammstedt's operation. Congenital hypertrophic pyloric stenosis is a relatively common condition occurring once in every 250–300 live births. The condition is found predominantly in males, with an increased incidence in the first-born. A history of vomiting is invariably present. It may commence at birth, but usually begins at 7–10 days of age. Dehydration and weight loss vary according to the severity and duration of vomiting. As a general rule, although operation cannot be delayed indefinitely, there is no urgency once the diagnosis has been made, provided the child is kept adequately hydrated by parenteral fluid administration. In the moderate and severe cases, delay is indicated whilst attempts are made to correct fluid and electrolyte balance. All cases should receive 0.45% sodium chloride in 2.5% dextrose for rehydration. If necessary to this may be added potassium so that 2 to 3 mEq/kg are given. In the *severe* case malnutrition is present as well as dehydration. If the haemoglobin is low, 5–10 ml/kg of blood should be used instead of 0.45% sodium chloride.

Anaesthesia: atropine (0.02 mg/lb) (0.04 mg/kg) should be administered particularly if suxamethonium is to be used.

The stomach should be emptied by means of a gastric tube. After oral administration of 125 mg chloral hydrate, and the fixation of the child to a 'crucifix', with adequate covering in 'gamgee' to avoid heat loss, the operative site (right upper quadrant of the abdomen) is infiltrated with 0.5% (3 mg/lb) (6.6 mg/kg) procaine and weak adrenaline solution (1:400 000).

General anaesthesia, however, may be used instead. Intubation should be carried out without anaesthesia because of the risk of vomiting or regurgitation of stomach contents. Intubation on the conscious subject constitutes no real problem in some of the cases as they are weak and ill. With early diagnosis, however, the patients are often very healthy and awake; intubation in a 6-week-old infant can be very traumatic, making prior anaesthesia necessary. The anaesthetic is best conducted with nitrous oxide/oxygen and a short acting relaxant as this gives the best operating conditions. With controlled ventilation throughout the child should be awake at the termination of the operation.

Familial dysautonomia (Riley-Day Syndrome). This rare condition of which 80% of cases occur in children of Jewish parents, is associated with retardation of growth and mental development. Sudden gross changes in blood pressure, with a tendency to severe hyperpyrexia and convulsions, and intractable vomiting may characterize the clinical picture. Other signs are recurrent pulmonary infections, marked indifference to pain, emotional upsets, faulty speech, diminished tendon reflexes, and skin blotching. When the child cries, tears are often absent. Excessive drooling and sweating may occur. The evidence suggests that the underlying defect is an enzymatic one, affecting the site and mode of action of acetylcholine, manifesting itself by acting primarily on the reticular activating substance and thalamic nuclei. Methoxyflurane and ether depress the blood pressure and cardiac rate in these patients, and it is suggested that a technique employing nitrous-oxide, oxygen and curare is probably best.

Anaesthesia for meningomyelocele surgery. The incidence of spina bifida cystica, with accompanying meningocele or meningomyelocele is 2.5 per

1000 live births in this country. In view of the good recovery of nerve function following early closure of the defect, surgery tends to be undertaken in the neonatal period. The average age at which operation is undertaken is 12.5 hours and the average duration of operation 65 minutes. In order to ensure adequate closure, extensive surgery, with, at times, removal of portions of vertebral column, is sometimes necessary. Particular care should be taken to conserve heat in these babies, both during the pre-operative and operative periods.

Anaesthesia: Schroeder and Williams (1966) recommend premedication with atropine 0.2 mg and vitK 1.0 mg intramuscularly 30–40 minutes pre-operatively. The neonates are intubated whilst awake and anaesthesia is maintained with an Ayre's T-piece, nitrous oxide, oxygen and halothane. The patients are placed in the prone position for operation, care being taken, by the use of padding, to allow free respiratory movement. An intravenous infusion is set up before surgery commences. The average loss at operation in 52% of cases was more than 10% of the blood volume (Schroeder and Williams, 1966) and in 8% exceeded 20%. Careful control and estimation of blood loss is therefore essential and replacement of warmed blood vital. Post-operatively these patients are nursed in the prone position.

Diathermy in small children constitutes a very real problem. It is difficult to find any one area of the body which is large enough for a diathermy electrode, and in addition, saline soaked electrodes may lead to body cooling. The problem can be overcome by lying the child upon paper-backed aluminium foil covering the full length of the body. The foil can be made to fit the body contours by lying the child and the foil upon a soft pillow. (This can be obtained from Allens Ltd., Iver Works, Lenborough Road, Buckingham, in rolls of 6, 12 and 50 yards. Domestic aluminium can be used but has only a quarter of the tear strength of the paper-backed foil.) No diathermy jelly is required.

The patient is in contact with the foil itself, the paper being on the other side in contact with the table covering. Care must be taken that the foil does not come into contact with the table or anything else which will conduct electricity. Connecting leads can be obtained from the manufacturers of diathermy machines. Owing to the risk of the foil tearing under the clip, the use of two leads is recommended.

Sclerema neonatorum. This condition, which can occur in newly born infants (particularly premature infants) is associated with an alteration in the physical characteristics of the subcutaneous tissues which become hard, and somewhat oedematous. Subcutaneous fat necrosis may occur. It may result from hypothermia, and in older infants may follow surgery. The primary cause may be due to an alteration of blood flow to the fatty tissues, associated with blood loss, stress, and hypothermia. It is sometimes associated with severe infection and systemic disease, especially of the gastro-intestinal tracts. If sclerema affects the chest it may form a sort of cuirass which impairs respiration and the baby may require ventilatory assistance. Unnecessary handling of the baby should be avoided as this may aggravate the condition. The anaesthetist may experience difficulty in opening the mouth of the established case.

The routine monitoring of the body temperature during anaesthesia may reduce the incidence of this complication. It should be noted that these patients are often treated with steroids.

Monitoring the paediatric patient

It has already been stressed that all children undergoing anaesthesia should have the body temperature monitored.

In addition to the routine monitoring of blood pressure, pulse rate and volume, and respiratory rate, the ECG may be employed. In order to facilitate the monitoring of respiration and heart rate the stethoscope is an invaluable aid. It may either be strapped to the chest wall, or, with a suitable attachment, be placed in the oesophagus behind the heart.

Geriatrics

The evolution of antibiotics, together with immense advances in anaesthetic techniques, has enabled surgeons to operate on elderly patients who, formerly, would have been considered inoperable. In the aged, excellent results now follow prostatectomy, the relief of strangulated hernia, and the pinning of a fractured femur.

As the life span of our population increases, so will the necessity of operation for elective and emergency surgery upon older patients. It must be acknowledged, however, that the degenerative processes of old age occur in all the systems of the body, though perhaps the heart, blood vessels and brain are predominantly affected.

The mortality rate in geriatric patients is considerably higher for emergency than for non-emergency surgery. Most of the deaths are associated with advanced carcinoma and the majority of the remainder with advanced intestinal obstruction. Concurrent degenerative disease and serious post-operative cardiac and respiratory complications increase the mortality rate. Errors in pre-operative preparation, in operative technique, in choice of operation and the lack of recognition of complications, also add greatly to mortality. Significant decrease in mortality arises from careful attention to hypovolaemia, water balance, electrolytes and heart failure. Improvement of pulmonary ventilation and drainage, early ambulation, the use of antibiotics and prophylactic anticoagulants all play an important part too. A successful outcome is helped by having an experienced anaesthetist and a short and non-traumatic operation, limited only to the correction of the patient's most threatening disorder. Throughout there should be prompt recognition and treatment of complications : for example, the importance of respiratory insufficiency and an ineffectual cough with retained secretions must be recognized. In aged patients, response to stress may be impaired. The release and utilization of cortico-steroids in older age groups are decreased, but as the response to ACTH remains unaltered, it is effective for treatment of adrenocortical insufficiency. The requirements for cortico-steroids for treatment of adrenal malfunction are less than for young persons. Heart failure may be present. The majority of old patients have diminished blood volume and are extremely sensitive to blood loss: when this necessitates massive replacement it predisposes to cardiac arrest in these cases. Great judgement and reasoned decisions are called for before deciding whether resuscitation should be carried out. Some should be allowed to die in comfort and with dignity. Many of the patients suffer from stiffening of the thoracic cage, decreased ventilation, and in some cases emphysema and chronic bronchitis. A decrease in arterial oxygen tension has been noted in association with old age and further hypoxaemia is likely to arise post-operatively. Dehydration, electrolyte depletion, malnutrition, vitamin B deficiency and anaemia may predispose to untoward effects of general anaesthetic agents: these must be treated with adequate fluid intake, hormone, vitamin and iron therapy. Vitamin C and nicotinic acid should be given routinely to these patients. Movement of all joints is impaired, there is increased brittleness of bone, and immobility of the jaws and cervical spine may make intubation difficult. The patients are often edentulous and thus difficulties may arise in maintaining an efficient fit with the face mask. Care must be taken with posturing these patients and every effort must be made before operation to ascertain the limitation of movement of the joints so that damage can be avoided.

Geriatric patients have a relatively low metabolic rate and their ability to detoxicate and eliminate drugs is impaired; the use of narcotic agents must therefore be carried out with caution. As a rule premedication is unnecessary and may indeed be harmful, particularly if opiates are used. Scopolamine is well-recognized as causing a confused state in old people and should be avoided. Meprobamate 800 mg or dichloralphenazone 1.3 g are satisfactory sedatives. If, however, restlessness is a feature in a geriatric patient, hypoxaemia must be considered and oxygen administered if possible.

The brain, and cerebral cortical tissue in particular, appears to be vulnerable to anaesthesia; consequently, cerebral hypoxia and hypotension must not be allowed. A well-administered general anaesthetic may be as good as, or better than, conduction anaesthesia. Adverse cerebral effects of general anaesthesia in old patients have been shown to be relatively uncommon, in present-day practice. It is likely that, with more advanced techniques, the hazards of anaesthesia in the elderly have been appreciably reduced; indeed, old age itself should not be a bar to its use, as anaesthesia has little lasting effect on physical activity, mental ability, or personality.

Accidental hypothermia

In emergency cases in the winter months it should be remembered that old people living alone without adequate heating can develop accidental hypothermia. The geriatric patient should have the oral temperature taken as a routine. Because temperatures may be as low as 28°C and the ordinary clinical thermometer will not record as low as this, special thermometers must be used. When treating this condition, it is inadvisable to use considerable external warmth, but rather to bring the body temperature up slowly, insulating the patient against further heat loss. Dehydration should also be corrected. Cortico-steroids and antibiotics should be administered together with oxygen, but thyroid hormone should only be given if myxoedema is present.

Preparation for anaesthesia

A thorough pre-operative examination should be carried out to ascertain the true nature of the patient's presenting disability. The haemoglobin and blood urea must be measured, and the urine examined for sugar. Where time allows the patient's nutritional state should be improved by vigorous therapy as outlined above, and heart failure and anaemia treated. Respiratory function should be improved by breathing exercises, ambulation and, if indicated, antibiotics. Where hypofunction of the endocrine system is present, hormone replacement therapy should be considered. Pre-anaesthetic medication with narcotic agents is best avoided. As a group, these patients are philosophical and not likely to be subject to psychical trauma but, physically, deafness may be a problem which interferes with efficient communication.

Anaesthesia

Because of decrease in functional activity, depletion of vital reserves and lack of adaptability of internal homeostasis, the geriatric patient will not tolerate violation of the basic principles of good anaesthesia. Poor and often friable veins, prolonged circulation time, impaired distribution, detoxication and elimination of drugs might favour the avoidance of intravenous induction agents. Nitrous oxide, cyclopropane, diethyl ether, halothane and trichloroethylene (with adequate oxygen) are all suitable anaesthetics. Muscle relaxants are rarely necessary except in small quantities in abdominal cases. Because the patients are usually edentulous, intubation is preferred by some, though with careful positioning of the mask, with the aid if need be of a mouth prop or other suitable arrangement, a gas-tight fit can usually be achieved. Nerve palsies and postural effects (often resulting from profound muscular relaxation associated with the use of neuromuscular blocking agents) must be avoided. Veins, arteries, and nerves are easily injured by pressure, resulting in thrombophlebitis, gangrene and nerve palsies. It should be noted that these patients are very sensitive to changes in posture and abrupt changes should be forbidden. The prevalence of postural hypotension in old people (more than 70 years of age) has been noted and it has been demonstrated that normal cardiovascular reflexes are absent in some elderly patients. Controlled ventilation should therefore be undertaken with care.

Hypotension in the elderly. From first principles it would appear to be unwise to allow the arterial blood pressure to fall during the course of general anaesthesia in the elderly. Rollason (1960) has studied the effects of hypotensive anaesthesia in patients undergoing retropubic prostatectomy. He used a variety of techniques including epidural block, ganglionic blockade, subarachnoid block, and halothane anaesthesia. He showed that ECG changes suggestive of reversible myocardial ischaemia occurred with pressures below 60 mmHg and that systolic hypertension predisposed the patient to these dangers. He suggests that the blood pressure should never be allowed below 60 mmHg in this age group and never below 80 mmHg in patients with systolic hypertension. He argues that the reduction of blood pressure will assist the oxygenation of vital organs in the majority of patients, whereas in a small minority the reduction of blood pressure will cause lack of oxygenation. He also states that the previous history of coronary or cerebral ischaemia is not an absolute contra-indication to the employment of hypotensive technique – morbidity and mortality appear to be no greater with hypotensive techniques than with the normotensive. Nevertheless, our opinion is that hypotensive techniques are unjustifiable in the elderly unless there is a very cogent reason for employing them, such as the reduction of blood loss which would otherwise be excessive and hazard the patient's life, or an operation impossible to perform with safety without its use.

Conduction techniques. Local infiltration should be employed whenever possible: it is particularly valuable for strangulated hernia. Full use should be made of blocks such as brachial plexus block, and intravenous regional techniques.

The operator must, however, bear in mind the fact that these patients detoxify local anaesthetic solutions less effectively than younger patients and the dose of the agents employed should be reduced accordingly.

Continuous epidural anaesthesia has its advocates who argue that general anaesthesia is unsuitable, because all the organs of the body are working with reduced efficiency. Employing a Tuohy needle, inserting it at T12–L1, passing the catheter tip up to T8–T9 for upper abdominal surgery, and to T10–T11 for the lower abdomen is satisfactory. A Tuohy needle at T12–L1 may be extremely difficult to insert in the elderly patient and, if a catheter tip at T8/9 is needed, the paraspinous thoracic approach is much better. Epidural analgesia is very suitable for prostatectomy. Following a suitable sedative agent one injection of 10–13 ml of 1.5% lignocaine with adrenaline is made into the T12–L1 interspace with the patient lying in the left lateral position and a 5–10° head down tilt adopted. The blood pressure must be carefully monitored. If chlorpromazine is included in the premedication the patient is usually lightly asleep. The risks of epidural block in the elderly are the accidental spinal block, and undesirably high extradural block because of the diminished extradural space. In view of this, the case of a more predictable technique such as subarachnoid block could be argued.

Anaesthesia for glaucoma: this is discussed on page 267.

Anaesthesia for thoracic surgery in the elderly. It should be remembered that the margin of cardio-pulmonary reserve is often small; indeed the total area of pulmonary vascular bed may have declined to a point where pulmonary arterial hypertension and cor pulmonale are present. The patients have respiratory insufficiency and an ineffective cough with retained secretions. In some cases a thoracic operation may be indicated to relieve the obstruction of an oesophageal neoplasm. Gross malnutrition, anaemia and lung infection are often present and will require vigorous therapy.

Anaesthesia for fractured neck of femur. This is, unfortunately, a common emergency procedure in elderly patients. Many of the patients are ill-prepared and in a poor metabolic state; in addition they may be suffering from shock. A sleep dose of thiopentone, following premedication with atropine, may be used for induction. Light general anaesthesia with nitrous oxide/oxygen/trichloroethylene, halothane, or ether is used for maintenance. Relaxants are generally avoided, except where intubation is carried out. This latter practice should, however, be considered in view of the likelihood of a full stomach and the possible difficulties associated with maintaining a gas-tight fit around the mask in an edentulous subject. The operation can be lengthy because of the difficulty with positioning the patient and the need to take multiple X-rays. Meticulous management is essential and, where possible, much benefit is to be gained by adequate and thorough pre-operative preparation. Rapid recovery is desirable too :

pulmonary embolism in the post-operative period is unfortunately common and early ambulation is of the greatest importance.

Post-operative care. The overall mortality from major geriatric operations is of the order of 14%. The absence of pre-operative complications reduces the mortality significantly. Similarly, the importance of efficient post-operative care cannot be over-stressed. Early movement and ambulation should be instituted. Recovery from anaesthesia should be rapid and provided cardio-vascular homeostasis is adequate, the patient should be enabled to sit up as early as possible and encouraged to breathe deeply. Post-operative oxygen therapy should be given to all these patients, at least for the first few hours, and the patient should be turned every half hour. Tracheal aspiration by catheter, breathing exercises, and gentle thumping of the chest wall should be instituted. If necessary antibiotic cover should be started. The blood pressure should be closely watched in the immediate post-operative hours and supported where necessary. Where ventilation is inadequate this should be improved by ventilator treatment in appropriate cases: in the first place, ventilation should be via an oro-tracheal tube, but if long term ventilation is required a tracheostomy may be performed. Cardiac dysrhythmias in the post-operative period are common, especially where pneumonectomy has been performed: treatment should be with digitalis or quinidine. Attention should be paid to urinary output and, where necessary, the patient should be catheterized. Prophylactic anticoagulant therapy is advocated by some. The problem of post-operative psychosis in the elderly, associated with confusion, can be reduced by the pre-operative correction of anaemia and fluid electrolyte imbalance and by instituting post-operative oxygen therapy.

5 *Anaesthesia and the Environment*

Civilization has spread to all corners of the earth – indeed to the space around the earth. In such environments, ambient temperatures and pressures are encountered which are of extremes unlikely, under normal circumstances, to be associated with human life, unless acclimatization or special environmental control is involved.

Low temperatures. The Polar plateau on the Antarctic continent is one example where there are not only very low temperatures but also a low barometric pressure. Nunn (1961) has devised anaesthetic equipment which will provide for general anaesthesia under these environmental conditions. Where skilled anaesthetic help is unlikely to be available a simple technique is clearly required. Because of open heating in huts, the agents used must be non-inflammable and, though the size and weight are of less importance than formerly because of modern means of transport, the apparatus must have a shelf life of at least 3 years and be able to withstand shock and fine drift snow. The equipment devised by Nunn carries 325 litres of oxygen, sufficient for five hours at one litre per minute flow : by using a reducing valve the oxygen flows through an air entrainment device giving a flow of 9 l/m of 30% oxygen, which then passes through a Fluotec vaporizer and thence via a Magill system to the patient. A non-return valve is placed between the patient and the vaporizer. The apparatus can be converted to a draw-over and can be used for controlled ventilation for short periods of time.

In climates with a low temperature, it is of great importance to have some system of allowing heat to reach the vaporizer, particularly in the case where agents with a high boiling point are used : it should also have temperature compensating devices incorporated within it. Special care should be taken when using pre-mixed nitrous oxide/oxygen mixtures in these environments (see page 245). The patients should be insulated against heat loss as it should be borne in mind that accidental hypothermia is particularly likely to occur in a cold environment, in the very young and the very old.

Low barometric pressures. Where the Polar plateau is concerned the barometric pressure is approximately 550 mmHg (equivalent to an arterial oxygen inhalation of 60–70 mmHg). Even at normal barometric pressure the inhalation of 21% oxygen during general anaesthesia shifts the lower arterial point to the upper bend of the oxygen dissociation curve, leaving the patient with no reserve in the event of temporary respiratory obstruction. The equipment must, therefore, be capable of delivering at least 30% oxygen. Not only will a 21% concentration of oxygen be insufficient to maintain adequate oxygenation of arterial blood at low barometric pressure, but weak anaesthetic agents such as nitrous oxide will become ineffective when used in the customary concentrations. Patients, unless acclimatized, will hyperventilate in an attempt to compensate for lack of an effective partial pressure of oxygen in the inspired air, and as a result will secrete an alkaline urine. With time, the oxygen carrying capacity of the blood will improve as a consequence of increased red cell production. Vaporizers with thermo-compensating devices, which depend on the expansion of air within a bellows, will function incorrectly when exposed to low environmental pressures unless the compensation bellows is filled with a liquid such as alcohol (e.g. Emotril). The concentration of vapour above a liquid is dependent upon the ambient temperature, not the pressure: therefore the number of molecules vaporized will be independent of ambient pressure. As the liquid is vaporized by means of a gas flow above the liquid, the actual concentration of the vapour within the gas will increase as the ambient pressure decreases but, because the ambient pressure is low the net effect will be for the partial pressure and for practical purposes the effect on the patients to remain the same, despite the fact that the actual concentration from the vaporizer will be higher than the setting. Because flowmeters, in part, depend on the density and viscosity of a gas, they will give inaccurate readings when used in environments with wide deviations from the normal ambient pressure.

High temperatures. From this point of view patient acclimatization is of great importance, and patients indigenous to the area take more favourably to anaesthesia and surgery. The unacclimatized may well suffer from salt and water loss, which has a direct bearing on the smooth course of events. Heat stroke may occur particularly if the patient is prevented from perspiring by the administration of atropine and by covering him with Mackintosh sheeting. Convulsions may also result from overheating the patient; should these occur the inhalational agent must be discontinued at once. A clear airway should be assured by intubation (if not already performed) and 100% oxygen administered. The convulsions can be controlled, either by the use of a non-depolarizing neuromuscular blocking agent, or by intravenous thiopentone, given with great caution to avoid depression of the cardio-vascular system. Hyperpyrexia should be dealt with by surface cooling. Salt and water imbalance should be corrected. Infections, such as malaria, will have to be treated.

Agents: liquids with low boiling point are extremely volatile and difficulty may be encountered in the administration of agents such as diethyl ether on an open mask. Suxamethonium may tend to lose its potency and should be stored in a cool environment, either as the powder (suxamethonium bromide: Brevedil M) or as solution (suxamethonium chloride: Scoline, Anectine); diethyl ether may decompose, and toxic decomposition products such as aldehydes and peroxides accumulate – these may cause convulsions if present in significant quantities.

High pressure. This is described under Hyperbaric oxygenation – page 221.

Malnutrition

Although this is, tragically, a major problem confronting medical men in underdeveloped and famine-stricken countries, true malnutrition from dietary deficiencies is rarely a prominent feature of patients presenting for operation in the United Kingdom. Old age may, however, be complicated by this condition. Inanition may accompany carcinomatosis, carcinoma of the oesophagus, and other lesions giving rise to intestinal obstruction, and because of poor tissue healing the patient may return to the operating theatre with a burst abdomen. Such a condition may be associated with varying degrees of ketosis, low plasma proteins, anaemia, low circulating blood volumes and electrolyte imbalance, including calcium deficiency with associated osteoporosis. Liver deficiency may also be found in cases of malnutrition and the patient may have reduced levels of cholinesterase.

As well as demonstrating undue sensitivity to depolarizing neuromuscular blocking, such a subject may have an altered response to non-depolarizing agents. The ability to detoxicate and eliminate anaesthetic agents may be impaired.

Obesity

Obesity is not an uncommon clinical feature, particularly in countries where malnutrition and poverty are rare. From the surgical and anaesthetic standpoint, obese patients present very real difficulties.

There is often an underlying disturbance of the cardio-vascular system with hypertension, myocardial disease, and heart failure. The respiratory system is particularly prone to involvement and its primary disorder is restriction of lung movement which may lead to mild bronchitis with sputum retention or, ultimately, to respiratory and cardio-vascular failure. Obesity may be associated with endocrine disease such as hypothyroidism, hypothalamic disorders such as Frolich's Syndrome, and disorders of the pituitary-adrenal axis. It may also be associated with metabolic disorders such as diabetes mellitus.

The effects of obesity on the respiratory and cardio-vascular systems are summarized in Fig. 5.1.

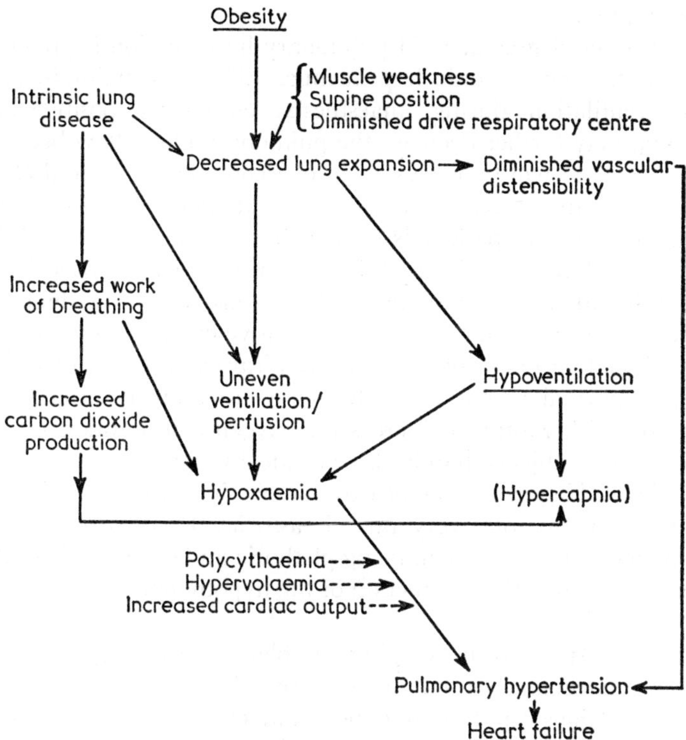

Fig. 5.1 The cardio-respiratory effects of obesity

In clinical practice it is relatively uncommon to encounter gross respiratory and cardiovascular decompensation, due to obesity. The cases usually encountered suffer from fatty infiltration of all muscles (including the heart muscle) that leads to bodily weakness and inadequate performance generally. Of particular importance is the cardiac and respiratory musculature, as with increasing deposition of adipose tissue the lung volume decreases, resulting in the collapse of poorly ventilated areas in the lung and, thus, hypoxaemia. It has been demonstrated that a somewhat similar situation can be produced in healthy adults who are made to breathe whilst chest movement is restricted by strapping the chest wall. Provided the respiratory centre and respiratory muscles remain adequate and there is no complicating respiratory disease, no more than mild hypoxaemia due to venous admixture will occur; there will be no carbon dioxide retention. However, if the patient is placed in the supine or Trendelenburg position, or develops respiratory weakness or lack of respiratory drive, then carbon dioxide retention will occur as well as hypoxaemia. Posture on the table, premedication with opiates, general anaesthetic agents and muscle relaxants will all predispose to hypoventilation.

Usually some degree of mild pulmonary hypertension is present in the obese, arising from chronic hypoxaemia. Efforts to maintain adequate alveolar ventilation during anaesthesia, employing positive pressure ventilation, may further decrease the pulmonary blood flow because high inflation pressure will be necessary to overcome low lung and chest wall compliance. The increased abdominal fat not only forces up the diaphragm when the patient is supine, but also makes intra-abdominal surgery very difficult as intra-abdominal pressure is increased in order to maintain adequate ventilation. Operations, therefore, tend to take long and this, in itself, increases post-operative complications. It has been confirmed that in obese patients the respiratory mechanism must work more than normal to maintain alveolar ventilation and that the mean oxygen cost of breathing is increased: oxygen consumption is therefore greater in these subjects than in those of ideal weight.

The Pickwickian syndrome of extreme obesity associated with alveolar hypoventilation, happily very rare, is associated with excessive somnolence and lethargy, the patient being plethoric and cyanotic. This disorder may be associated with malfunction of the hypothalamus.

Preparation. Apart from causing problems during operation, obese patients are particularly prone to post-operative hypoventilation, respiratory complications (sputum retention and chest infection), and cardiovascular complications (phlebo-thrombosis). Where it is possible to delay an operation, much is to be gained by dieting and weight reduction, with a regimen employing a 1000 calorie diet enforced under strict supervision. The underlying endocrine and metabolic disorders must also be treated.

Pre-operative breathing exercises should be taught in order that the patient's ventilation may be improved and respiratory disorders such as asthma should be energetically treated. Respiratory depressants must be avoided in the premedication.

Anaesthesia. When possible, spinal or epidural anaesthesia may be a better choice for operations below the level of T10, but it must be recognized that difficulty may arise with the actual spinal puncture. Where spinal or epidural anaesthesia is employed, it should be possible to localize the maximum relaxant effect without intercostal or diaphragmatic weakness. In all cases where not contra-indicated, conduction anaesthesia should be seriously considered, bearing in mind the difficulties associated with such a technique in obese subjects.

The first problem confronting the anaesthetist about to give a general anaesthetic to an obese patient is the difficulty in finding a suitable vein. Very often the only ones available are on the anterior aspect of the wrist and these are usually very fragile. It is of the greatest importance to have a stable access to the venous system throughout anaesthesia, and much anxiety can be avoided by a venous cutdown and cannulation. In view of the prolonged circulation time and possible cardiovascular instability, induction with thiopentone should be carried out with caution.

The next important factor is the maintenance of the patient's airway, bearing in mind that obese patients have thick necks, lack mobility of the cervical spine and, not uncommonly, have large tongues. In view of the fact that the majority of patients requiring general anaesthesia will be undergoing major surgery (e.g. cholecystectomy), oro-tracheal intubation should be performed. Intubation is best carried out using suxamethonium, with the application of 4% lignocaine to the larynx. Maintenance with nitrous oxide, 30–40% oxygen with the addition of small quantities of halothane is usually adequate. We believe that if the decision has been taken to use a general anaesthetic, ventilation should be controlled in any procedure lasting more than a few minutes. Because it is possible to encounter weakness in the respiratory muscles, despite reversal of the non-depolarizing blockers with neostigmine, depolarizing neuromuscular blocking agents should be used in minimal doses, and relaxation achieved by supplementing where necessary with inhalational agents. The plasma cholinesterase level of obese patients is elevated: it is, therefore, possible that greater quantities of depolarizing agents may be required than is usual and the attendant risk of 'dual block' must be recognized. Any tendency to bronchospasm should be treated promptly with antispasmodics.

Post-operative. Respiratory inadequacy in the post-operative period is a common sequel, particularly if there is a large painful upper abdominal wound, or if the patient has been depressed by opiates. As early as possible the patient should sit and be encouraged to breathe adequately, using a Ventimask to provide extra oxygen. The close supervision by a physiotherapist is essential, and ventilatory support should be offered if any doubt exists as to whether the patient is breathing adequately.

6 *Anaesthesia for the Patient with Cardiovascular Disease*

The evaluation of the patient

Two preliminary procedures are of the utmost importance: a careful history and a meticulous clinical examination. Evidence of coronary artery disease, hypertension and cardiac failure should be looked for in particular, for these factors will greatly influence the response of the patient to anaesthesia for surgery. The presence of pulmonary hypertension will also be an important feature, for such patients are extremely sensitive to general anaesthesia, whether it is carried out with spontaneous or controlled ventilation. The electrocardiogram is of little use, in itself, in helping the anaesthetist to decide on the management of his patient. In particular, a normal electrocardiograph at rest is of no value in predicting the severity of coronary artery disease. However, it serves as a useful baseline, and reference to previous electrocardiograms may be of value in patients with coronary artery and myocardial disease. Attention should be paid to the blood electrolytes, particularly potassium and sodium, for low levels of these ions may be associated with diuretic therapy. Hypokalaemia may give rise to altered response to neuromuscular blocking agents. An X-ray examination of the chest should be performed.

Special attention should be paid to the patient's current drug therapy, particularly if he is on antihypertensive or anticoagulant drugs. Since compensation for the cardiac effects of anaesthetic drugs relies largely on an intact sympathetic nervous system, drugs which interfere with adrenergic effects, such as the antihypertensive agents, may give rise to severe reactions when general anaesthesia is incautiously superimposed. Many general anaesthetic agents, such as thiopentone and halothane, give rise to vasodilation and decreased cardiac output, these effects being increased in the presence of antihypertensive agents. Patients on antihypertensive agents are often sensitive to changes in posture, more particularly if this is done under general anaesthesia; similarly lack of the normal response to the Valsalva manoeuvre may make itself apparent if these patients are subjected to IPPV. Further details regarding the management of the patients on antihypertensive agents are given on page 7.

Risk. Patients with hypertension, valvular heart disease and non-rheumatic heart disease, who are not in failure, present slightly greater risk than patients without these abnormalities. Coronary artery disease carries a significantly higher mortality than other forms of heart disease. The mortality following anaesthesia and surgery may be as high as 40% in patients who have suffered a myocardial infarction less than three months prior to anaesthesia, and only about 14% if longer than three months prior to anaesthesia. Almost 40% of cases suffering from myocardial infarction following surgical operations have pre-operative evidence of heart disease, hypertension or diabetes, and almost half of these patients have abnormal pre-operative electrocardiographs. Clearly, the more extensive the surgical operation the greater is the risk likely to be in association with coronary artery disease. A history of angina at rest undoubtedly is associated with an increase in mortality. Provided normal oxygenation and adequate cardiac output are maintained, patients with coronary artery disease respond relatively well to anaesthesia: the occurrence of dysrhythmias may, however, severely impair the cardiac output.

The anaesthetist who is relatively unskilled ought not to involve himself with such poor risks as those patients with heart disease. The handling of the severe cardiac case calls for a thorough knowledge of the pharmacological properties of anaesthetic and ancillary drugs, and the physiological derangements they may cause. With a skilled anaesthetist, the severe cardiac patient is possibly under optimal condition during general anaesthesia, for blood pressure and electrocardiograph are carefully monitored and maximal oxygenation is achieved.

Anaesthetic. It is, on the whole, better to avoid opiates in the premedication as undue respiratory depression may occur: however, if sedation is required for an apprehensive patient, promethazine, the barbiturates, or chloral are satisfactory. Atropine is said to provoke acute cardiac failure in conditions associated with a restricted cardiac output, though it is our opinion that it is not contraindicated in such conditions as mitral stenosis. If drying agents are required then other agents such as hyoscine, may be chosen.

The patients should be oxygenated prior to induction and this should be carried out in a posture to which he is normally accustomed: the sudden adoption of the fully supine position for a subject who is normally used to several pillows may well provoke pulmonary oedema. (Should pulmonary oedema occur during general anaesthesia, venous tourniquets may be applied to the limbs, and frusemide 20 mg given intravenously:

IPPV with high oxygen concentration should also be instituted). As patients with cardiovascular disease may have a prolonged circulation time, intravenous agents should be given slowly and cautiously, remembering that almost all intravenous agents may lead to some fall in blood pressure. Similarly, intubation should be carried out smoothly, with full relaxation. Some anaesthetists use suxamethonium for this purpose giving a non-depolarizing agent for maintenance. The prior application of topical anaesthetic agents to the larynx and trachea will minimize the cardiac effects of intubation, and will reduce the chances of the patient straining on the endotracheal tube, with resultant impairment of cardiac function. All cardiac patients receiving general anaesthesia should have the central venous pressure monitored in addition to arterial blood pressure: ideally, the electrocardiograph should also be monitored. If dysryhthmias lead to impairment of cardiac function then these should be treated. Facilities must be available for the adequate replacement of fluid and blood, and full oxygenation and carbon dioxide elimination should be ensured by artificial ventilation with oxygen enriched mixtures. Oxygenation: It cannot be overstressed that full oxygenation must be ensured during cardiac operations. An already diseased myocardium is particularly vulnerable to oxygen lack.

During the course of closed operations for mitral stenosis, arterial oxygen tensions may be below 100 mmHg just prior to valvotomy with the lung collapsed, even when 50% oxygen is delivered to the patient. After re-expansion of the left lung, some patients may still have arterial oxygen tensions below 100 mmHg when breathing 50% oxygen. Oxygenation is only really adequate throughout the operation when 90% oxygen is administered to the patients. If such high concentrations of oxygen are employed unconsciousness must be ensured by use of agents other than nitrous oxide, e.g. halothane or a neuroleptic technique. However despite this theoretical danger of hypoxaemia, most anaesthetists employ nitrous oxide/oxygen mixtures in their techniques. In choosing a relaxant, gallamine and D-tubocurarine are probably best avoided because of their effects on pulse rate and blood pressure.

Pulmonary hypertension

These patients are extremely sensitive to all forms of general anaesthesia and as it is very difficult to predict the outcome of any particular case, they should receive conduction anaesthesia whenever possible. If general anaesthesia cannot be avoided, then the patients should be handled with the greatest of care. Mild pre-operative sedation is helpful, avoiding atropine. Following a period of pre-oxygenation, general anaesthesia should be induced with inhalational agents such as cyclopropane or halothane. Many of these subjects react extremely badly to intravenous induction agents and it is our opinion that they should not be employed.

When an adequate depth of anaesthesia has been achieved, the trachea and vocal cords should be thoroughly sprayed with 4% lignocaine or prilocaine, and induction continued until about three minutes have elapsed from the application of the topical agent to the respiratory passages. An endotracheal tube, well lubricated with 2% lignocaine jelly, can then be passed. We feel that spontaneous ventilation is best maintained unless neuromuscular blockade has to be established. The use of IPPV, unless very skilfully applied, can prove catastrophic. Some anaesthetists prefer to carry out IPPV manually rather than mechanically. In particular, one must avoid too high inflation pressures and allow time for an appreciable expiratory pause. Depolarizing agents such as suxamethonium are probably best employed if relaxation is required for only a few minutes, rather than having to reverse neuromuscular blockade with atropine and neostigmine. Full oxygenation should be maintained throughout the operative and immediate post-operative periods and IPPV via an indwelling endotracheal tube may be required for the first 12–48 hours post-operatively. As soon as possible the patient should be propped up in a sitting or semi-recumbent position.

Polycythaemia

Many patients with cardiac and respiratory disease suffer from polycythaemia, and severe hypoxaemia has been reported in relation to general anaesthesia in these cases. The evidence suggests that this condition is associated with alteration in the ventilation/perfusion relationship, together with a low diffusing capacity in the lung. Pre-operative venesection and myelotherapy are advised in severe cases.

Ischaemia and anaesthesia

Generalized occlusive vascular disease may increase the vulnerability of certain organs to the effects of general anaesthesia : in particular, cerebrovascular and coronary artery disease may lead to central nervous and cardiac sequelae from general anaesthesia. Consequently, the anaesthetist should at all times ensure that oxygenation of the patient is adequate and the lowering of the arterial blood pressure should not be permitted. The development of cardiac dysrhythmias may be a manifestation of the adverse effects of general anaesthesia on a diseased myocardium, and will result in a lowering of the mean diastolic filling pressure, which is necessary for adequate coronary perfusion. Unless corrected, such dysrhythmias may well result in coronary insufficiency and acute cardiac decompensation.

Pre-oxygenation should precede induction of anaesthesia. Care should be taken to avoid hypotension, particularly if induction is carried out with an intravenous agent. The possibility of a prolonged circulation time in these patients should be considered. Provided that lowering of the blood pressure, reduction of cardiac output and dysrhythmias do not occur, the conditions under general anaesthesia should be optimal for these patients, as adequate oxygenation and careful monitoring of the patient are ensured. Ventilation should be such that hyperventilation with resultant reduction in the carbon dioxide tension is avoided – normocapnia should be aimed for.

Coronary artery replacement

Recently there has been a move towards replacement of diseased portions of the coronary arteries with vein grafts. Many of the patients suffering from coronary artery disease are introspective, highly intelligent individuals: consequently, liberal sedation, both the night before and as an immediate pre-operative medication, is essential. The main problems arise through the development of dysrhythmias. Attention should be paid to the blood chemistry during anaesthesia. Digitalis may be given and liberal coronary vasodilator therapy should be employed, both pre-operatively (at induction isosorbide dinitrate 5 mg sublingually) and during the operation (nitro-glycerine 0.4 mg intramuscularly every half hour, unless this unduly affects the blood pressure). It is essential to monitor the arterial and central venous pressure: to ensure an adequate oxygen content of the inspired mixture: to control ventilation: and, following extubation, to carry out oxygen therapy until the patient's cardiovascular state has stabilized. It may be necessary to support ventilation artificially in the post-operative period as with other open-heart surgery.

Anaesthesia for internal mammary implant surgery: like the Beck operation this procedure has been used to improve blood supply to an ischaemic myocardium though it has largely been superseded by coronary grafts.

Dysrhythmias

The regular beat of the heart can be modified in a great variety of ways, both in health and disease. Symptoms arise in patients with cardiac dysrhythmias either because the rate is too slow or too rapid, or because of the underlying disease. Only after a careful examination and an exact electrocardiographic diagnosis should treatment, with drugs or electric countershock, be prescribed. It is imperative to ask about previous digitalis therapy since over-dosage can cause a variety of dysrhythmias, particularly when the total body potassium is low, as it may be after diuretic therapy.

Dysrhythmias arising as a result of digitalis therapy. Five types of dysrhythmias can arise: sinus bradycardia, ectopic ventricular beats, atrial tachycardia with block, nodal tachycardia and ventricular tachycardia. The first step in treatment should be to stop digitalis and estimate the serum potassium. (Oral potassium 20–100 mEq/day may be prescribed in the form of potassium effervescent tablets (6.5 mEq) or 'slow K'.)

Complete heart block. Usually a ventricular rate of about 30 per minute is present. Isoprenaline 30 mg (Saventrine) tablets up to six times per day are frequently prescribed and steroids are also employed. Oral drugs are not particularly effective and the long-term management of patients with recurrent Stokes-Adams should include consideration of electrical pacing of the heart. In the un-paced patient who suffers a Stokes-Adams attack, apart from the normal resuscitative measures, isoprenaline 1 mg/500 ml in 5% dextrose may be given intravenously at a rate of 15 drops (1 ml)/min approx.

Cardiac dysrhythmias during anaesthesia

In the absence of underlying cardiac disease, most of the dysrhythmias occurring during anaesthesia can be traced to excessive adrenergic stimulation. Precipitating factors include pre-operaive apprehension, atropinization, surgical stimulation, carbon dioxide retention, adrenaline infiltration, the presence of thyrotoxicosis or phaeochromocytoma.

The administration of atropine in the presence of hypercarbia may give rise to serious dysrhythmias. They have also been described in relation to the stimulus associated with dental extraction, and to halothane anaesthesia, where the role of adrenaline has been proved. The importance of adequate carbon dioxide elimination in reducing the incidence of cardiac dysrhythmias must be stressed. Hypercarbia causes a rise in plasma catecholamines. The common dysrhythmias in patients under halothane anaesthesia are ventricular extrasystoles, nodal rhythm, and bradycardia: ventricular extrasystoles are provoked by stimuli under light anaesthesia with halothane, but do not generally occur during deep halothane in effectively ventilated patients.

Should dysrhythmias occur immediate attention should be paid to the factors outlined above and any hypoxia or carbon dioxide retention should be corrected. Certain general anaesthetic agents such as chloroform, trichloroethylene, cyclopropane, and halothane, are associated with a relatively high incidence of dysrhythmias, but opinions vary about their correct management in association with these agents. We hold the view that if irregularities persist after attention to such details as arterial blood pressure, carbon dioxide elimination, adequate oxygenation and the deepening of anaesthesia (cyclopropane), it is better to discontinue the administration of the agent in question and maintain anaesthesia with either nitrous oxide, oxygen and relaxants, or diethyl ether. Recently there has been increased interest in β-adrenergic blocking agents:

E

propranolol (Inderal) corrects many dysrhythmias: in view of possible bradycardia and hypotension, 0.5 mg should be administered intravenously over a period of one minute, followed by further doses of 0.5 mg at two minute intervals, probably not exceeding a total dose of 1.5 mg. Propranolol is contraindicated in patients with bronchial asthma or bronchospasm associated with chronic bronchitis, cardiac failure (in patients not already digitalized), heart block, and in the presence of metabolic acidosis. It has been employed for the correction of dysrhythmias occurring in the presence of hypothermia; however, until further information is available, it would appear unwise to administer more than 0.5 mg to the hypothermic patient.

A derivative of propranolol, practolol (Eraldin) is possibly more effective: this is given intravenously in doses of 5 mg up to a total of 20 mg but, although this agent may be cautiously given during halothane anaesthesia, its safety during other anaesthetics has not yet been evaluated.

Another anti-dysrhythmic substance, oxprenolol hydrochloride (Trasicor), is currently being evaluated. It is suggested it may be administered slowly, intravenously, in doses up to 2 mg *always* after 0.6–1.2 mg atropine given intravenously.

A further β-adrenergic blocking agent (Alprenolol) may be given in doses of 5 mg intravenously.

Practolol, oxprenolol and alprenolol have less negative inotropic effect, than propranolol, and all carry an intrinsic sympatho-mimetic effect. They are specific to the heart and do not carry the disadvantage of broncho-constriction which is associated with the use of propranolol. All these three β-adrenergic blockers can cause a fall in cardiac output and rate with a rise in venous pressure in patients receiving nitrous oxide, oxygen, halothane anaesthesia.

Atropine 0.3–0.6 mg may be used for the treatment of bradycardia developing during anaesthesia.

Direct current shock therapy

Direct current shock to the heart has been employed to reverse atrial fibrillation, atrial flutter and ventricular tachycardia to normal rhythm. A sustained normal rhythm is achieved in approximately 40% of cases of atrial fibrillation so treated. Originally most workers preferred to intubate their patients and control ventilation, but, now that the procedure is better understood and the risks appreciated, intubation appears to be unnecessary.

Anaesthesia: premedication varies, some preferring not to give vagolytic drugs. Pethidine and promethazine appear to be satisfactory as premedicant agents or 100–250 mg of pentobarbitone may be administered after premedication with pethidine and atropine. Alternatively

5–20 mg of diazepam may be administered slowly, intravenously, to produce a tranquillized and sleepy patient. Induction of anaesthesia may be with thiopentone, methohexitone, propanidid or althesin, though in the gravely ill, with a low blood pressure and cardiac output, an inhalational induction is better carried out. Nitrous oxide/oxygen mixture with halothane (the oxygen being in excess of 30%), appears to be satisfactory for both induction and maintenance of anaesthesia. In very severe cases it may be preferable to dispense with general anaesthesia.

Pulmonary oedema has been reported. This is thought to be partly due to too much electrical energy discharge over a diseased myocardium. All patients should receive anticoagulants and lignocaine or quinidine prior to defibrillation, although with acute dysrhythmias this may prove impractical.

Anaemia and blood dyscrasias

The normal healthy adult has approximately 15 g of haemoglobin per 100 ml of blood, thus permitting the transport of adequate quantities of oxygen to the tissues under normal conditions. A gradual reduction in the quantity of haemoglobin is met by a compensatory increase in cardiac output. A sudden reduction of circulating haemoglobin, such as may occur with haemorrhage, may not necessarily be met with an increase in cardiac output, particularly if there is an appreciable reduction in circulating blood volume.

Patients with anaemia are unduly sensitive to general anaesthetic agents both intravenous and inhalational, and extreme caution should be exhibited with their use. Should transfusion be required pre-operatively to bring the haemoglobin up to an acceptable level, 'packed cells' should be transfused and the venous pressure monitored. What constitutes an 'acceptable level' will vary with the urgency of operation and the duration of the deficiency. Anaemia is never an absolute contraindication to anaesthesia, each case having to be considered on its merits.

Even in the absence of anaemia the oxygen carrying capacity of the blood may be impaired should methaemoglobinaemia or carboxyhaemoglobinaemia exist. It is said that more than 5 g per 100 ml of circulating reduced haemoglobin are necessary for cyanosis to be recognized. In severe anaemia this physical sign may be absent even in the presence of severe hypoxaemia.

Sickle cell haemoglobinopathy

This condition is found in the blood of certain American, West Indian or West African Negroes, and other pigmented races, the sickle cell being a peculiar elongated and sickle-shaped red blood corpuscle. Research has shown that sickling occurs only in erythrocytes containing the abnornal haemoglobin known as haemoglobin S, the occurrence of which is determined by the inheritance from either or both parents of a dominant gene. The homozygote suffers from sickle cell anaemia and the heterozygote is the asymptomatic healthy carrier with sickle-cell trait. In some cases the phenomenon is associated with a severe haemolytic anaemia; in others, periodic occlusive vascular crises occur with malaise, pyrexia, and abdominal pain due to splenic infarcts. The haemolytic attacks are associated with the deformation of the erythrocyte due to crystallization of haemoglobin S, which is insoluble when it is reduced: indeed, any conditions which give rise to an increased amount of reduced haemoglobin within the circulation may provoke an attack. Mortality is greatest where there is existing debility such as severe anaemia. Operations and dental anaesthesia should be avoided where possible. Occasionally, unnecessary laparotomies have been carried out because of abdominal pain, and the patients have subsequently been shown to have been suffering from this condition. Any Negroes or other members of the pigmented races should be screened: the 'Ortho Sickledex' test is a useful screening test for sickle cells before anaesthesia. If the test for sickle cells is positive, the abnormal haemoglobin should be identified by further tests. The sickle cell trait does not, in itself, contraindicate anaesthesia, as haemolysis does not occur with normal clinical concentrations of oxygen.

Pre-operative management. The anaemia should be treated by transfusion and folic acid if necessary, but great care must be taken to avoid metabolic acidosis from large transfusions of stored acid citrate dextrose blood. To avoid aplastic anaemia and the occasional occurrence of megaloblastic anaemia, folic acid therapy may be instituted and all infections, including tonsillitis and malaria, should be treated. Fresh blood should be given whenever possible, as not only is stored blood excessively acid, but the oxygen dissociation curve is shifted to the left, giving rise to defective oxygen transport. If the haemoglobin is below 10 g/100 ml, patients should have either 11 ml/kg packed cells every twelve hours for 4–10 days, or an exchange transfusion of 12–24 ml/kg packed cells. This regimen should be adopted in all patients with more than 40% haemoglobin S and, as the marrow will react to transfusion by becoming functionally depressed, repeated transfusion is necessary. If possible the operation should be postponed for 10 days, but, if time is short, haemoglobin S can be reduced to 40% or less in four days using the above regimen. Sickling can be reduced by alkalosis induced by sodium bicarbonate.

Anaesthesia. Should an operation prove necessary, this should where possible be performed under conduction anaesthesia. Hypotension and hypothermia should be avoided at all times, and it is probably wise not to use tourniquets, though if the limb is effectively exsanguinated prior to the application of the tourniquet, harm is less likely to accrue. Throughout the course of anaesthesia and in the post-operative period hypoxia, acidosis and stasis should be avoided. Low molecular weight dextran (40 000–70 000) may facilitate peripheral blood flow and 30% oxygen, at least, should be given throughout anaesthesia and for 24 hours post-operatively.

Recent work has shown that Arvin (Malayan pit viper venom), when administered intravenously, may have a place in the treatment of sickle cell crisis. It acts at the fibrin-fibrinogen level, as it is an anti-thrombin.

Bleeding tendencies

Careful questioning prior to surgery should elicit a history of easy bruising, or abnormal bleeding after tooth extraction. Where any suspicion of coagulation defect is raised, it should be pursued before surgery is undertaken, for replacement therapy may make the operation safe. Liver disease may reduce prothrombin, factors X and XII, and other related substances.

Platelet deficiency. Thrombocytopenia may follow virus infections and respond to ACTH or cortico-steroids. Platelet-rich plasma, platelet concentrate, or if associated with anaemia, fresh blood should be given to allow operation in the thrombocytopenic patient. Such transfusions have a temporary haemostatic effect, usually for a few days, but they are as a rule less effective with repetition and the formation of platelet anti-bodies may be stimulated by them.

Anticoagulant therapy. The anaesthetist is likely to encounter a patient on anticoagulant therapy quite frequently. From time to time he will have to give an anaesthetic to such a patient with vascular disease affecting either the cerebral vessels or the coronary arteries, but as long as the prothrombin level is not below 20%, major surgery can be undertaken with safety. The level should be checked carefully in the post-operative period to avoid too great a variation: in addition the sudden stopping of anticoagulants will tend to cause an 'overswing' towards vascular thrombosis. If the operation involves the use of heparin (open heart surgery) the patient must have been weaned off oral anticoagulants pre-operatively.

Haemophilia and allied disorders

Haemophilia is the commonest of the constitutional blood coagulation defects. It occurs in approximately 2–4 people per 100 000 of the population, but each one of them constitutes an almost continuous and life-long responsibility to his doctor. Haemophilia is due to a deficiency of factor VIII, and the somewhat similar Christmas disease, to that of factor IX. A level of anti-haemophilic-globulin (AHG) above 25% is compatible with reasonable haemostasis and if the haemophiliac is subjected to trauma, such as a surgical operation, the level of AHG must be kept above 25% until the risk of bleeding is past. It is therefore of importance that all haemophiliacs should be treated in hospital under the direction of a haematologist.

The administration of 1000 ml of plasma will raise the AHG levels in a haemophiliac from nil to 10–15%. As this quantity may be insufficient to raise the level without giving large volumes of fluid, AHG concentrates are often essential. If anaemia is present blood transfusion may be necessary. With the high levels of AHG needed for major surgery, provided they are achieved before operation and maintained by at least daily doses until healing is complete, the surgeon should not feel restricted in what he would do to a patient, but it should be borne in mind that 5% of haemophiliacs have antibodies to AHG and therefore great care is necessary pre-operatively. For this, full co-operation should exist between the anaesthetist, surgeon, haematologist and nurse.

Dental treatment. It is not uncommon to find a young haemophiliac child who has multiple cavities at an early age. For there to be any prospect of success, these cavities must be tackled shortly after eruption of the teeth (age 2 years) or on the first diagnosis of haemophilia. If these can be prepared and restored at this time and if a proper diet is followed, it is reasonable to expect that extraction can be postponed for several years or avoided completely. When it is considered that an extraction for these children usually involves parenteral administration of AHG, as well as considerable physical and mental discomfort, the advantages of conservation (using a high speed drill under general anaesthesia) can be appreciated.

Anaesthetic management: injections should be reduced to a minimum and premedication confined to the oral or rectal route: fine bore needles should be employed for intravenous injections. Any trauma during laryngoscopy and intubation carries with it the risk of haematoma formation in the floor of the mouth and laryngeal region, respiratory obstruction and many other serious consequences. Nasal intubation must not be employed, owing to the danger of haemorrhage: instead, careful laryngoscopy, avoiding damage to the lips and pharynx, should be followed by oro-tracheal intubation. For operations in the mouth a nylon reinforced latex tube (with cuff if the age of the child allows) may be used, as it is virtually unkinkable and can be moved to any part of the mouth. No injections should be made within the mouth. The throat may be gently packed off with either a marine sponge or ribbon gauze soaked in saline. One of the required conditions is adequate relaxation of the jaws and, later, a rapid return to consciousness. Acrylic resin splints or caps should be made to cover the sockets of teeth which have been extracted and the sockets themselves packed with Col-Pak.

Epsilon-aminocaproic acid (EACA) therapy: good results have been reported following the use of this substance in classical haemophilia and Christmas disease. The administration of EACA by mouth at the rate of 24 g/day in four or six divided doses, begins 12 hours pre-operatively. The therapy is maintained until 24 hours after the removal of sutures, usually 6–7 days post-operatively. During the period of operation and 24 hours post-operatively the EACA is given by intravenous infusion.

Primary capillary haemorrhage is a rare condition, although apart from haemophilia and Christmas disease, it is probably the most common of the hereditary haemorrhagic states. The essential abnormality of this condition, which includes von Willebrand's disease, is prolongation of the bleeding time. As far as treatment is concerned, the patients fall into two main groups; those with an uncomplicated capillary defect, and those in whom the defect is associated with an abnormality of blood coagulation. All types of surgery should be carried out in hospital, with treatment aimed at combating anaemia and shock, using blood transfusions if necessary. Local reduction of haemorrhage can be achieved by removal of sepsis, local pressure, and the use of absorbable dressings such as Calgitex and Oxycel. It should be remembered that many of these patients may be on steroid therapy.

Fibrinolysis. This uncommon condition occurs in such situations as massive blood loss, cardio-pulmonary by-pass, abruptio placentae, anmiotic fluid transfusion, intra-uterine retention of a dead foetus, and surgery of the prostate or pancreas. It is sometimes present in chronic hepatic insufficiency. The increased fibrinolytic activity associated with severe injury probably arises because of occlusion of blood vessels at the level of anoxaemic capillaries. The transfusion of double or triple strength plasma, fresh blood, or fibrinogen can be administered to raise the level of fibrinogen to more than 200 mg/100 ml. EACA is of value when increased fibrinolytic activity is proven by laboratory tests and clot observation. EACA causes inhibition of even the normal fibrinolytic process and may preserve sufficient fibrin to permit clotting in such conditions as haemophilia and von Willebrand's disease. A 'loading' dose of 4–6 g intravenously should be followed by 1 g/h or alternatively 0.06 g/kg body weight can be given intravenously every four hours. The 40% solution is diluted in an intravenous infusion. Great care should be taken to ensure that aggregations of blood are removed from the surgical wound and cavity, before closure, when this substance is used, as clot lysis does not occur. Aprotinin (Trasylol) can be given when fibrinolysis has occurred.

Estimation of blood loss during surgery

The principle indication for transfusion of blood is haemorrhage which, if the loss is allowed to continue unreplaced, will result in lowered blood volume, diminished oxygen carrying capacity, and cardiac output. This will result in a reduction of the amount of oxygen available to the tissues under anaesthesia. A slow haemorrhage of even up to 1.5 litres may occur with only a slight increase in pulse rate or fall in blood pressure, in the normal fit adult male. However, if oligaemia is not corrected in such patients they are liable to sudden post-operative hypotension. Although there is a compensatory increase in plasma volume following blood loss, there is no significant increase in the number of red cells and, without blood transfusion, the red cell count does not return to normal for several weeks. This may result in varying degrees of hypoxaemia, which tend to prolong post-operative recovery and, in patients already possessing a diseased myocardium, may lead to cardiac and circulatory disturbances and possible cardiac failure.

It has been suggested that patients benefit most when the blood loss is replaced by blood given as a loss occurs. It is also believed that even minimal blood loss retards convalescence, and that all blood loss, in poor risk patients, should be replaced with equal quantities of whole blood. Some teach that blood loss in the normal fit adult male, lightly anaesthetized, will only require to be replaced when the loss exceeds 500 ml. We believe that it is unsound to take a figure in an arbitary manner such as this, as the need for replacement is dependent on many factors; amongst these are the type and duration of operation, the response of the patient to the operative procedure, the experience of the anaesthetist, his familiarity with the expected requirements based on the need of patients in the past and the likelihood of any further loss. There is a definite relationship between the amount of blood lost, the nature of the surgical procedure and the dexterity of the surgeon. Accurate replacement of blood loss during operative surgery depends on the accurate measurement of blood loss as it occurs. Armed with this knowledge the anaesthetist and surgeon are in a strong position to influence the cardiovascular homeostasis of their patients. They must, of course, relate this loss to the pre-operative status and constitution of the patient, to the anticipated repsonse of the particular individual to haemorrhage and his reaction to the operative procedure.

Methods of measurement

Subjective estimation by visual assessment is extremely untrustworthy and should certainly not be relied upon in any but the fittest adult patients for the simplest of operations. Such a method should never be used in cardiac, thoracic, traumatic, or paediatric surgery. Blood loss in trauma can be readily underestimated; accumulation of blood or plasma in the soft tissues and post-operative oozing can neither be predicted nor determined by haematocrit change or visual estimation. The method has the advantage of being inexpensive, rapid and continuous but in differentiating between 500 and 1500 ml loss observers are extremely inaccurate. Blood loss as estimated by the surgeon is always less than that actually measured.

Gravimetric

Patient weighing. A large weighing machine can be used to measure the pre- and post-operative weight of the patient. Unfortunately the blood balance cannot be assessed concurrently during the course of operative procedure, as allowance must be made for drains, dressings, infusions, insensible water loss and the removal of tissue. The method is dependent upon the sensitivity of the weighing machine.

Swab weighing. It is customary to assume that 1 ml of blood weighs 1 g. However, the average specific gravity of red corpuscles is 1.029 and of plasma 1.027. (The discrepancy between the assumed and actual specific gravity is a source of error, but a correction can be applied to reduce this). The method originally necessitated the use of dry swabs, although swabs may be moistened with known quantities of saline : these must be weighed as soon as possible after contamination with blood, so that the loss by evaporation is minimized. Furthermore, there is the advantage that, as there is inevitable loss on to the gowns and drapes, this loss cannot be included in the final balance.

Electrolyte conductivity. LeVeen and Rubricius (1958) introduced an automatic blood loss meter, based on electrolyte conductivity. This method has the advantage of giving a continuous reading, but is dependent on the constancy of the electrolyte content of the blood during the period of estimation.

Colorimetric method. Blood can be extracted by various means from the swabs and the concentration of the resultant solution can be used to determine the actual blood loss. This method (Thornton *et al.*, 1963) assumes constancy of the blood haemoglobin concentration during the course of the estimation and it can be modified for use during transurethral bladder surgery. Until recently, extraction has been facilitated by manually washing the swabs, but during the last few years washing machines have been used in conjunction with flow through meters giving a continuous record. The rinsing of the blood-contaminated swabs is carried out in a known volume of tap water, to which has been added sufficient ammonium hydroxide to give a 1 in 1000 dilution, and a defoaming agent. During operation, swabs, blood from suction apparatus, towels, etc., are added and the concentration of the resultant solution determined. With a knowledge of the patient's haemoglobin concentration, a value for the blood loss is readily calculated:

$$\text{Blood loss in ml} = \frac{\text{Hb (g/100 ml) washing fluid} \times \text{volume washing water}}{\text{Hb (g/100 ml) of patient}}$$

where Hb is the concentration of haemoglobin Bond (1969) has discussed the factors influencing the accuracy of this technique.

Radioactivity of blood loss. Radio-isotopes may be employed in the estimation of blood loss by measuring the activity of blood on swabs collected during the course of an operation: this involves the injection, intravenously, of a small but known amount of isotope. There are serious disadvantages, however, as the technique demands time and expensive apparatus, and there is leakage, if tagged albumen is used, of tracer into non-vascular compartments. It becomes increasingly inaccurate as transfusion occurs and, if red cells are used, the patient's cells have to be taken and labelled pre-operatively.

This radio-isotope technique at present appears to have little to offer over existing gravimetric or colorimetric techniques.

Blood volume measurements

Most of the methods employed depend upon the injection of a known quantity of tracer substance and the subsequent measurement of its dilution.

Radio-isotopes

Plasma method. ^{131}I or ^{125}I are used for tagging albumen. This method carries certain disadvantages, in that there is a tendency for albumen to leak into non-vascular compartments: Heath and Vickers (1968) have evaluated this technique for clinical practice.

Red cells method: the tagging of red cells affords greater accuracy than tagging plasma protein, as it is possible to measure the red cell volume of a patient pre-operatively using red cells labelled with ^{51}Cr and the post-operative red cell volume can be measured using red cells labelled with ^{32}P. The use of two isotopes in the same patient at the same time is practicable and safe as, in the ^{51}Cr method, radiation is counted in a scintillation counter and in the ^{32}P method beta particle emission is measured in a Geiger-Mueller counter. Thus one count interferes minimally with another. Measurement in the change of blood volume is dependent on the haematocrit and inaccuracies can arise when the circulation is disturbed, in conditions of severe oligaemia: then correction must be made for trapped plasma and for the whole body/venous haematocrit ratio. The method cannot be relied upon to give concurrent blood loss values during the course of an operative procedure, as it requires technical staff and is relatively expensive. Investigations have shown that erroneous results can be obtained when inadequate dilution and mixing result from the injection of the tracer into a circulation suffering vasomotor instability.

Dye method

Techniques have been employed using the intravenous injection of certain dyes such as Evans blue, to measure blood volume. These dyes must neither be catabolized nor rapidly lost from the circulation. They carry many disadvantages, such as colouring the patient's blood, and subsequent disadvantages when further measurements are contemplated within a short space of time.

Measurement of blood loss by suction

In cardiac, vascular, and thoracic surgery, considerable haemorrhage may occur which is removed from the operation field by suction and the material contained in the jar on the apparatus: inaccuracies can arise as a result of the large area of cross section of the jar. These can be reduced by having a measuring cylinder in the suction line containing a small quantity of defoaming agent or by weighing the suction bottle.

Comparison of methods

Comparison of measurements of blood loss between swab weighing and the colorimetric method, indicate that the general adoption of the swab weighing method can be advocated because of its simplicity. However, it does not include loss on to the drapes, so the blood loss estimated from patient weighing is consistently greater than the loss as determined by swab weighing. Some of this difference can no doubt be attributed to loss of fluid on to drapes, perspiration, and loss of water.

A comparative study of blood loss measured by swab weighing, colorimetric and blood volume studies in the same patients show that the blood loss estimated by blood volume studies is greater than when measured by other methods (Thornton *et al.*, 1963). The assumption must, be made therefore, that the actual blood loss during a surgical procedure is more than can be measured by swab weighing, colorimetric or any other method dependent on measuring blood lost to the exterior of the patient. This 'concealed' haemorrhage, revealed by red cell volume studies, does not appear outside the body. It presumably consists of leaking of blood into the tissue spaces around the operation site or in the incision, and as a result of the immobilization of blood in vessels proximal to ligatures. Although this blood is within the body confines it is unavailable blood and is lost to the circulation.

The colorimetric method described for measuring blood loss compares well with swab weighing, and provides a practical and simple method for use during the course of an operation in which blood loss on the gowns and drapes can be included in the final measurement. Red cell volume studies serve to remind us that there is additional bleeding into the operation site, during the operation and immediately following it; this amount should be anticipated and taken into account when estimating blood loss measured by other methods. It must also be remembered that swab weighing estimates only the minimal blood loss and is the minimum amount of whole blood that need be replaced.

Accurate replacement of whole blood loss acts as a prophylaxis against circulatory collapse and also decreases post-operative morbidity. Less blood is required to prevent hypotension than to correct it; therefore, ideally, blood should be replaced as it is lost, thus helping to maintain cardio-vascular homeostasis. In order to facilitate this state of affairs, accurate and up to date balance sheets must be kept and account must be taken of the fact that 540 ml of citrated blood contains only 420 ml of whole blood. Stick-on labels can be used so that the amount of transfused whole blood given at any one moment can be readily determined, if bottles are used. If Fenwal bags are used then the blood given can be determined by hanging the bag on a spring balance.

It should be borne in mind that blood transfusion itself carries a definite morbidity and mortality. There are approximately 4 deaths per annum in the United Kingdom from transfusion arising from homologous serum jaundice and a significant number of cases of infection due to the transfusion of blood and its products. Mismatched blood and transfusion reactions contribute further to the morbidity of blood transfusions.

In most instances it would appear to be unnecessary to transfuse blood or blood products during surgery, unless the total blood loss is likely to exceed 10% of the blood volume of a patient with a normal pre-operative haemoglobin. In the hands of an experienced surgeon, a cholecystectomy or nephrectomy is unlikely to loose more than 400 ml, but usually loses much less. On the other hand an abdomino-perineal resection of rectum is likely to lose at least 1000 ml, and a prostatectomy about 500 ml, (Thornton, 1971). It is the practice of many anaesthetists to establish an intravenous infusion of 5% dextrose or Ringer-lactate solution for most major operations. This enables blood to be easily administered if it be required.

Blood loss after trauma

The decision as to whether a blood transfusion is necessary after severe injuries depends on many matters. Most of the blood loss occurs shortly after the trauma, and as well as the obvious quantity of blood shed from external injuries, there may be considerable concealed internal haemorrhage. This alone can convert a healthy person into one with marginal blood volume, in whom any further bleeding might well prove disastrous.

Fractures always cause concealed haemorrhage, which might not be considered in spite of swelling at the fracture site. As much as 1000 ml of blood or more can be lost into the tissues after a fracture of the femur, and double this after a fractured pelvis. Damage often occurs in internal organs such as the spleen, liver and kidneys, from which several litres of blood can escape. This should always be considered if, once obvious blood loss has been corrected, the arterial and central venous pressures remain depressed.

Haemorrhagic 'shock'

Slow blood loss is tolerated better than rapid loss, as the plasma volume has time to expand in response to the loss and the total blood volume is not greatly changed. Red cell replacement takes place at a much slower rate but oxygen carrying capacity of the blood is compensated for by an increase in the cardiac output; thus the individual who is suffering from anaemia is less able to withstand acute haemorrhage.

With acute haemorrhage, the central and sympathetic nervous systems increase their activity and initiate mechanisms to support the circulation. Thus there is increased secretion of adrenaline and nor-adrenaline, of gluco-corticoids and mineralo-corticoids, and of the anti-diuretic hormone (ADH). There is diminished secretion from intestinal and salivary glands, and reduced output of urine. Such acute haemorrhage leads to depletion of the venous reservoirs, diminished venous return to the heart and, eventually, failure to maintain an effective arterial blood pressure.

Compensatory circulatory changes which result from this haemorrhage lead to a reduction of skin, muscle, renal, splanchnic and coronary blood flow. However, the blood flow to the intercostal muscles and the diaphragm remain unaltered. These compensatory mechanisms help to maintain the cerebral circulation for some while. After losses in excess of 10% of the blood volume (the total blood volume amounts to about 77 ml/kg lean body weight), the vasoconstriction of the capacitance vessels no longer provides an adequate central venous pressure and venous return, and cardiac output and tissue perfusion fall. Though the blood pressure is sustained by cardiac acceleration and constriction of the resistance vessels, further exsanguination results in a fall together with increasing reductions in cardiac output, tachycardia and intensification of vaso-constriction.

The physiological dead space can increase to 70%–80% of the tidal volume: it is thought that this is a direct result of the decreased pulmonary blood flow. In a subject in whom the tidal volume has not been depressed by narcotic agents, the response to this increase in dead space is met by an increase in ventilation with resulting hyperpnoea: this 'air hunger' characterizes the patient suffering from severe blood loss. Under anaesthesia and the influence of morphine, alveolar ventilation may become reduced leading to severe hypoxaemia in a patient breathing air. Pain, shivering, and hyperpnoea with associated muscular activity lead to increased oxygen consumption. This increased oxygen extraction at the periphery leads to an increase in oxygen desaturation of mixed venous blood. There is no evidence of increased shunting within the lungs of these patients, provided that they are not under the influence of an anaesthetic nor have pathological disturbances of the lungs: however, the passages of grossly desaturated mixed venous blood through the normal degree of shunt can lead to a further intensification of the arterial hypoxaemia.

In these shocked patients the flow of blood to vital centres, such as the brain, becomes of paramount importance and the arterial blood pressure is an increasingly unreliable guide to the amount of available oxygen. Vasoconstriction and subsequent redistribution of blood away from non-vital tissues will tend to maintain the blood pressure, but the supply of oxygen may be seriously imperilled. Vasopressors may further reduce flow, indeed the central venous pressure can be a more sensitive index of reduction of circulating blood volume than the arterial blood pressure alone.

The available oxygen is at its highest when the haematocrit is 42%. When the haematocrit is above 42%, the increased viscosity increases peripheral resistance and tends to lower cardiac output. However, haemodilution invariably follows haemorrhage, the 'half-time' being in the order of 24 hours: 25% dilution for two litres of blood loss occurs in from two to twelve hours.

Breathing under normal circumstances, approximately 1.5 litres of oxygen are stored in the body of a 70 kg man, 400 ml of this is in the lung, 300 ml in arterial blood, 600 ml in venous blood and 300 ml in the muscles and tissues. It will thus be seen that haemorrhage can seriously deplete the body stores of oxygen. Should transient obstruction or depression of ventilation occur in association with haemorrhage, hypoxaemia may rapidly ensue as these stores are reduced. Oxygen administration can, however, increase the oxygen store of the body even though red cell depletion is present, as nitrogen can be displaced from the lung store by oxygen. The stores can be increased by up to 2 litres and this way reduce the risk of hypoxaemia arising as suggested above. Evidence of the value of the administration of oxygen is demonstrated by the survival rate of bled dogs after halothane and ether anaesthesia: a twofold reduction in mortality occurred when they breathed an oxygen-enriched mixture, thirty per cent of oxygen proving adequate for this purpose (Freeman, 1963).

Irreversible shock can be described as deterioration in the clinical picture associated with haemorrhage, when the shock becomes unresponsive to treatment. It arises as a result of intense vasoconstriction, producing ischaemic anoxia in the tissues. If transfusion is delayed, the constricted arterioles become less and less responsive to adrenaline. Although the capacitance vessels (large veins and vessels) continue to maintain their tone for very much longer than the resistance vessels (arterioles), engorgement and stagnation of flow occur even though blood catecholamines continue to rise. Such anoxic changes also produce haemorrhage and the absorption of endotoxins from the bowel, which, because of failure of the reticulo-endothelial system in the spleen and liver, cannot be detoxicated, and their presence in the circulation potentiates the pressor responses of catecholamines.

Early replacement of blood loss reduces the chance of the shock becoming irreversible.

Management of the oligaemic state

The management of blood loss will depend on the response of the patient to the loss and the magnitude of the loss, but, as a general rule, red cells should be replaced where evidence suggests that the oxygen carrying capacity of the blood has fallen significantly.

Plasma expanders. Plasma or plasma substitutes may further reduce the haematocrit, though this disadvantage may have to be weighed against the advantage of promoting blood flow to the periphery, particularly if dextrans of a low molecular weight (LMWD) are used, e.g. Rheomacrodex, or Lomodex 40 (mol. wt. = 40 000). Dextrans should not be given to patients with a coagulation defect. LMWD 40 000 does not interfere with blood grouping, but as the molecular weight increases, dextrans are more apt to interfere with this. Macrodex or Lomodex 70 (mol. wt. = 70 000) remains in the intravascular compartment for a longer period of time than LMWD. Approximately 60% of LMWD is excreted within 6 hours, whereas dextrans with a higher molecular weight are excreted at the rate of about 20% in 24 hours. There is still argument concerning which molecular weight dextran to use in the oligaemic state: LMWD is removed from the circulation more rapidly than dextrans of higher molecular weight, but as it prevents clumping and sludging of red cells in the smallest vessels, it is possibly the one of choice. In general, not more than 1–1½ litres of dextran solution should be used in 24 hours (20 ml/kg).

Pooled human plasma is the ideal plasma expander, although two dangers remain. Stored plasma has a high content of potassium and rapid transfusion is known to cause cardiac arrest. There is still the possibility of homologous serum jaundice, though this has been greatly reduced by limiting the number of donors contributing to each bottle. The pre-requisites of blood replacement are an efficient venous cannula and the monitoring of arterial and central venous pressures.

Posture. The head down tilt has been the traditional approach to the management of low blood pressure, whether it results from oligaemia or not. Recent work has shown that the adoption of this position in the shocked state does not improve the circulation to the brain, and may indeed lead to impairment of the cerebral circulation. The patient should be nursed in the *horizontal* position with the *legs elevated.* Patients should be given oxygen by mask, and, if necessary, adequately ventilated (using a ventilator) to overcome any alveolar hypoventilation. A tidal volume in excess of normal is required because of the increased alveolar dead space associated with haemorrhage. Always provided that the venous return is not impeded by an inadequate expiratory pause or a high mean intrathoracic pressure, a negative phase if often beneficial in these patients. Acid-base balance should be corrected: metabolic acidosis is treated by the administration of sodium bicarbonate or THAM, as this improves the cardiac output and results in an increase in the arterial oxygen tension. Some workers have, in addition, artificially raised the osmolarity of the extracellular fluid by the administration of hypertonic solutions during, or prior to, transfusions with blood. 10% glucose, 2.7% sodium bicarbonate, and 1.8% saline are the solutions employed. Ringer's lactate solution has also been found beneficial when used in addition to the blood replaced.

Vasodilators. In an effort to improve the amount of available oxygen to the tissues, deliberate vasodilation has been advocated by some and promoted by the use of halothane or diethyl ether. Both agents promote peripheral flow by causing vasodilation: whereas halothane leads to a fall in cardiac output and blood pressure, ether tends to cause a rise in blood pressure and an increase in cardiac output. No deleterious effect appears to result from the administration of halothane, provided high oxygen concentrations are administered. Other workers have advocated the use of ganglion and alpha-adrenergic blocking agents, arguing again that peripheral blood flow is enhanced. Chlorpromazine 10–25 mg intravenously has been employed to this purpose, and phenoxybenzamine may also be used in a slow drip of 1 mg/kg over a 1–2 hour period. Similarly trimetaphan may have a place because of its rapid onset and short duration of action. Large quantities of steroids have also been employed because of the associated α-adrenergic blocking action. Although vasoconstriction is an undesirable consequence of trauma and haemorrhage, the abolition of vasoconstrictive reaction to injury, important as it is in the control of surgical shock, carries with it serious and perhaps dangerous risks to the patient. It must be fully realized that the cerebral and cardiac complications are likely to ensue when vasoconstriction is abolished in the presence of a reduced circulating blood volume.

The use, therefore, of vasodilator agents should be allowed only if replacement of circulating blood volume is carried out at the same time. The venous pressure should be monitored throughout, as the arterial blood pressure is a most unreliable guide to the adequacy of replacement under these circumstances.

Regimen of management

(1) Lay the patient flat and, if possible, arrest the haemorrhage
(2) Elevate the legs
(3) Clear the airway
(4) Administer oxygen
(5) If there is evidence of underventilation, ventilate the patient artificially
(6) Insert a reliable venous cannula
(7) Monitor arterial and venous blood pressure
(8) Commence an infusion of hypertonic saline and glucose or Ringer's Lactate solution
(9) Transfuse with warmed blood supplemented by plasma expander as soon as possible (see below)
(10) Correct metabolic acidosis
(11) Consider the possibility of deliberate vasodilatation
(12) Consider the administration of cortisone 50 mg/kg as a vasodilator
(13) Replace calcium. 1 g calcium gluconate per 1000 ml blood transfused
(14) Consider the administration of digitalis. (Digoxin 0.25 mg intravenously)

It should be stressed that the treatment of oligaemic shock should be carried out side by side with the treatment of the basic lesion.

In many cases the management outlined above will be of little or no value, unless the haemorrhage is stopped. This also applies to bony injury, where manipulation and immobilization often lead to a dramatic improvement in the patient's condition. Little purpose would be served in waiting for an improvement in blood pressure prior to surgery where surgery is required (e.g. ruptured ectopic pregnancy). In many cases hypotension will not only be due to blood loss but also to neurogenic shock; for example reduction of a fractured pelvis under general anaesthesia, with the placing of the patient in slings, is usually followed by an immediate improvement in the patient's condition. Operation, therefore, should not be unnecessarily delayed, as such delay carries a high mortality. The patient should be placed under the care of the specialist responsible for the major injury, i.e. where a crush injury of the chest is the major injury – the thoracic surgeon; where head injury – the neurosurgeon; where abdominal injury – the general surgeon. This is because attenion to the major injury usually brings about immediate improvement in the patient's condition: if no improvement occurs, then it is extremely likely that the obvious lesion is not the only one. Should surgery be considered necessary in these circumstances, the patient should go straight to the anaesthetic room from the casualty department. Transfusion, and the administration of oxygen, and possibly Entonox, will have already commenced, light general anaesthesia should be induced, ventilation controlled and the operation carried out.

General anaesthesia. Pre-oxygenation is an essential and immediate emergency measure to be taken on receipt of the patient within the hospital. It must be fully recognized that the stomach may be full, and adequate precautions taken to cope with regurgitation and vomiting during induction. The anaesthetic should be induced on a trolley or table with the facility of lowering the head, using intravenous induction agents with caution and not commencing anaesthesia until an adequate intravenous infusion has been secured: many authorities prefer to use cyclopropane (50%) and oxygen for induction purposes in these patients. As soon as unconsciousness is achieved suxamethonium is administered and a cuffed endotracheal tube passed. Anaesthesia may be maintained with 5–10% cyclopropane/oxygen, or nitrous oxide/oxygen with controlled ventilation, using a non-depolarizing agent to maintain relaxation. The judicious use of halothane may have a place in promoting peripheral blood flow.

Massive blood transfusion

The transfusion of blood carries with it risks for the patient. Unless adequate time has been allowed for detailed cross-matching, there is the chance that the blood may be incompatible; the blood will almost certainly have been stored and have a low oxygen carrying capacity (blood is normally stored between 4–6°C, and if left at room temperature for more than one hour cannot be replaced in a blood refrigerator for further use); if it contains acid-citrate-dextrose as an anti-coagulant, it may have a particularly low pH, further exacerbating an already established metabolic acidosis within the patient. The risks increase as the quantity of transfused blood mounts. The transfusion of large quantities of cold blood will lead to a reduction in the body temperature of the patient, with an increase in the tendency to bleed, and the heart action will also be impaired. Citrate will accumulate in the body, particularly if its detoxication and destruction are impaired by the effects of hypothermia upon the liver, thus reducing the amount of available ionized calcium, and giving rise to dysrhythmias and a low cardiac output. There is, however, no evidence of increased bleeding associated with low levels of ionized calcium. Not only hypothermia but also metabolic acidosis will tend to cause further depression of cardiac activity. In 15 days the potassium concentration of stored blood rises from 4 mEq/l to the region of 25 mEq/l: thus, it will be seen that large quantities of potassium may be delivered during the course of a massive transfusion of stored blood. Furthermore, should hypoxia and the retention of carbon dioxide occur, this will lead to the out-pouring of adrenaline and the release of potassium from the liver.

The complications of massive blood transfusion are thus manifold and far-reaching and can develop into an almost irreversible situation. The risk of cardiac arrests during massive blood transfusion (3000 ml or more/hour) may be reduced significantly by warming the stored blood to body temperature before transfusion. In many cases, owing to the rapidity of replacement, it may be difficult to predict the quantity required, in which case equipment has been developed to allow the warming of blood concurrently with replacement. It has been shown that with blood flowing through a coil of plastic tubing in a water bath at 37°C, with the initial temperature of the blood at 4.0°C–5.8°C, an end temperature of 30°C–35°C is achieved at a flow rate of 150 ml/min. Other devices have been developed for warming blood e.g. a thermostatically controlled heating blanket placed around the transfusion bottle, a thermostatically controlled water bath, or high frequency electromagnetic waves together with insulation of the bottle with a polystyrene cover after warming. If the temperature is kept below 40°C there is little risk of haemolysis. Besides taking every precaution to prevent hypothermia, attention must be paid to metabolic acidosis by the administration of bicarbonate or THAM (see page 162). The toxic effects of citrate can be reduced by giving calcium chloride, using 5–10 ml of 10% calcium chloride intravenously for every 500 ml of citrated blood transfused, over and above 1.5 litres: great care must be taken to administer the calcium slowly. ECG control will greatly facilitate the management of massive blood transfusion, and serial readings of arterial and venous pressures give a good indication both for transfusion requirements and of myocardial depression caused by citrated blood. There is negligible haemolysis when conventional methods for rapid delivery of blood are employed, even though a needle as small as 18 gauge is used.

Central venous pressure monitoring

Measurement of central venous pressure can nearly always throw additional light during the following situations:

Massive blood or fluid replacement especially in small children or cardiac cases
Acute circulatory failure of obscure origin
Periods when cardio-vascular dynamics are unstable
Anuria or oliguria with a normal arterial pressure

Central venous pressure monitoring reflects the rate of return of blood to the right side of the heart and can be an accurate guide for body fluid replacement. A central venous pressure of about 0.5 cm water in the presence of a low arterial blood pressure usually indicates *hypovolaemia*, whereas a central venous pressure above 14 cm in the presence of a low arterial blood pressure indicates *cardiac failure.* In conditions of cardiovascular instability, such as may occur in association with peripheral vasoconstriction, the central venous pressure will indicate the 'physiological balance', as distinct from an indication of the true blood loss. It must be remembered that a normal arterial blood pressure and central venous pressure can exist in the presence of a reduced blood volume, because compensatory vaso-constriction has occurred. As the introduction of general anaesthesia and consequent vasodilation might be catastrophic in such a situation, a knowledge of blood volume might be helpful. As the patient's condition improves, and vasodilatation occurs, the central venous and arterial pressures will fall, thus indicating a need for further transfusion. Full interpretation of the venous pressure must, however, be done in conjunction with other clinical signs.

Technique of central venous pressure monitoring: a catheter, with as wide a bore as possible, should be inserted using full aseptic precautions into the antecubital, internal or external jugular, subclavian, saphenous, or femoral veins, using either the percutaneous technique through a wide bore needle, or a venous cut-down. The latter routes may only be employed when the antecubital approach is not possible.

Subclavian venepuncture. Most authorities hold the view that either side of the neck is satisfactory for this technique, although there are sound reasons to prefer the vein on the right side because of its more medial position and straighter course, and the presence on the left of the frail thoracic duct and the left pleural dome.

The patient should lie supine, with the arms adducted, the head rotated to the opposite side, and in the Trendelenberg position to facilitate the puncture and avoid air embolism. An aseptic technique should be employed, the operator wearing sterile gloves. A three inch long needle, no smaller than 20 gauge should be attached to the syringe.

Infraclavicular route: the operator should face the patient and press his left index finger into the triangle between the sternal and clavicular heads of the sterno-mastoid muscle. With his right hand, the operator inserts the needle immediately below the clavicle and slightly medial to its mid-point. The needle is directed parallel to the chest wall upwards, backwards, and medially towards the tip of the left index finger, advancing slowly and exerting a strong backward pull on the plunger to induce a negative pressure in the barrel. At a depth of 4 cm (range 2–8 cm) a double click (costoclavicular ligament and then the vein wall) and a flow of dark blood herald a successful venepuncture.

Supraclavicular route: this approach carries less risk of pleural or arterial puncture than the infraclavicular route. It has the advantage of definite cutaneous landmarks, a shorter distance from skin to vein, and is more accessible to the anaesthetist during surgery. The operator stands alongside the patient's head, facing the feet; the angle between the upper border of the clavicle and the medial margin of the sterno-mastoid is defined. The needle is inserted at the tip of this angle, at 45 degrees from both the horizontal and sagittal planes, and slowly advanced in a direction 15 degrees forward of the coronal plane, then progressively deviating away from the pleural dome, until at an average depth of 1.0 to 1.5 cm (range 0.5–4.0 cm) a slight loss of resistance and the appearance of dark blood in the syringe indicates success.

With both routes great care must be taken to avoid repeated and deep thrusts with the needle as serious complications such as pneumothorax may result. Failure on one side should be followed by chest X-ray and no attempt should be made on the other side. During the introduction of the cannula the patient should be apnoeic and the hub digitally occluded at all times except when introducing the catheter which should itself be connected to a prepared and filled drip set. The risk of catheter embolism must be reduced by at no time withdrawing the catheter through the needle. Confirmation of the position of the catheter should be made by employing radiography.

Internal jugular venepuncture. Percutaneous catherization of the internal jugular vein should be carried out using the same aseptic technique as outlined above and with the patient in a 20–30 degree head-down tilt to reduce the chances of air embolism and to distend the internal jugular veins.

(1) This method is preferable in patients who are under general anaesthesia. As the internal jugular vein has to be felt under the sternomastoid muscle the patient should have good muscular relaxation. The head is turned away from the side on which the catheterization is to be carried out. The internal jugular vein can usually be palpated slightly laterally to a line joining the medial edge of the clavicular head of the sterno-

mastoid to the mastoid process and should be distinguished from the carotid artery. Venepuncture is made at a point where the vein is clearly felt under the muscle, using an 8 inch (20 cm) size 1614 Bardic Intracath without a stillette (in the adult). The needle is inserted through the skin slightly cephalad and medial to the position where the vein is most easily felt, at an angle of 30–40 degrees to the skin surface, and is advanced caudally and laterally. The deep cervical fascia is usually pierced with a definite loss of resistance and a similar loss of sensation is felt as the vein is entered. It is quite often necessary to insert the needle through the substance of the sternomastoid if the internal jugular vein is felt some way lateral to its medial edge.

(2) An alternative technique may be employed in cases where the method described has failed or where the jugular vein is not palpable. As it does not depend on muscular relaxation, it can be used with local analgesia in conscious patients. The patient is again postured as already described. The triangular space between the sternal and clavicular heads of the sterno-mastoid, with its base on the medial end of the clavicle is identified. The terminal part of the internal jugular vein lies behind the medial edge of the clavicular head of the muscle. The needle is inserted at the apex of this triangle at an angle of about 30–40 degrees to the skin surface and advanced caudally and laterally towards the inner border of the anterior end of the first rib behind the clavicle. Although entry into the vein is often felt, passage through the deep cervical fascia may not be so evident. The tip of the catheter should lie within the thorax as near to the confluence of the superior and inferior venae cavae as can be accurately determined (preferably by using radiography, the ECG or pressure measurements with an electromanometer). The importance of checking the position of the tip of the catheter cannot be overstressed as it has been clearly shown that otherwise no reliance can be placed on the measurements obtained. The pressure transmitted should be connected to a column of saline, so that the zero point corresponds with the junction between the manubrium and the sternum : the actual zero level can be fixed by having a hinged arm with a spirit level, attached to the stand upon which the venous column is fixed. Alternatively, various methods have been devised to correct for changes in zero with alterations of patient posture (Frostad, 1968). A three-way tap can be turned to connect either the patient to the manometer or to a saline reservoir, which may be allowed to drip slowly to maintain the potency of the vein. The normal central venous pressures lies between +2 and +5 (cmH_2O).

Reduction in blood loss

Under the following circumstances it may be desirable to ensure that there is a dry operation field :

neurosurgery – to aid the removal of vascular tumours
peripheral vascular surgery, e.g. operations for coarctation of the aorta
operations associated with severe haemorrhage, such as for the removal of tongue or jaw
certain operations performed by plastic and orthopaedic surgeons
certain ENT operations, e.g. the fenestration procedure

In addition it may be desirable to reduce blood loss in patients of rare blood group, and where Jehovah's Witnesses or other objectors to blood transfusion on religious grounds are the patients. Consideration should not be given to hypotensive techniques until the following more simple measures to reduce bleeding have been applied, wherever possible:

the application of tourniquets
the infiltration of the tissues with adrenaline or octapressin (Felypressin) solutions
the use of posture
adequate carbon dioxide elimination (it has been shown that bleeding from the cut skin during cyclopropane anaesthesia is inversely proportional to the depth of anaesthesia). Hyperventilation through soda lime reduces blood loss
the employment of equipment with minimal resistance for ventilation

The technique of hypotensive anaesthesia is probably justifiable when an operation is required to correct some disorder which is making the patient's life miserable, and when the success of that operation is put in hazard because the surgeon cannot obtain a sufficiently clear field in which to exercise his skill. In certain cases where blood loss may be excessive, the hazards of hypotensive anaesthesia must be weighed against the hazards of unreplaced blood loss on the one hand and of massive blood transfusion on the other. Blood transfusion carries a risk to life variously estimated at between 0.1%–0.3%, with a significant proportion of these deaths due to serum hepatitis: non-fatal reactions occur in about 5% of transfusions. When deliberate hypotension was practised by a cross section of 300 anaesthetists in Great Britain, the mortality rate directly attributable to the hypotension was 0.2%, with a complication rate involving the brain, heart and kidneys of 3%. There is no doubt that in expert hands hypotensive anaesthesia carries a low morbidity and mortality but the dangers of reducing blood flow to the brain cannot be overstressed and herein lies the greatest objection to the hypotensive technique. There is some evidence that blood pressure below 100 mmHg with elevation of the head predisposes to cerebral injury and thrombosis. However, Enderby (1961) reporting on the mortality and morbidity following 9107 hypotensive anaesthetics had only one case of cerebral thrombosis. In the past, cerebral blood flow has generally been considered to be regulated extrinsically, i.e. that it follows the changes in systemic blood pressure quite passively: this view has been challenged and it is now shown that when blood pressure falls the cerebral vessels dilate. Cerebral blood flow is maintained at a constant level over a fairly wide range until, when the blood pressure reaches about 50 mmHg the flow begins to fall. It is also particularly sensitive to carbon dioxide. With a raised arterial carbon dioxide tension (in the region of 70–80 mmHg), cerebral flow is linearly related to blood pressure. A reduction in carbon dioxide tension, however, leads to a reduction in cerebral blood flow: at normal levels of blood pressure cerebral blood flow is directly related to arterial carbon dioxide tension. At low systolic blood pressures the intrinsic control of cerebral vessels is lost and there is no response to changes in arterial carbon dioxide tension. Certain anaesthetic agents, e.g. thiopentone reduces cerebral blood flow.

Coronary arterial flow is largely independent of blood pressure down to about 70 mmHg systolic pressure. Below this level, the work load of the heart has to decrease in proportion to the hypotension, if the coronary flow is to keep pace with the oxygen requirements of the heart. Animal experiments have shown, that although the coronary flow is independent of blood pressure down to 70 mmHg, this is not true if the blood pressure is lowered very rapidly. It takes time for collaterals to open up, particularly if athero-sclerosis is present.

Evidence appears to point to the fact that an abnormal ECG under induced hypotension is only transient.

There is an intrinsic regulation of renal blood flow and this will maintain renal flow in the face of severe falls in the blood pressure. There are, however, two exceptions: diseased kidneys do not necessarily behave in this way and, furthermore, rapid changes in blood pressure are not followed by equally quick compensatory changes.

The vital capacity is little altered by hypotensive techniques in normal subjects, whereas in patients with orthopnoea and dyspnoea the vital capacity increases – in some more than 30%. This increase is linked with the severity of the symptoms, not with the degree of hypotension. The VD/VT ratio is also increased.

Hypotensive anaesthesia

Deliberate reduction of the blood pressure can be achieved by controlling peripheral resistance. Blockade of vaso-constrictor fibres to resistance vessels causes a fall in peripheral resistance and thus a fall in blood pressure: blockade of vaso-constrictor fibres to capacitance vessels causes vaso-dilation with decreased venous return, a consequent decreased cardiac output and a further fall in blood pressure.

Drugs acting centrally. Central depressants, such as anaesthetic agents, cause depression of the vasomotor centre. (Reserpine is thought to have a specific effect on the vasomotor centre as well as a peripheral action).

Spinal subarachnoid and epidural anaesthetics. Any local anaesthetic drug used to paralyse the pre-ganglionic fibres produces vaso-dilatation but, if the extent of block is small, hypotension may not occur. High subarachnoid block has been used to achieve this effect.

Ganglionic blocking agents. Transmission through autonomic ganglia is by the release of acetyl-choline at the pre-ganglionic nerve endings, activating receptors on the cell bodies of post-ganglionic neurones. Competitive ganglionic blockers effect both sympathetic and para-sympathetic ganglia, so that para-sympathetic effects of dryness of the mouth, constipation, difficulty with micturition and blurring of vision may occur. Though most drugs in this group, which includes quaternary ammonium groups, are badly absorbed when taken orally, they may be used parenterally during anaesthesia. The blocking action of these drugs may be due to an action like that of acetyl-choline and so compete with acetyl-choline, or potentiate its effect. Certain anti-cholinesterases compete at receptors to block transmission. Ganglion blocking agents include hexamethonium, pentamethonium, pentolinium, and trimetaphan.

Adrenergic blockade. Post-ganglionic transmission is dependent on the release of noradrenaline from storage granules. Adrenergic transmission may be blocked at the post-ganglionic (pre-receptor) site, or at the final receptor site. Pre-receptor adrenergic 'blockers' include reserpine, bretylium, guanethidine and methyldopa. At the receptor site, adrenergic alpha-receptor blockers include phentolamine, dibenamine, phenoxybenzamine, chlorpromazine and some other phenothiazines. Three different characteristics are significant: reserpine depletes noradrenaline from the storage granules and the available pool due to inhibition of the transport mechanism; bretylium prevents the release of noradrenaline by the nerve impulse; and guanethidine depletes noradrenaline stores, possibly because of the release of active noradrenaline from the pool. Thus the adrenergic blockers act specifically on sympathetic transmission, sparing the parasympathetic system.

Methods of producing hypotension during anaesthesia. In surgery ganglion blocking agents are particularly suitable for producing hypotension.

Phenactropinium (Trophenium): phenactropinium is of short action, with a specific ganglion blocking effect, which is readily controllable by altering the rate at which it is infused. A concentration of 2 mg/ml (in an intravenous infusion) with an initial drip rate of 100–120 drops per minute may be given, followed by the drip rate being slowed to 40–60 drops per minute when the systolic blood pressure is within 10 mmHg of that required.

Trimetaphan (Arfonad): trimetaphan in a 0.1% solution (500 mg in 500 ml) may be given at the rate of 40–60 drops per minute in an intravenous infusion until the systolic pressure is between 70–80 mmHg and thereafter maintained at the rate found necessary. Unlike phenactropinium, trimetaphan releases histamine. Tachyphylaxis often, and tachycardia occasionally, occur with it and its use should be avoided with asthmatic patients. With Trophenium and Arfonad there is usually little difference between the predictability and the adequacy of the hypotension achieved, occurrence of post-operative complications and the duration of blood pressure recovery on stopping the administration. Both drugs are associated with rapid onset of hypotension and short duration of effect. However, a few patients are resistant to the hypotensive effects of trimetaphan and other additional drugs may require to be given.

Pentamethonium (C5) and *hexamethonium* (C6): with these the dose tends to be dependent upon age and pre-operative blood pressure, with a total dose range from 50–150 mg. The patient can be premedicated with omnopon and scopolamine in normal doses, together with either chlorpromazine, promethazine, or promazine. Following induction of anaesthesia the patient is placed in the horizontal position and controlled hyperventilation is carried out using D-tubocurarine as a neuromuscular blocking agent. The blood pressure is adjusted to not less than 80 mmHg systolic, by positioning the patient and giving hexamethonium the dose being related to age and pre-operative blood pressure and to the initial response to hyperventilation. (The average dose of hexamethonium bromide is 40 mg and hexamethonium tartrate 35 mg). Halothane can be used as an accessory hypotensive agent in association with ganglionic blockers, because of the occasional failure of large doses of hexamethonium and trimetaphan, in particular, to produce useful degrees of postural hypotension in a small proportion of patients. Procaine amide (Pronestyl) (25–50 mg) or phenoxybenzamine (Dibenyline) (12.5–100mg) given intravenously may be of value in these refractory cases, though the latter has no effect in reducing the tachycardia commonly associated with this technique: β-'blockers' have been used to reduce this tachycardia, but great caution must be displayed in their use in these particular circumstances.

Pentolinium (Ansolysen): this may also be employed as a sole hypotensive agent (average dose 8 mg) given in divided doses; up to 20 mg may be required in refractory cases or as 0.5% infusion.

Controlled ventilation, using halothane as the hypotensive agent is employed by many: the effect of halothane is due, in part, to a direct relaxing action on smooth muscle, though mainly to reduction in cardiac output, particularly if carbon dioxide elimination is excessive. Premedication may be with pethidine and promethazine, occasionally giving chlorpromazine in addition. Atropine should be avoided as it tends to prevent blood pressure fall. After induction with thiopentone and intubation under suxamethonium the patient is positioned, an intravenous needle is inserted and ECG electrodes applied. No nitrous oxide is administered, but apnoea is produced with halothane and oxygen, and intermittent positive pressure ventilation using larger than normal tidal volumes. D-tubocurarine may be given as this will not only provide adequate neuromuscular blockade but will enhance the hypotensive effect of the halothane. A gradual fall in blood pressure ensues. Because increased mean airway pressure associated with IPPV decreases the venous return, associated with lack of venoconstriction, this leads to a fall in the blood pressure. The arterial blood pressure is stabilized at the minimum systolic pressure consistent with reduced arterial bleeding and the maximum halothane concentration. Good peripheral perfusion is evidenced by warm, pink extremities. Care must be taken with the selection of cases, avoiding those patients with evidence of cardio-vascular and neuro-vascular disease. The blood volume must be maintained throughout the duration of anaesthesia and the hypotensive technique. It is essential to monitor the ECG, pulse rate, blood pressure, pulse pressure, blood loss and ventilation, at the same time observing closely the patient's colour, capillary refill time and the warmth and dryness of the skin. It must be remembered that blood pressure in the head is some 16–20 mmHg less than in the brachial artery, the blood pressure reducing by 2 mmHg for each inch above the heart level. The technique of deliberate hypotension is only for the experienced, namely for those who are fully aware of the consequences of mismanagement.

Sodium nitroprusside: this substance has a direct vasodilator effect on vascular smooth muscle, giving rise to a fall in peripheral resistance and an increase in the volume of the venous vascular compartment. The effect is quickly reversible because of the rapid detoxication and breakdown in the body. Sodium nitroprusside is usually administered in the form of an intravenous infusion of 0.005% solution. A tachycardia is frequently associated with the use of this drug, and the pulse rate may be controlled by the cautious use of a β-adrenergic receptor blocking agent. Tachyphylaxis is not uncommon and the need to give increasing doses may indicate the development of an associated metabolic acidosis. Great care should therefore be taken in regard to not exceeding the maximum safe dose which is probably of the order of 200 mg in the adult.

There is no evidence that induced hypotension increases the risk of reactionary haemorrhage, provided the surgeon is meticulous in ligating all potential bleeding points.

Hypotensive anaesthesia in the elderly. Rollason and Hough (1960) came to the conclusion that hypotension in the elderly is not absolutely contra-indicated, even in cases of known coronary or cerebro-vascular disease, provided that the blood pressure is not lowered below 60 mmHg, the anaesthetist is skilled, and surgical advantages are likely to ensue from the technique. They argue that the benefits to the surgeon of an avascular field must be weighed against the possible risks to the patient. Our views are not in accord with this: we would not deliberately produce the hypotensive state in someone with known coronary or cerebro-vascular disease.

Vasoconstriction

The local infiltration of the operative site with solutions containing vasoconstrictors, such as adrenaline, is not an uncommon practice in surgery. Adrenaline may also be added to the local anaesthetic solutions to prolong their effect and to minimize the absorption of toxic local agents into the systemic circulation.

The increased sensitivity of the heart to the effects of endogenous and exogenous adrenaline, during anaesthesia, has been known for many years: it was a well-recognized hazard associated with chloroform anaesthesia. Adrenaline and noradrenaline, particularly in the presence of carbon dioxide accumulation, may precipitate severe ventricular disturbances during cyclopropane anaesthesia. Halothane is thought to be intermediate between cyclopropane and chloroform in its effect in 'sensitizing' the heart to the action of adrenaline. Ventricular dysrhythmia has been reported even when adrenaline solution was used to irrigate the bladder. During reconstructive operations of the vagina under halothane anaesthesia, following the injection of adrenaline solution to these highly vascular areas, dysrhythmias leading to cardiac arrest have also occurred. Isoproterenol and ephedrine given intravenously to patients under halothane anaesthesia result in a high incidence of ventricular dysrhythmias. As an alternative, phenylephrine may be used as a local infiltration during halothane anaesthesia. The dose should be limited to 0.1 mg per kg body weight. Infiltration with 1.5 mg% of phenylephrine is as effective as 2.0 mg% of adrenaline in reducing bleeding. The use of topical or subcutaneous adrenaline during methoxyflurane anaesthesia appears to be acceptable. A synthetic polypeptide, octapressin (Felypressin) with vasoconstrictor properties, appears to give good haemostasis during vaginal surgery, and to cause no cardiac dysrhythmias when used in the presence of halothane: the solutions may vary from 5 pressor units/ml of normal saline to 5 pressor units/100 ml normal saline, the dose varying from 0.75 to 15 pressor units. Using such a dosage it would appear that octapressin is compatible with halothane, methoxyflurane, and cyclopropane anaesthesia. Results, however, would appear to be more satisfactory in vaginal than ENT surgery. Some authorities appear to advocate the routine IV administration of β-receptor 'blockers' prior to the injection of adrenaline in patients receiving halothane anaesthesia. We do not subscribe to this practice.

The monosemicarbazone or adrenochrome (Adrenoxyl) was claimed to reduce capillary permeability and bleeding time, but most workers can find no evidence of reduction of blood loss during e.g. radical mastectomy. Ethamsylate (Dicynene) is said to have similar properties.

There would appear to be no correlation between the arterial carbon dioxide tension and bleeding and clotting times.

Pressor agents

A fall in blood pressure occurring during the course of general anaesthetic should be met with a quick reappraisal of the technique. The anaesthetist should consider the following questions:

Has the blood loss been inadequately replaced? A tachycardia might suggest this.

Is ventilation adequate and has the patient received adequate amounts of oxygen during the course of anaesthesia? Is the patient being excessively hyperventilated?

What is the colour of the patient? Is he sweating? What is the capillary refill time?

Is the agent which is being employed likely to cause a fall in blood pressure? For example, the administration of halothane to a subject who has received D-tubocurarine may cause a fall in blood pressure: indeed D-tubocurarine may sometimes cause a fall in blood pressure in its own right. Have relatively excessive amounts of the agent been given?

Is the anaesthetic too 'light'? Certain surgical manoeuvres, such as traction on the oesophagus during a vagotomy, may produce a profound fall in blood pressure, if the patient is in a 'light' plane of anaesthesia.

Is the heart rate excessively slow? This situation sometimes arises during the course of mitral valvotomy and it is our experience that small quantities of atropine, administered slowly intravenously, often reduce the vagal tone and improve the blood pressure. If halothane is being used bradycardia may necessitate the administration of intravenous atropine. Are dysrhythmias present?

If the patient is receiving intermittent positive pressure ventilation are the inflation pressures excessive? Excessively high inflation pressures with an inadequate expiratory pause may well reduce the blood pressure. This is particularly the case in those subjects who suffer from pulmonary hypertension, have a reduced blood volume, or have been receiving anti-hypertensive agents.

What is the posture of the patient? (N.B. The 'supine hypotensive syndrome' of pregnancy results from presence of the gravid uterus on the inferior vena cava).

Where blood loss has occurred, this should be replaced, bearing in mind the fact that the normal fit young adult may withstand the loss of at least 500 ml. Massive blood transfusion results in hypothermia, metabolic acidosis, potassium and citrate intoxication and may well cause a fall in blood pressure; excessive transfusion may do the same by over-loading of the heart. Attention should be given to calcium replacement, the administration of bicarbonate, and warming the blood.

Table 6.1 *Pressor agents* (*after Benazon, D. 1962*)

Agent	*C.N.S.*	*Heart* *rate*	*irritability*	*force*	*cardiac output*
adrenaline	stimulates	increases	increases	increases	increa
noradrenaline (Levophed)	no change	reflex bradycardia	increases	increases	reduc
phenylephrine	no change	reflex bradycardia	probably increases	slightly increases	little chang reduc
methoxamine (Vasoxine)	no change	no change or bradycardia	little change	no change	reduc
ephedrine	stimulates	increases	increases	increases then decreases	increa
methylamphetamine	stimulates	increases	increases	increases	increa
mephentermine (Mephine)	stimulates	little change	increases	increases	increa
metaraminol (Aramine)	no change	little change	increases	increases	little chang
angiotensin (Hypertensin)	little change	reflex bradycardia	little change	inconstant fleeting positive inotropic effect	no ch or sli fall
isoprenaline	stimulates	increases	increases	increases	incre

Hypotension may follow a fall in cardiac output, peripheral resistance, or both. Where excessive blood loss and replacement are concerned, there are advantages to be gained by monitoring venous pressure. A knowledge of the central venous pressure, together with the systemic arterial pressure, will give a guide to the cause of the low blood pressure.

Should the anaesthetist be satisfied that attention has been paid to such detail, then consideration should be given to the question of whether pressor agents should be given. They are of possible value in the presence of normal blood volume associated with an expanded vascular bed, e.g. after spinal anaesthesia and spinal blockade. Although it is known that mexthoxamine, phenylephrine, and noradrenaline act directly on the vessel wall, and may be of value in this respect, it is preferable to fill the

	coronary	*external iliac*	*pulmonary*	*sup. mesenteric*	*renal*	*Veins*	*Total effect*
	increased	–	vc	–	vc	vc	vd
	increased	vc	vc	vc	vc	vc	vc
	increased	vc	vc	vc	vc	–	vc
	no change	vc	vc	vc	vc	–	vc
	increases	vc	–	vc	vc	–	vd
	probably increased	vd	vd	vd	vd	–	vd
	increased	vd	vd	vd	–	–	vd
	increased	–	vc	vc	vc	–	vc
	mild effect	vc	no change or mild effect	vc	vc	mild effect	vc
ge	no change	vd	no change	vd	vd	no change	vd

vasoconstriction vd = vasodilatation

Table 6.1—*continued*

Agent	*Duration*	*Dose*
adrenaline	short	i.v. infusion 2 ml 1/1000 in 500 ml 5% dextrose
noradrenaline (Levophed)	short	i.v. infusion 4 mg added to 1 litre 5% dextrose
phenylephrine	short	i.v. intermittent 0·15–0·5 mg i.v. infusion 10 mg in 500 ml 5% dextrose vials contain 1 ml 1% soln.
methoxamine (Vasoxine)	sustained 1 hour	i.v. intermittent 1–5 mg i.m. 10–20 mg vials contain 20 mg in 1 ml
ephedrine	sustained several hours	vials contain 32 mg suitable for i.m. 15–25 mg for i.v.
methylamphetamine	sustained several hours	i.v. 2–5 mg. i.m. 10–15 mg vials contain 30 mg in 1·5 ml
mephentermine (Mephine)	sustained (approx 1 hour)	i.v. 3–5 mg doses i.v. infusion 150 mg in 500 ml 5% dextrose vials contain 15 mg/ml
metaraminol (Aramine)	sustained (20 minutes – 1 hour)	i.v. 25–100 mg in 500 ml 5% dextrose i.m. 2–10 mg vials contain 10 mg in 1 ml
angiotensin (Hypertensin)	short (2–4 min)	single dose 5–20 μg i.v. or 1 mg/l dextrose rate varying from 1–10 μg/min. initial drip rate 1 μg/min normally not more than 2 μg/min
isoprenaline	short	10–20 μg i.v. or 2 mg in 500 ml dextrose

expanded vascular compartment by intravenous infusion. Pressor agents may also be of some value in coronary artery insufficiency, except for vasopressin and angiotensin, which are known to constrict the coronary arteries. Care, should, however, be taken in these patients, as the agents may increase the excitability and oxygen requirements of the cardiac muscle.

Isoprenaline is a β-adrenergic receptor stimulant which, in normal subjects, increases the rate and force of contraction of the heart and dilates peripheral blood vessels. In a shocked patient, with a raised venous pressure, its use may sometimes lead to a reduction in heart rate and a rise in blood pressure as a result of rise in cardiac output. The drug is usually infused by a pump at a rate which varies from 1 to 10 μg/min (concentration of solution 1 to 10 μg/ml). The aim is to give a dose which is adequate to reduce central venous pressure without causing undue tachycardia.

It is our firm conviction, that pressor agents are rarely required and, indeed, their exhibition may well be harmful. There is now strong evidence that the administration of pressor agents to a subject who is 'shocked' can indeed perpetuate poor peripheral blood flow, with resultant tissue hypoxia and metabolic acidosis, so that further impairment of cardiac action results therefrom.

Benazon (1962) has reviewed the pharmacology and clinical application of pressor agents in detail. Table 6.1 gives the effects of various pressor agents.

Water and electrolyte balance

Disturbances of electrolyte and water balance may arise from a deficiency in intake, or from excessive losses. The latter may arise through an increased loss of fluids and electrolytes normally lost from the body, or a loss through abnormal channels. A deficiency of intake of a duration of two or three days does not usually impose a great upset to the normal individual, as the loss which occurs over this time is largely water loss from the skin, lungs, and faeces. The kidney has the ability to retain water and sodium, and the normal reaction to general anaesthesia and surgery is characterized by a reduction in urinary output in urine and sodium, as a result of an increased production of ACTH, ADH and of adrenal cortical steroids (17-hydroxy corti-costeroids and aldosterone).

Water

The total body water averages about 60% of body weight. At birth it comprises about 75% decreasing to 65% by one month. Whereas the total body water amounts to approximately 60% of the body weight between the ages of 17–39 years in the male and 50% in the female, it decreases to 50% and 45% respectively at about the age of 60 years. The amount of water is proportional to the lean body mass with less water in fat. 55% of the water is contained in the intracellular space and the remainder in the extracellular space (45%). The extracellular space is made up of the plasma (7.5% of the total body water), the functional extracellular space (20% of the total body water), and two pools which pay little part in the losses and dislocations of fluids in surgical patients, namely dense connective tissue (cartilage, ligaments, and tendons) and bone. Each of these two latter pools comprises 7.5% of the total body water. Finally, there is the transcellular fluid, which is water passing through cells in order to become extracellular and includes water on the way to the gastro-intestinal tract. The transcellular fluid amounts to only 2.5% of the total body water. The functional extracellular fluid (previously called the interstitial lymph) can be considered as being contained in a chamber with a gelatinous matrix which is capable of expanding and contracting rapidly, and is readily permeated by crystalloids which are in equilibrium with the capacitance side of the vascular compartment. It acts as a reservoir in or out of which water and sodium can be mobilized for the circulation.

The normal adult intake of water amounts to approximately 30 ml water/kg/day or 2500 ml for a 70 kg individual. This intake is made up of the water content of food (800 ml/day), the product of catabolism (350 ml/day), and drink (1500 ml/day). The normal output balances this intake, 400 ml/day being lost via the lungs, 500 ml/day by the skin, and 100 ml/day in the faeces, the remainder being lost via the kidney.

Water depletion occurs when water is unavailable and when it is withheld during or after surgical operation, or therapeutically as in the management of raised intracranial pressure. Inability to swallow because of coma, painful conditions such as quinsy, or carcinoma of the oesophagus also lead to diminished intake. Increased loss of water occurs with raised body temperature (sweating), hyperventilation (from the lungs), or in such conditions as diabetes mellitus, and Addison's disease (kidneys). Water depletion is characterized by dry mouth, furred tongue, sunken cheeks, difficulty in swallowing or chewing, lowered intraocular tension, inelasticity of the skin, weight loss, and, with extreme loss, lowered blood pressure. As thirst acts as a stimulus for replacement, water depletion (without sodium depletion) is uncommon in the average adult surgical patient. It is more likely to occur in infants, or in association with prolonged unconsciousness, or with lesions of the pharynx or oesophagus. Plasma sodium and chloride tend to rise, the rise in plasma urea tending to be slow if exogenous nitrogen is not being given. When the water deficit amounts to 10% of the body weight mental impairment occurs, and death ensues when a loss of approximately 20% of the body weight (14 litres) has been reached. The kidney endeavours to maintain a normal composition of the extracellular fluid by excreting a hypertonic urine which contains high concentrations of urea, sodium, potassium, and chloride. The pure water deficit can be calculated approximately from the following relationship:

$$\text{Water deficit} = \text{normal body water} - \text{actual body water}$$

$$\text{Actual body water} = \frac{\text{normal body water} \times \text{normal plasma sodium (140 mEq/l)}}{\text{actual plasma sodium}}$$

The normal body water is calculated from a knowledge of the patient's weight prior to the occurrence of the deficit (i.e. 60% of the body weight in kg).

Treatment: about $\frac{1}{3}$ of the deficit should be replaced in the first 4 hours using fluids containing sodium concentrations of 30–75 mEq/l and the remainder of the deficit can be corrected by using 5% dextrose or 1/5 normal saline over the next 36–48 hours together with the replacement of the normal requirements. The use of 5% dextrose alone should be avoided as it is easy to convert hypernatraemic water depletion into water intoxication.

Water intoxication is associated with an increase in the total body water without a comparable increase in the body sodium. Such intoxication is likely to occur in acute renal failure, which may result from hypotension occurring with surgery, injury, or myocardial infarction. Intoxication with water may arise post-operatively where excessive production of anti-diuretic hormone (ADH) reduces the ability of the kidney to compensate for excessive intravenous intake of solutions such as 5% dextrose. Water intoxication is associated with headache, muscle cramps, pulmonary oedema, systematic oedema, convulsions, and even coma. There is a fall in plasma protein, sodium, and bicarbonate, with a rise in plasma potassium.

Treatment: 50–100 ml 5% or molar (5.85%) saline can be given slowly intravenously, there being no danger of the patient if the plasma sodium is below 120 mEq/l. Such therapy is usually associated with a rapid improvement in the patient's condition and causes a brisk diuresis.

Sodium

The total body sodium amounts to approximately 52.0 mEq/kg, $\frac{1}{3}$ of this quantity being stored in bone. 75% of total body sodium is exchangeable. Food contains little sodium, which has to be added to the diet as salt. The kidney is the principle regulating mechanism, for when the intake is high the concentration of sodium in the urine may rise to 300 mEq/l, and when the intake is low sodium may disappear from the urine completely. In health the total body store of sodium as well as the plasma concentration is maintained within relatively narrow limits. The blood level does however tend to give an inaccurate reflection as to the total body store.

The plasma sodium concentration lies between 135–140 mEq/l. A low plasma sodium may be associated with excessive loss of sodium or, more usually, is dilutional. A high plasma sodium may be caused by water depletion. Most patients who are chronically ill (except Addison's-type diseases) have raised sodium stores. Trauma, in particular, retains sodium, and if sodium intake continues leads to an increase in sodium stores. The daily requirement for sodium amounts to 1.0–2.5 mEq/kg/day in the normal individual. Sodium deficiency arises from increased loss as may be found with sweating, vomiting, diarrhoea, effusions and exudates, in Addison's disease, with diuretics, and along with an osmotic diuresis, such as may occur in association with diabetes mellitus.

Decreased intake may occur in the treatment of cardiac failure, the use of ion-exchange resins, in conditions associated with an inability to swallow, and post-operatively, particularly if water is given alone in the first few days.

Treatment: a normal plasma sodium is often taken as an indication that significant depletion of sodium stores has not occurred. However, a normal value may be present even when sodium stores are depleted. If clear signs of extracellular fluid volume depletion are present, even in the presence of a normal plasma sodium, isotonic solution should be given. Signs of a normal extracellular fluid volume are rapid capillary refill, a warm periphery, and a blood pressure which is maintained with the patient sitting upright. Under such conditions it is unlikely that extracellular fluid volume is depleted or attempts to give sodium will be beneficial. If very low levels of plasma sodium are present (below 120–125 mEq/l) in patients free from cardiovascular disease it is reasonable to use hypertonic (1.8%) saline when signs of extracellular depletion of fluid are present. Once plasma levels above 125 mEq/l are restored isotonic saline should be substituted.

Hypernatraemia. Sodium retention may occur with over transfusion of isotonic or hypertonic sodium containing solutions, such as may be associated with the uncontrolled infusion of 8.4% sodium bicarbonate. Excessive oral intake of sodium in an unconscious patient especially when associated with a high protein diet is a further cause. Inability to secrete sodium when the intake is normal may result from excessive amounts of cortico-steroids, and may occur with Cushing's disease and Conn's disease (primary aldosteronism). Essential hypernatraemia may occur with head injury, frontal lobe lesions, and in diabetic coma. Relative water depletion may lead to a rise in plasma sodium even when the sodium stores are depleted.

Symptoms of hypernatraemia apart from those of the usually accompanying disease include mild oedema of the lungs; hyperosmolality causes confusion, dullness and apathy, leading to coma. When water deficiency is not a feature the plasma and extracellular volumes, the haemoglobin and the plasma proteins are normal. The plasma sodium and chloride are raised in essential hypernatraemia (sodium may be as high as 180 mEq/l). The urine is well concentrated with a specific gravity above 1020. The excretion of sodium and chloride is below 20 mEq/l in hyperaldosteronism, and there is absent excretion of sodium and chloride in essential hypernatraemia. The sodium retention type of hypernatraemia is differentiated from hypernatraemia of water deficiency by clinical evidence of dehydration in the latter and the relatively high volume of the urine in the former. Sodium retention, that is causing oedema is differentiated from water intoxication by the clinical history and the low plasma concentration of sodium associated with water intoxication.

Treatment of hypernatraemia: the chief risk is that the patients may receive large infusions of 5% dextrose rapidly, and it is possible to change hypernatraemic water depletion into water intoxication. Therefore sodium should always be included in the repleting fluid (30–75 mEq/l in children : 75 mEq/l in adults).

Potassium

The total body potassium amounts to 57 mEq/kg body weight. The normal exchangeable potassium amounts to 85% of total body potassium. Most foods contain high concentrations of potassium and the average intake in an adult amounts to 60–100 mEq/day. The kidney is the chief regulator but cannot cut off completely the output of potassium. Potassium excretion continues despite no intake. The normal loss by the kidney (60–110 mEq/day) balances the input. There is a small loss in the faeces (10 mEq/day). Gastro-intestinal fluids contain up to 10 times the concentration in plasma. The blood level is in the range of 3.5–5.0 mEq/l. The plasma potassium may be above the normal lower limit of 3.5 mEq/l even in the presence of a large deficit in the total body potassium. In contrast to the retention of sodium associated with acute and chronic illness and trauma, a loss of as much as 100 mEq of potassium may be found in the first 36–48 hours after a major operation.

Potassium deficiency can result from a decreased intake, either because of inability to swallow (coma, debility, carcinoma or stricture of the oesophagus), potassium-free fluids given in parenteral fluid therapy, or decreased absorption as may occur with steatorrhoea, or with overdosage of potassium-binding resins (Resonium-A). Excessive loss may also give rise to potassium depletion. Such excessive loss may be associated with primary hyperaldosteronism (Conn's syndrome), secondary hyperaldostonism (malignant hypertension, congestive heart failure, hepatic failure), Cushing's syndrome, cortico-steroid therapy, potassium losing nephritis, treatment with diuretics, and aspirin intoxication. Loss occurs with diarrhoea, vomiting, fistulae, ileostomy, and gastric and intestinal aspiration. Potassium is also lost from the extracellular fluid during the treatment of diabetic coma. Potassium depletion produces characteristic symptoms and signs. The effect on the heart muscle may make itself apparent by a raised heart rate, extrasystoles, cardiac dilatation and even heart failure. The ECG findings are very variable, but prolonged QT interval, depression of the ST segment, broad and flat T waves which may become inverted, and A-V block have been seen. Well marked U waves may be found. Muscle weakness and hypotonia are present particularly in the alkalotic patient. In extreme circumstances, paralysis of the arms, legs and respiratory muscles may occur. Abdominal distension and paralytic ileus are sometimes associated with low potassium levels, though many of the characteristic symptoms and signs may be absent despite low plasma potassium levels. A low potassium level, although well recognized as creating an altered response to neuromuscular blocking agents in some patients, does not always do so. However, caution should be taken in the administration of such drugs to a patient with a low plasma potassium – a test dose of non-depolarizing neuromuscular blocking agent may be given prior to the injection of the full dose to judge the patient's response. Intravenous potassium may correct a prolonged response to a neuromuscular blocking agent in a potassium depleted patient.

If the plasma potassium is below 3.5 mEq/l a potassium deficiency is probable and below 3.0 mEq/l a potassium deficit is certain, particularly if the plasma bicarbonate is above 30 mEq/1 (hypokalaemic alkalosis).

Treatment of hypokalaemia: intravenous potassium equilibrates extremely rapidly with the extracellular fluid and if the circulation is normal, equilibration is 95% complete in one circulation time. The penetration of this potassium into cells is also rapid if cellular deficiency of potassium is present. The liver, lungs, heart and skeletal muscle take up potassium under these circumstances more rapidly than the brain and red cells. A considerable improvement in muscle power can take place even after the intravenous administration of small quantities of potassium (far less than required to replenish the total body store). When administering potassium intravenously a concentration of not more than 1.5g KC1 (20 mEq) in a 500 ml intravenous infusion should be given at a rate not exceeding 15 mEq/h up to a total quantity of 50 mEq/24 h for the prevention of depletion. When established depletion has occurred a total of 8 g KC1 (107 mEq) may be given in 24 hours. Relatively large quantities of potassium are given post-operatively to patients who have received diuretic therapy prior to cardiac surgery. Normally, however, it is customary not to give potassium on the day of the operation or when a urine volume of less than 500 ml has been passed in 24 hours.

Potassium intoxication occurs when the plasma potassium exceeds 5.5 mEq/l. Diminished excretion of potassium arising from oliguria or anuria, chronic azotaemic kidney disease, hypopituitrism, Addison's disease, or overdosage with aldosterone antagonists (spironolactone) all cause an increase in the whole body potassium. It may also rise when there is an increased catabolism of endogenous protein (trauma, diabetic coma, etc.), and when excessive amounts of potassium are given by mouth or intravenously particularly in the presence of oliguria or renal failure. Potassium intoxication is aggravated by hypoxaemia and acidosis.

Patients with hyperkalaemia may be listless, with mental confusion, numbness and tingling of the extremities. The heart rate may be slow, with an irregular rhythm or heart block, and if the potassium intoxication is not treated cardiac arrest may ensue. With levels of potassium above 6.5 mEq/l the ECG may show enlarged and pointed T waves, widened QRS complex and increased PR interval with loss of P waves. In renal failure the raised potassium is associated with a raised blood urea and lowered plasma bicarbonate. In adrenal failure there is only a moderate rise in blood urea associated with a fall of sodium and chloride concentration in the plasma.

Treatment of hyperkalaemia: if the plasma level is above 7 mEq/l immediate treatment with 10 ml calcium gluconate given slowly intravenously is advised. This should be given with 25 g of intravenous glucose and 15 units of soluble insulin. An infusion of 50 ml (8.4%) molar sodium bicarbonate at a rate of 1 ml/min should also be given.

Fluid and electrolyte balance in relation to surgery and trauma

Amongst the many responses of the patient to trauma and surgery is the stimulation of the anterior and posterior pituitary to produce adrenocorticotrophic hormone (ACTH) and antidiuretic hormone (ADH). The adrenal cortex responds by secreting cortisol and aldosterone which lead to retention of water and sodium by the kidney, the urinary sodium falling below 50 mEq/l. Further water retention arises from the action of ADH, and there is also as much as 600–1000 ml of water produced as a result of the catabolism of mixed tissue with a high fat content. Water retention is further aggravated if water containing no sodium e.g. 5% dextrose, is given. There is therefore a tendency towards hyponatraemia in the post-operative period.

In addition to these metabolic responses, protein breakdown leads to the excretion of 2.5 mEq potassium for each gram of nitrogen excreted. If more than 2.5 mEq potassium are lost for every gram of nitrogen this suggests that it is a response to water depletion and must occur if cells are to give up water. Operation may be associated with a loss of as much as 50–100 mEq potassium in the first 24 hours post-operatively, the loss then falling to about 25 mEq/day in the starving patient. If no potassium is given a deficit of some 200 mEq can arise within a few days. In addition, repeated measurement of the 18 or 20 minute 'radiosulphate' space in relation to surgery has demonstrated large contractions of the volume of the space (Shires *et al.*, 1961), a loss of as much as 3–4 litres has been claimed, varying with the degree of trauma involved. Shires and his co-workers, on the basis of this evidence, have advocated the administration of large volumes of 'balanced salt' solutions. Undoubtedly there is likely to be a pool of traumatic oedema and sequestered fluid at the operation site, but there is by no means general agreement that any benefit is to be obtained by expanding the extracellular compartment other than to witness an increased urinary output post-operatively. Some, in fact, still hold the other extreme view that no sodium-containing fluids should be given during surgery. However, the current trend is to give moderate amounts of fluid during operation in addition to the replacement of other estimated losses.

Not more than 1–1.5 litres should be given during operation, and not more than 2.5 litres should be given in excess of replacement in the first 24 hours, including the hours of operation. Such a regimen will give a positive sodium balance post-operatively if Ringer lactate solution is given. It would seem reasonable therefore to give in addition to measured losses (other than urine):

On the day of operation:	Ringer-lactate 5 ml/kg/h of operation + 1 litre 5% dextrose + 0.5 litre isotonic saline
Following 24 hours:	1.5 litres 5% dextrose + 0.5 litre isotonic saline
Next 24 hours and each subsequent 24 hour period:	2 litres 5% dextrose + 0.5 litres isotonic saline (75 mEq/day sodium), adding 4 g potassium chloride (50 mEq potassium) a day to the 24 hour replacement

Intravenous potassium is not administered in the first 48 hours post-operatively unless there has been established post-operative potassium depletion or potassium intake has been inadequate pre-operatively.

There is still a large body of opinion that feels that the normally healthy adult does not require any special regimen operatively or post-operatively, provided abnormal losses such as haemorrhage do not occur. Such patients should be allowed to take fluids by mouth as soon as possible.

Some gastro-intestinal operations will, by their very nature, require aspiration of bowel contents during the post-operative period. If this is likely to be necessary for a significant time, the loss of water and electrolytes will have to be accurately measured and replaced intravenously. An alternative to intravenous therapy in certain operations, such as vagotomy and pyloroplasty is the aspiration of gastric contents and the replacement of these into the small intestine through a tube.

Abnormal losses may be self-evident, manifesting themselves as vomiting or diarrhoea. However, severe salt and water depletion may occur through loss via the skin, particularly in association with hypyrexia, and hot environments, leading to such excessive loss, may result in depletion of extracellular fluid volume and circulating blood volume, reduction of blood pressure and peripheral circulatory collapse. Other losses may be contained within the confines of the body – these, which may be considerable, are to be found in association with pancreatitis and strangulation of gut.

Pyloric Stenosis. The continued loss of chloride and hydrogen ions, together with water, leads to the development of a metabolic alkalosis, and excessive aldosterone production, with an attempt by the kidney to retain sodium and hydrogen ions in the body. Such retention may be associated with an excessive loss of potassium through the kidney, which can provoke profound effects upon the myocardium and may also alter the response of the motor end plate to neuromuscular blocking agents.

Gastro-intestinal obstruction. The normal secretions of the gastro-intestinal tract are shown in Tab. 6.2. Of the total quantity of 8100 ml only 200 ml per day are normally lost to the body. Excessive loss from the gastro-intestinal tract represents loss of isotonic fluid, as the electrolyte content of gastric mucus, hepatic and jejunal juice is predominantly made up of sodium and chloride ions. Loss of potassium from the gut mainly occurs in diarrhoea, and potassium loss from the kidneys is secondary to the loss of anion from the stomach. Another significant cause of loss of potassium from the body is in association with diuretic therapy. Prolonged loss of fluid and electrolytes from the gastro-intestinal tract causes a reduction of the circulating blood volume and results in the clinical signs of shock i.e. poor peripheral perfusion, with blue, cold extremities and poor capillary refill. The clinical signs largely result from arteriolar (resistance vessel) and venous (capacitance vessel) constriction, in an attempt to compensate for the depleted blood volume.

Table 6.2 *Secretions of the gastrointestinal tract*

Secretion		*Amount*
saliva		1400
gastric		2500
bile		500
pancreatic juice		700
intestinal		3000
	Total	8100

Loss from the gastro-intestinal tract, if it occurs in the post-operative period, can be generally observed and measured. Biliary fistula, paralytic ileus and bowel obstruction should be treated with drainage or suction, measuring the loss in terms of volume and electrolyte content, and treated volume for volume with accurate electrolyte replacement, over and above the normal regimen for such individuals, i.e. about 2000 ml/day. If it is not possible to replace the fluid and electrolytes into a lower level of the gastro-intestinal tract, the solutions should be given intravenously.

Where, however, the loss has occurred at home over a period of 24–48 hours or longer, the problem is less easy as such loss cannot be accurately quantitated. The principles of management of these cases depend largely on the clinical picture. The initial observations should take into account the state of the circulation, venous tone, the colour, temperature and texture of the skin, and the blood pressure. These clinical observations should be supplemented by serial measurements of the haematocrit, the blood haemoglobin, and the volume, specific gravity and electrolyte concentration of the urine. The blood urea and serum creatinine levels are other useful guide lines. Although not essential, indeed sometimes misleading, observations of the serum electrolytes can serve as useful baselines.

Patients may require large amounts of solutions of electrolytes, and perhaps plasma, to restore their circulating blood volume. In order to assess the response of the patient to treatment, the central venous pressure is a most useful and essential measurement, particularly in the elderly patient with incipient myocardial failure. Repeated observations of haematocrit and central venous pressure, together with the arterial blood pressure, should be carried out during the intravenous infusion of electrolyte solution and plasma. Continuous suction, by either intra-gastric tube or intra-duodenal Miller-Abbott or Cantor tube, will allow decompression of the abdomen, prior to surgery. Fluid collected by suction should be measured, both for volume and electrolyte content, and the equivalent replaced along with the intravenous infusion. There is no doubt that, provided strangulation of the bowel can be excluded from the diagnosis, a deliberate delay of surgery in order to restore the circulating blood volume will decrease the morbidity associated with these conditions. The maintenance of fluid balance charts is essential throughout this therapy.

In calculating the daily requirements of fluid, calories, and electrolytes, in a patient with no abnormal losses, Tables 6.3 and 6.4 are a guide.

Water and electrolyte depletion in children

In the first few months of life infants have a greatly increased turnover of water, and the total body water is greater than that of adults when

Table 6.3 *Daily fluid, electrolyte, and calorie requirements*

Daily intake per kg body wt.	
calories	25
fat	2 g
carbohydrate	2 g
protein	1 g
water	25 ml
sodium	1·0–2·5 mEq
potassium	0·7–0·8 mEq
chloride	1·0–2·5 mEq
calcium	0·5–1.5 mEq

Table 6.4 *Electrolyte content of commoner intravenous fluids*

isotonic 0·9% saline	154 mEq/l sodium, 154 mEq/l chloride
8·4% sodium bicarbonate	1000 mEq/l sodium, 1000 mEq/l bicarbonate
1 gram potassium chloride	13·4 mEq/l potassium, 13·4 mEq/l chloride
Hartmann's Ringer-lactate (compound sodium lactate injection B.P.)	131 mEq/l sodium, 5·0 mEq/l potassium 111 mEq/l chloride, 29·0 mEq/l lactate 4·0 mEq/l calcium
4·3% glucose 0·18% sodium chloride	31 mEq/l sodium, 31 mEq/l chloride
5·5% glucose	200 cal/1/l
aminosol 10%	160 mEq/l sodium, 0·5 mEq/l potassium 120 mEq chloride, 300 cal/l
intralipid 20%	2000 cal/1 1
fructose 20%	800 cal/1 1
ammonium chloride (molar 1/6)	167 mEq/1 chloride
sodium lactate (molar 1/6)	167 mEq/l sodium
aminosol – ethanol fructose	50 mEq/l sodium, 0·15 mEq/l potassium 40 mEq/l chloride, 875 cal/l
aminosol-glucose	50 mEq/l sodium, 0·15 mEq/l potassium 40 mEq/l chloride, 300 cal/l

compared on a weight basis. Up to a weight of 25 kg the daily intake of water should be 70 ml/kg and that of sodium and potassium 2 mEq/kg each. If water has to be given by the intravenous route it should be given as 0.18% sodium chloride in 4% dextrose i.e. as 1/5 isotonic saline in dextrose. 1 g of potassium chloride (13.4 mEq potassium) should be added to each 500 ml of infusion fluid but potassium should be omitted until 48 hours after surgery. In the first week of life the fluid and electrolyte intake should be reduced by multiplying the quantity to be given by $\frac{\text{age in days}}{7}$. Hypernatraemia should be treated by replacing the calculated water deficit by the slow infusion of $\frac{1}{3}$–$\frac{1}{2}$ isotonic saline and not 5% dextrose. Children are particularly prone to gross water and electrolyte depletion in conditions like acute apprendicitis – the depletion may be severe and may amount to as much as 10–15% of the body weight. Isotonic sodium chloride 40 ml/kg may be given in 40–60 minutes. Very ill patients can with advantage receive instead 20 ml/kg of plasma or dextran 70 in saline, and 20 ml/kg of normal saline, Ringer-lactate, or 1/16th molar sodium lactate. Metabolic acidosis should be treated by the administration of sodium bicarbonate on the basis of: mEq sodium bicarbonate = Base deficit in mEq/1 × 0.3 × body weight in kg. Further replacement of the calculated deficit of water should continue with 1/5 or ½ isotonic saline with the objective of correcting the deficit of water in 6 hours.

Post-operative phlebo-thrombosis

Phlebo-thrombosis, arising as a result of venous stasis, can lead to pulmonary embolism in the post-operative period. As delay in the emptying of the deep veins during intermittent positive pressure ventilation has been noted, it is suggested that, in order to try and reduce the incidence of this deep vein thrombosis, patients should be ambulant prior to operation. Hydration should be adequate. During surgery a 10°–15° head down tilt may be used, or, if this is not possible, the legs should be bent at the hip joints; the diathermy pad although in firm contact with the skin should not be so tightly applied as to obstruct the venous circulation; the calves should be kept clear of the table by foam rubber supports behind the ankle and when the foot of the table is bent, great care must be taken to ensure that the knee joint is distal to the break, so that no pressure is exerted on the back of the calf or knee joint. If intermittent positive pressure ventilation is employed, then the mean intrathoracic pressure should be kept as low as possible, by using, if desired, a negative phase. During the course of long operations either the anaesthetist should attempt to massage the legs at regular intervals or a ripple mattress should be employed to encourage venous flow. An electrical stimulating device has been devised in which a Galvanic stimulus is applied to the leg muscles throughout the operation: the use of this or similar devices, will no doubt prove itself if the incidence of post-operative venous thrombosis is thereby decreased. Work on the use of 40 000–70 000 dextrans claims that, if given during and immediately post-operatively, they will significantly lower the incidence of phlebo-thrombosis. Post-operatively the patients should be kept in the 10° head down position until they are fully conscious, as this will encourage the limb blood flow, and deep breathing and leg movements should be started as early as possible. There is considerable discussion concerning the prophylaxis of this complication and this includes the possible use of anticoagulants in the post-operative period.

Cardio-pulmonary by-pass

Surgery within the heart, under direct vision, requires the interruption of normal cardiac function and the replacement of the pumping activity of the heart by artificial means. It is more straightforward with modern equipment to by-pass both the lungs and heart than the heart alone. Cannulation of the major veins as they enter the heart, and thus the diversion of venous blood into an oxygenator and the return of that blood, now oxygenated, to the systemic side of the circulation by the use of a mechanical pump, constitutes the basic essentials of cardio-pulmonary by-pass. Prior to the sophistication of modern equipment, use was made of the patient's own lungs in several techniques, the most important of which was the Drew Technique (Drew *et al.*, 1959), incorporating hypothermia to a body temperature of 10°–15°C, so-called deep hypothermia, thus allowing protection against hypoxia for longer periods than at normal body temperature of 37°C. Two pumps were incorporated in the system, one taking on the function of the left ventricle, pumping blood from the left atrium into the systemic circulation via the femoral artery, after it had passed through a heat exchanger to lower its temperature. Once body temperature had fallen to below 28°C and heart function was failing, a further pump returned right atrial blood into the pulmonary circulation and allowed adequate circulation to continue, while further cooling to 10°–15°C occurred. The brain was able to withstand total circulatory arrest for up to 45 minutes at this temperature, thus allowing surgery within the dry heart to be undertaken for his period. Should further time be required, the pumps could be restarted, the body perfused for a period, the oxygenation of tissues improved and a further time of circulatory arrest could then allow an extended period of intracardiac surgery. Once the intracardiac repair was completed, the process was reversed; warming replaced cooling and normal cardiac function was returned as the temperature rose. This technique continues to be used in a limited field and by a limited number of workers, for specific types of heart lesions. It has recently formed the basis, in some centres, for major open heart surgery in infancy.

In the majority of cardio-thoracic centres the complete cardio-pulmonary by-pass system is now commonly used. Venous blood is drained from the patient by cannulae placed in the right atrium, or introduced into the superior and inferior venae cavae via the right atrium. Blood flows along the venous tubes into the machine by gravity and first passes through an artificial oxygenator.

There are several types of oxygenator, though they all basically depend on the same principle of oxygenation as the human lung, namely the exposure of as thin a film of blood as possible to an atmosphere containing oxygen.

Bubble oxygenator. Venous blood and oxygen enter the bottom of a vertical column and mix to form a froth of blood : oxygenation progresses as the froth ascends the column. The blood returns to the liquid phase, free of bubbles, by passage through antifoam chambers and settles out as arterial blood. Presterilized, disposable plastic bubble oxygenators of the Temptrol, Rigg, or Travenol type are in common use today. They are effective for most operations, require little preparation and the amount of fluid required in them in preparation for the by-pass procedure, the so-called priming volume, is generally less than that needed for a disc oxygenator of comparable output.

Rotating disc oxygenator. Blood passes along the lower part of a horizontal cylinder and is picked up on stainless steel vertical discs which rotate through the blood, picking up a thin film and exposing it to an oxygen atmosphere, where oxygenation occurs. As the blood passes down the cylinder progressive oxygenation occurs. This equipment is expensive, time consuming, both in preparation and cleaning, and for most operations has few advantages over the bubble oxygenator. Examples of the disc oxygenators are the Kay Cross oxygenator and the Melrose oxygenators.

Screen oxygenator. This is seldom used nowadays as expense and high priming volumes alone probably preclude its general acceptance. The principle of the oxygenators is the downwards passage of a thin film of blood over a series of screens in an atmosphere of oxygen.

Membrane oxygenator. Future oxygenators may be of this kind. As before, thin films of blood pass along channels, separated only from the oxygen atmosphere by a thin membrane. This is an attempt to reproduce conditions within a normal lung with a membrane, similar to the alveolar membrane and capillary wall separating the gaseous from the liquid phase. Technical problems, up to date, have been the manufacture of membranes thin enough to allow rapid diffusion of gases, without running the risk of small holes in the membrane allowing gas bubbles to enter the blood stream and with them the dangers of systemic gas embolization. Membrane oxygenators are not yet generally available, they are expensive, and their future place in perfusion work cannot yet be assessed. Their value may lie in the use of cardio-pulmonary by-pass for periods of days rather than hours in the management of acute cardiac or pulmonary failure as a supportive therapy while normal processes effect healing.

Artificial lungs are not as efficient as normal lungs and high percentages of oxygen are needed to oxygenate the volumes of venous blood in a cardio-pulmonary by-pass. 90–100% oxygen is usually employed.

Anaesthesia has to be maintained throughout the period of cardio-pulmonary by-pass. If volatile agents are used then small concentrations of powerful agents, such as halothane, can be introduced into the oxygenators with the oxygen. The high concentration of oxygen required precludes the use of an effective concentration of nitrous oxide. Carbon dioxide may also be added to the oxygenator, to maintain a normal or above normal level of carbon dioxide tension in the arterial blood. This encourages good peripheral circulation by increasing vasodilatation.

The arterialized blood is returned to the patient by an arterial pump, usually a DeBakey type of roller pump, which gives a virtually continuous rather than pulsatile, flow of blood back to the systemic circulation: the arterial blood is returned to the arterial system via a cannula inserted in the femoral artery or into the aortic arch. In order to achieve an adequate circulation in the patient, a flow of at least 2.4 l/m^2 should be achieved at normal body temperature (37°C). This figure can be lowered if hypothermia is used in association with cardio-pulmonary by-pass; as a lowered temperature lowers oxygen requirements, flows may be decreased. Hypothermia of a moderate degree, to temperatures of 28°–30°C, may protect the patient from the damaging effects of a poor perfusion and may also lessen the trauma to blood caused by passage through the heart-lung system. The patient's post-operative progress may, however, be less troublesome if the body temperature remains normal throughout perfusion. To effect a fall in body temperature, or to maintain a normal temperature, the heat exchanger through which water at varying temperatures can be circulated is incorporated in the system, either as a separate entity in the returning arterial line or as an integral part of the oxygenator system, as in the Temptrol Bag. Water at varying temperatures can be circulated through the exchange to effect changes in the temperature of the blood by conduction without direct contact of blood and water. The modern heart-lung machine has certain extra refinements. Pumping systems are incorporated to remove blood from the operative field, thus effecting economy in blood usage, and separate pumping systems may be present to allow separate perfusion of the coronary arteries when the aortic arch is clamped and the aorta open during aortic valve surgery. Reservoirs for blood and bubble-traps to ensure the complete exclusion of any gas bubbles from the arterial blood are also used.

Priming of pump oxygenator systems. In the early days of open heart surgery fresh heparinized blood was used to prime the machine, i.e. to fill the oxygenator, pumps, heat exchanger and tubing. Fresh blood is required to overcome the acidity and high potassium content of routine stored blood. Heparin was used in a dosage of 30 mg per litre. Heparinized blood was later replaced by edlugate (EDTA) blood, or freshly drawn acid citrate dextrose blood. The EDTA or ACD blood has to be heparinized prior to priming the machine and perfusion into the patient, using the same dosage as before. In addition 10 ml of 10% $CaCl_2$ per litre is also added.

Fresh blood has disadvantages in the priming system, as it has in any major blood transfusion. Gadboys *et al.* (1962) described the homologous blood syndrome, constituting changes of a functional and histological nature in certain organs of the body following extra-corporeal circulation with a heart lung machine. Evidence has since accumulated, suggesting that this condition, often clinically most severe in the lungs, is related to the use of large volumes of donor blood in this type of surgery. Though this blood may be compatible by the usual cross-matching methods, it may contain antigen systems capable of setting up reactions in the body similar in nature to a tissue-host reaction. (Nahas *et al.*, 1965).

A reduction in the quantities of fresh blood in the heart-lung machine should go some way towards preventing the patient's exposure to such hazards. Two ways in which this may be effected are a decrease in the priming volume of perfusion systems and the replacement of blood by other substances. Modern oxygenators have a smaller priming volume than in the past and substances other than blood are commonly in use. Plasma substitutes such as low molecular weight dextrans have been used, though the excessive use of such solutions (more than 20 ml/kg, body weight) may increase post-operative haemorrhage, and the hypertonic nature of such solutions results in the attraction of further fluid into the vascular system with a resultant further dilution.

Haemodilution techniques today depend commonly on the use of crystalloid solutions (such as 5% dextrose in water), or electrolyte solutions (such as Hartmann's solution), to replace a proportion of the blood required for priming the machine. On mixing with the patient's circulation such solutions result in a reduction in oxygen-carrying capacity. The amount of such solutions used depends on several factors, all of which are related to the resulting oxygen carrying capacity of the perfusing fluid. A safe level is calculated, and with good blood flow rates being maintained throughout perfusion, there is no evidence of metabolic upset or oxygen lack.

Following perfusion, the haemodiluting fluid passes rapidly from the patient's circulating volume into tissue spaces and can be replaced by blood or fluid from the heart-lung machine. Such dilution even to levels of 40–50 ml/kg body weight, results in few problems, and may completely replace blood in the heart-lung prime. Clotting mechanisms, though diluted, do not result in increased post-operative bleeding; indeed blood damage is lessened by the dilution and the fall in viscosity, which results in a lower perfusion pressure but an improved peripheral circulation.

The management of cardiopulmonary by-pass

Pre-operatively, a full assessment of patients submitted to cardio-pulmonary by-pass must be made by the anaesthetist. Thorough haematological and biochemical examination is necessary in addition to a physical examination.

Both drug therapy and cardiac rhythms may require stabilization. The effects of prolonged diuretic therapy should be appreciated and suitable potassium supplements given in appropriate doses as required. Any infections and bad teeth must be treated before surgery and physiotherapy also plays an important part. Prophylactic antibiotics may be prescribed, though the indiscriminate use of such drugs may hazard post-operative management by the introduction of resistant organisms or yeast infections.

Such patients may fear the anaesthetic more than the operation. The anaesthetist must reassure them, explain what is to happen to them before and after operation, and prescribe suitable sedation if necessary. The anaesthetic management of cardio-pulmonary by-pass calls for specialized knowledge on the part of the anaesthetist. It is beyond the scope of this book to deal with the details of such knowledge.

The anaesthetist may be responsible for the running of the perfusion in addition to the anaesthetic, with the heart-lung machine run by a pump technician, directly responsible to medical personnel, commonly the anaesthetist; or the anaesthetist, himself, may run the machine. In either situation, such cases require the presence of more than one anaesthetist and there will be present in the theatre one or more skilled technicians responsible for the monitoring equipment. Close co-operation with blood gas technicians and chemical pathologists will also be necessary throughout the operation. Clearly such a number of people must work as a team, with close co-operation which will have to be carried on into the post-operative period.

The anaesthetic for open heart surgery is generally along the lines followed for any cardiac operation. Premedication need not be limited, except in the very ill, or in patients with pulmonary hypertension. Induction of anaesthesia may be intravenously with thiopentone (3–4 mg/kg), methohexitone (1 mg/kg) or diazepam (0.2–0.3 mg/kg); circulation time may be slow, and so induction may be prolonged. Intubation is effected with the aid of a short-acting depolarizing relaxant or a long acting non-depolarizing relaxant such as pancuronium (0.075–0.1 mg/kg): this has the advantage over D-tubocurarine that hypotension and cardio-vascular upset are minimal.

Maintenance of anaesthesia is by agents having minimal cardio-vascular effects. Nitrous oxide/oxygen mixtures may be sufficient with muscle relaxants or may be supplemented by intravenous analgesics or low concentrations of volatile anaesthetics such as halothane (0.5%). Neuroleptic techniques are very suitable for open heart surgery as they cause little upset to ill patients and can be carried on throughout the perfusion. If an inhalation technique is being used, some alternative method, or modification of the anaesthetic will be required during perfusion when the patient's lungs are out of use, as the artificial oxygenator is dependant upon a high oxygen intake, thus preventing the use of nitrous oxide. Halothane in concentrations of 0.5–1% is usually adequate, though the cardiac depressant action must be considered in patients whose myocardium may be severely damaged.

Position. Most open heart operations are carried out with the patient supine: the heart is approached through a mid-line incision with sternal splitting (though a right or left thoracotomy incision may be used). The positions of the arms depend on the siting of intravenous or intra-arterial infusions.

Monitoring of various physiological parameters is necessary during open heart surgery. In addition to the usual intravenous infusion, a cannula is placed in a major vein to measure central venous pressure: this may be introduced into a vein percutaneously at the antecubital fossa and advanced centrally, or by a subclavian or internal jugular vein puncture; or the surgeon, on opening the chest, may introduce a cannula directly into an innominate vein. The arterial pressure of the patient is measured by an arterial cannula introduced percutaneously or by arterial 'cutdown' into the radial, brachial, or femoral artery. This cannula may also be used during operation and in the post-operative period for arterial blood sampling.

Temperature is measured in the pharynx, oesophagus and skin by suitable probes and electric thermometers and, in addition, rectal and muscle temperatures may be used. Electroencephalography may be used to provide an assessment of cerebral function. Heart rhythm is monitored throughout operation on an electrocardiograph, and electrolytes and blood gases are measured at regular intervals during operation and the post-operative period. As patients with heart disease do not tolerate blood loss well, it is important to maintain a normal blood volume. Blood loss is therefore measured by swab weighing, suction loss measurement and colorimetric methods (see page 126). The use of a central venous pressure measurement in conjunction with arterial pressure measurement will give a more accurate picture of the physiological state of the circulation than the blood balance, which is only a guide to the patient's condition.

Prior to cardio-pulmonary by-pass the patient must be heparinized to prevent clotting in the heart-lung machine. Heparin 3 mg/kg (300 iu/kg) body weight is administered and this is repeated in a dosage of 1.5 mg/kg hourly throughout perfusion. During perfusion, anaesthesia is maintained by inhalational agents into the oxygenator or by intravenous agents. Oxygenators, though not as efficient as normal lungs for oxygenation, allow rapid respiratory alkalosis to develop, but this may be overcome by the use of 3–7% CO_2 added to the oxygen. Hypercapnia has been deliberately used to enhance tissue perfusion. At the end of perfusion the action of heparin is reversed with protamine, administered in a dosage of 4–6 mg/kg body weight. The adequacy of this reversal of the heparin may be assessed by heparin-protamine titration tests.

Post-operative care

The post-operative management of open heart cases is seldom straightforward as the clinical picture can change rapidly from many causes. In addition to expert clinical care the availability of biochemical data at short notice can make significant differences to the morbidity and mortality.

Cardiovascular

The maintenance of an adequate cardiac output is the most important single feature of post-operative management. It is not a feature of the cardiovascular system alone but may be dependent on the proper functioning of the respiratory system, good cerebral function and a normal biochemical picture. How cardiac output may be affected is summarized in the following paragraphs.

Poor myocardial function. This may be related to long-standing disease, to operative trauma, or to a temporary biochemical upset. Treatment depends on the cause. Biochemical upsets of an electrolyte or metabolic nature should be treated. Failure of response should lead to the use of cardiac stimulants, usually in the form of intravenous infusions, of which the most commonly used are isoprenaline 4 mg in 500 ml or adrenaline 4 mg in 500 ml. Such drugs are given by infusion in doses as required – usually in drops per minute or by a slow rate infusion pump. Digitalization will commonly have been effected prior to an operation in acquired heart disease, but where no digitalis has been previously given, rapid digitalization may be undertaken.

Hypovolaemia. Blood loss balance and replacement in conjunction with central venous and arterial pressure measurements should not allow hypovolaemia to occur. Some patients will, however, have an improved cardiac action with a higher than normal central venous pressure. In some centres, left atrial pressures are measured in addition to central venous pressures in an attempt to assess the different functions of the right and left sides of the heart.

Dysrhythmias. Cardiac dysrhythmias are a common cause of diminished cardiac output. The dysrhythmias encountered are legion; they may be regular atrial, nodal or ventricular rhythms or irregular rhythms due to atrial fibrillation or multifocal extrasystoles.

Digitalis activity may fluctuate following surgery, particularly in association with biochemical changes. Potassium levels, though apparently normal in the serum, may be very low in the body as a whole, particularly in patients on long term diuretics. Potassium supplements pre-operatively may improve the total body levels, and large amounts may be required post-operatively. Dysrhythmias are commonly associated with changes in potassium levels, and doses of 2–3 mEq are given intravenously, as potassium chloride may abolish ventricular dysrhythmias. Potassium loss in the urine may be heavy after open heart surgery and will be required to be replaced, initially in an intravenous infusion. 6 g of potassium chloride, containing 80 mEq of potassium are added to 500 ml of intravenous fluid and given as required. Doses as high as 20 mEq/h may be required. Patients receiving large doses of potassium should be electrocardiographically monitored throughout. It is such monitoring and a constant watch on serum and urinary potassium levels that allows such apparently large doses of potassium to be given safely.

Other drugs used to combat dysrhythmias are lignocaine, procaine and procaine amide; of these lignocaine is the most satisfactory as it causes the least cardiac depression. It is most effective in combating ventricular dysrhythmias in a dosage of 1 mg per kilogram initially intravenously, followed, if required, by a steady infusion of 1 mg/kg/h. Fast heart rates, particularly of ventricular origin, and extrasystoles may be treated with β-adrenergic blocking drugs. The most acceptable of these at the present time are Practolol or Trasicor.

Hypoxia. This may be caused by several mechanisms (see below) and itself may cause dysrhythmias, affecting cardiac output and causing the development of metabolic acidosis, a potent factor in dysrhythmia production and falling cardiac output. Such a situation can be self perpetuating and requires effective, early treatment.

Cardiac tamponade. Tamponade may develop following open heart surgery, due to inadequate drainage of the pericardial or mediastinal spaces. Arterial pressure falls, the pulse rate and venous pressure rise and peripheral circulation is poor, with resultant metabolic acidosis. Cardiac output falls and the situation becomes a vicious circle. Re-exploration of the wound is the early and effective treatment.

Respiratory system

The patient undergoing open heart surgery is liable to the complications associated with any thoracotomy, namely pulmonary collapse, pneumothorax, haemothorax and pleural effusion. In addition, certain changes occur post-operatively in the lungs following cardio-pulmonary by-pass. These changes are part of the homologous blood syndrome (see above) and consist of multiple small areas of pulmonary infiltration, oedema and consolidation, becoming maximal in about 48 hours and slowly resolving thereafter. Such changes result in areas of lung being perfused with blood, but not being ventilated, thus causing a right to left intrapulmonary shunt which manifests itself as a low arterial oxygen tension with an increasing alveolar-arterial oxygen gradient. Arterial desaturation will be further aggravated by ventilation-perfusion changes similar to those following any cardiac surgery. This aspect of the desaturation can be treated by oxygen therapy but the desaturation resulting from right to left shunting will not respond fully to increasing the oxygen percentage in the inspired gases. Some desaturation must be accepted. Too high an inspiratory concentration of oxygen may itself prove damaging to respiratory function.

After all but the most straightforward open heart surgery, ventilation is commonly maintained by a mechanical respirator. Adequate oxygenation is ensured, the work load of respiration is removed, the patient can be given adequate analgesia in the form of strong narcotics, or a nitrous oxide/oxygen mixture such as Entonox may be used in the ventilator. Initially, ventilation is maintained through an endotracheal tube and if spontaneous respiratory activity is achieved within several days, as is the common pattern, tracheostomy and its attendant problems can be avoided.

Renal problems

Post-operative renal problems are minimal in the presence of a good cardiac output and following a good perfusion. Urinary output following surgery is a very good indication of cardiac function and should be measured hourly, until the cardiovascular state is stabilized. Oliguria may occur temporarily and can be overcome by the intravenous administration of 50 ml of 20% mannitol, though progression to a severe renal failure may occur: treatment of such a patient follows the established lines of acute renal failure.

Cerebral damage

This is more commonly related to embolization than to a generalized cerebral hypoxia: such emboli may be gaseous or particulate in form. Gaseous emboli are likely to arise from air remaining in the heart or major vessels following surgery, while particulate matter may arise from the heart-lung machine, though efficient filters should preclude this. From the site of the surgery blood thrombi or calcium particles from acquired heart valve damage, may occur. Treatment is symptomatic and expectant.

Haemorrhage

Post-operative bleeding may prove an embarrassment in a small proportion of cases. The commonest cause is surgical, thus requiring re-exploration in a proportion of cases. Medical causes, secondary to the perfusion, may be related to falls in the levels of various clotting factors or to the incomplete reversal of heparin. Full haematological co-operation is required to establish a cause. This is commonly not found and the empirical treatment with freshly drawn blood may prove the quickest and most effective treatment. Specific treatment for low fibrinogen levels with fibrinogen infusions, and for the rare complication of fibrinolysis with EACA (Epsiloaminocaproic acid) or Trasylol may be needed.

An intensive care atmosphere and expert surgical, anaesthetic, biochemical and haematological co-operation are essential for the minimal morbidity and mortality in such cases.

Anaesthesia for aortic aneurysm

Aortic aneurysms are commonly a manifestation of generalized vascular disease. Patients requiring surgery may therefore have poor myocardial activity and a diminished circulation to essential organs. Planned surgery for aortic aneurysms is likely to be generally straightforward from the anaesthetic standpoint, though the surgery must be considered of a major type. Aortic aneurysms may present as a sudden emergency, with sufficient leaking into surrounding tissues to make the patient severely shocked. Pre-operative preparation will be minimal and anaesthesia undertaken without a full medical history. Such patients may be normally hypertensive, and on hypotensive drugs. Digitalization may be present and the patient's fluid balance may have been disturbed by regular diurectic therapy.

Pre-operative. Where possible, a full blood and biochemical profile will have been obtained, an ECG taken and full aortography will have delineated the site and extent of the lesion. The commonest site for degenerative aneurysms is distal to the renal arteries and, in such cases, clamping of the aorta below the renal arteries will not impair the function of any major organs.

If the aneurysm is sited elsewhere a more complex situation exists as major organs will not tolerate the period of lack of circulation during aortic occlusion. In such cases, the viability of such organs as the liver and kidneys must be protected by hypothermia to levels of 30°C, or by the use of a temporary by-pass from above the lesion to below it. Such a by-pass may take the form of a woven graft sewn in above and below, or the transfer of arterial blood from the left atrium, through plastic tubing and a pump to the vascular tree distal to the aneurysm, commonly into the femoral artery – the so-called left atrio-femoral by-pass. Complex lesions involving aortic arch vessels and the ascending aorta may require cardio-pulmonary by-pass and deep levels of hypothermia. The mortality from such surgery is high.

Operative management. Straightforward anaesthetic techniques, with controlled respiration, are usually applicable, though care at induction with the shocked unprepared patient is necessary. Efforts to improve the general status of the patient may prove ineffective prior to surgery; indeed blood and fluid loss during, and prior to, surgery may be large. Assessments of the cardiovascular state should be made throughout the operation by the measurement of arterial and venous pressures, assessment of blood loss and monitoring of the ECG and body temperature.

Large blood transfusions may be necessary over a short period of time, so all fluids should be warmed to 35°–37°C prior to infusion to maintain a normal body temperature, thus preventing myocardial failure. 10 ml of 10% calcium chloride should also be given with each litre of transfused blood, to offset the low calcium level caused by the citrate anticoagulant. Large volumes of citrated blood, unless fresh, will be very acid and a regular assessment of the metabolic state by blood gas analysis can be helpful throughout the operation. Where metabolic acidosis is present, particularly in shocked cases, sodium bicarbonate should be infused in sufficient quantities to maintain a normal bicarbonate level in the blood.

Cross clamping of the aorta will result in a deficient blood supply to the distal arterial tree. Oxygenation and metabolism will therefore both be impaired and acidosis will develop. The release of aortic clamps, following repair of an aneurysm, may allow quantities of acid metabolites to be washed into the venous system and these may adversely affect cardiac function with dysrhythmias and hypotension. Slow release of clamps, with the resulting slower release of metabolites, may prevent such dangers to the myocardial function. Hypotension can be minimized by attention to blood balance throughout surgery, and by the prophylactic administration of sodium bicarbonate prior to the release of the aortic clamps.

Post-operative management is simplified in an intensive care atmosphere. Ileus is commonly present, the fluid balance may be upset and renal function impaired. Also, the age group of patients with degenerative lesions will be high, and ventilatory support following such a major procedure may be considered valuable for a short period, post-operatively. The use of infusion of intravenous alcohol (10% in 5% dextrose) and the use of low molecular weight dextran, may be beneficial, both if peripheral circulation is impaired and as a good sedative.

Anaesthesia for carotid endartercectomy

Patients with carotid artery stenosis may have an impaired cerebral circulation, though unilateral disease, with normal anastomoses in the Circle of Willis, will cause little fall in cerebral blood flow to the affected side. Obstruction to a major vessel will not result in a significant fall in flow until the obstruction is 80% complete (Brice *et al.*, 1964).

Patients with carotid artery disease commonly have bilateral disease, with a history of systemic hypertension and other evidence of cardio-vascular disease. Anaesthesia for such patients must be planned to prevent any fall in cerebral blood flow, or hypotension, and to ensure adequate oxygenation throughout. Premedication will be generally light and the induction of anaesthesia will be by small doses of intravenous agents. The site of the surgery makes endotracheal intubation mandatory, the intubation being accomplished with the aid of a short acting depolarizing relaxant such as suxemethonium chloride, or a longer acting non-depolarizing relaxant if ventilation is to be controlled throughout the procedure. D-tubocurarine has some ganglion blocking activity and may cause hypotension, consequently pancuronium or gallamine could be a wiser choice. Maintenance of anaesthesia can be by inhalation agents, if hypotension does not occur, as the mild hypercarbia associated with inhalation techniques may prove beneficial to cerebral blood flow. The use of controlled respiration with nitrous oxide/oxygen mixtures is satisfactory so long as hypocarbia is not pronounced. In unilateral disease, however, a 'cerebral-steal' syndrome may result from hyperventilation, resulting in cerebral vasoconstriction on the normal side of the brain and thus an increased blood flow to the affected side. Neuroleptic techniques are also satisfactory for such cases.

In total obstruction of the carotid artery, the vessel can be clamped above and below the lesion without any further impairment of blood supply, but, if the obstruction is incomplete and particularly if disease is bilateral, the surgical and anaesthetic management may be more complex. The brain must be protected from hypoxia by the insertion of a temporary by-pass from below to above the lesion whilst the vessel is clamped; or alternatively the metabolic requirements of the brain must be lowered whilst the vessel is clamped. Oxygen requirements are lowered by hypothermia, and by surface cooling the patient to 30°C (pharyngeal temperature) sufficient protection to allow up to ten minutes clamping of the carotid artery will be available. However, surface hypothermia would appear to be a more complex and time-consuming procedure than the use of a temporary by-pass shunt.

Carotid artery surgery is carried out successfully in the absence of either hypothermia or shunts, an overall brain circulation being dependant on the anastomoses produced by the Circle of Willis. The benefits of hypocapnia or hypercapnia for such procedures have been advocated to improve the blood supply to the affected region.

As clamping of major arteries, particularly in the presence of generalized disease, may predispose to clot formation, an intravenous injection of 1–1.5 mg heparin per kilogram bodyweight may be given, prior to clamping the artery. Blood loss is usually minimal and complications are few, if hypotension is avoided. Early ambulation, if cerebral function allows, should be encouraged.

Anaesthesia for cardiovascular investigations

It is customary for a large proportion of these investigations to be carried out in the X-ray department, and the advent of image intensifiers and television monitoring has removed to some extent the dangers of working in darkness. In some centres general anaesthesia is commonly used, while in other units, only in selected cases undergoing heart catheterization. Certain vascular investigations, such as trans-lumbar aortogram, will be carried out in uncomfortable positions, e.g. prone, so general anaesthesia is employed for such cases. The presence of an anaesthetist is not always requested for such procedures, but the necessary equipment must be ready. The anaesthetist may be called upon at a moment's notice to deal with a crisis, emotional or cardiovascular, therefore the anaesthetic and resuscitation equipment must be in good condition and readily available. Unless the X-ray department has its own anaesthetic technician it is easy for maintenance of the machines to be overlooked.

The majority of cardiac catheterizations are carried out under sedation with local infiltration or nerve blocks of the area where the catheter is to be introduced, usually the saphenous or brachiocephalic veins. The drugs used for sedation are many, from Omnopon or morphine to chloral, barbiturates, diazepam or neuroleptic technique. In the poor risk patient, particularly with a fixed cardiac output, the actions of strong narcotics may be greater than expected : caution is required in prescribing for such patients.

Where general anaesthesia is required, it should be the object of the anaesthetist to maintain a steady state in the patient's cardiovascular and respiratory activity. Pressure and flow measurements and oxygen studies on samples from all heart chambers may take a long time. It is impossible with drugs and techniques presently available, to achieve such a steady state in comparison with the patient's usual pre-operative state, so the results from cardiac catheterization and cardio-angiography must be assessed in this light. For instance, neuroleptanaesthesia and diazepam usage may result in falls in the pulmonary vascular pressures.

General anaesthetic techniques of all kinds have been described for cardiovascular investigations. Oxygen percentages in the inspired atmosphere, the choice of main anaesthetic agent, the question of intubation, the question of spontaneous or controlled ventilation – these have all been discussed: the patient's physiological state must influence the choice of drugs and the technique used. Careful intravenous induction in adults, and induction by volatile agents in infants and children, followed by a technique allowing adequate oxygenation and minimal cardiovascular depression, will be satisfactory. A light level of anaesthesia is all that is required.

During anaesthesia for cardiovascular investigations certain parameters should be regularly observed. A continuous electrocardiograph should be available and the pulse rate, blood pressure and respiration monitored. The investigations may supply much of the information and also the blood specimens must be readily available to allow a check to be kept on the patient's blood gases, and the metabolic state. In infants and children the patient's temperature should be monitored and any fall prevented by using water blankets, electric blankets or radiant heat. Though blood loss in adults is not significant, it may be so in infants with small total blood volumes; consequently cross matched blood should be available for such cases. As catheters must be kept patent, care should be taken that an excess of fluid is not used for this purpose, with the danger of overloading the circulation.

The hyperosmolar solutions used for cardioangiography may be distressing to the patient, causing hot flushing, chest pain, coughing or apnoea, and in some centres, general anaesthesia will be used for angiography, while sedation is used for cardiac catheterization. The hyperosmolarity of contrast media can attract sufficient quantities of extravascular fluid into the circulation to cause pulmonary oedema, with resulting hypoxia and cardiac embarrassment.

Major complications of cardiac catheterization and cardio-angiography amount to about 4% each and mortality to about 1 in 200 cases. Since the cardiovascular state may be poor, care must be taken with drugs, as those used in the medical treatment of heart conditions may predispose to problems for the unwary, viz: β-adrenergic blockers may have a greater effect under anaesthesia. The safe dosage of local anaesthetics must be strictly adhered to, e.g. lignocaine 3 mg/kg, should not be exceeded: this is most likely to happen in infants, weighing only several kilograms.

Many failures under sedation may be associated with an inadequate description of the nature of the investigation and the equipment in the X-ray room pre-operatively: even the noise occurring during the taking of multiple picture angiographs can be very frightening to the unprepared.

Coronary angiography

Investigations are carried out under light general anaesthesia, following the lines above. Modern catheterization techniques, allowing selective catheterization of the coronary vessels and the use of high speed cine-radiography, means that the heart does not have to be slowed by a Valsalva manoeuvre or by the intravenous or intra-aortic injection (via the catheter) of acetylcholine or neostigmine. Coronary circulation may be very poor in these cases so that serious dysrhythmias may commonly occur : full resuscitation equipment must always be available.

Translumbar aortography

With the patient prone and the needle introduced into the abdominal aorta through the back, general anaesthesia is the common practice. Endotracheal intubation with controlled ventilation overcomes the problems associated with the prone position, as supports to allow free abdominal movements are inadmissible for good quality films to be obtained.

Cerebral angiography

Such patients may be cerebrally disorientated and have serious brain disease. Carotid artery puncture is carried out under local or general anaesthesia, whilst vertebral angiography is achieved with general anaesthesia. This should be simple, of a light plane, but deep enough to prevent coughing and straining; hypotension should be avoided and the airway ensured by the insertion of an armoured endotracheal tube. As the head may be moved considerably during these procedures there is a risk of a disturbance of the airway, possibly leading to raised intracranial pressure. Hypocarbia, associated with controlled respiration, may assist in the production of good X-ray films.

Cardiac arrest

In any case of unexpected sudden death, resuscitation in the form of cardiac massage and ventilatory support should be immediately carried out. The value of such measures is without question, though time is the essential factor, as only three minutes is available from the time of arrest until an adequate circulation must be restored if irreparable cerebral damage is to be avoided. Any person in immediate contact with the patient must be capable of rendering the basic treatment whilst more definitive aid is being sought. All medical, nursing and other persons should be conversant with the details of external cardiac massage and artificial ventilation, in the form of mouth to mouth respiration.

Ventilatory support. External cardiac massage does not provide adequate alveolar ventilation. In the absence of mechanical aids to ventilation in the form of airways, intubation equipment or self-inflating bags, ventilation by mouth-to-mouth, or mouth-to-nose methods must be initiated. Ideally, the patient should be ventilated with an oxygen-enriched atmosphere, though expired air, containing 15–16% oxygen, will ensure adequate oxygenation of the patient's blood if alveolar ventilation is adequate.

Mouth-to-mouth ventilation depends for its success on the intermittent inflation of the patient's lungs by the resuscitator's positive pressure exhalation. A clear airway is essential. Any debris within the mouth and pharynx should be removed. The neck is then flexed by a hand behind the neck and the head extended, thus further improving the airway. The nose is closed by the free hand and the resuscitator's mouth is applied to the patient's open mouth and the patient's lungs expanded by the resuscitator's expired breath. Passive expiration of the patient's lung occurs when the resuscitator's mouth is removed for inspiration to occur and the next cycle to start. This sequel is repeated 12–15 times per minute and should be synchronized with external cardiac massage if this is being undertaken. As an alternative, the patient's mouth may be closed throughout the procedure, the patient's nose being used as the upper airway. Such form of ventilation can prove adequate for long periods, though a method of manually ventilating the patient's lungs by self-inflating bag and face mask or a Water's circuit (see page 23) should be available in all wards, and all staff should be practised in its use. Once ventilatory support is established it must be maintained, until resuscitation is abandoned, or until spontaneous ventilation is adequate. After successful resuscitation, ventilatory support, in the form of intermittent positive pressure ventilation with a mechanical lung ventilator, may be maintained for prolonged periods.

External cardiac massage. No special equipment is required, so that an effective circulation may be established as soon as the diagnosis of cardiac arrest has been established. Closed chest cardiac massage is as effective in the presence of ventricular fibrillation as it is in cardiac asystole.

The principle of external cardiac massage is the maintenance of a cardiac output by the rhythmical compression and relaxation of the heart by the displacement of the sternum towards the back-bone. The patient is placed in the supine position on a hard surface, and the operator kneels at the side of the patient, facing the head. The heel of one hand is placed over the lower half or third of the sternum and the other hand placed on top: the sternum is displaced towards the patient's spine by about 1–1½ inches, thus compressing the heart beneath, then the pressure on the sternum is released and the process repeated sixty to eighty times per minute. Effective massage is tiring and a second operator's assistance should be available. The cardiac masseur and the mouth-to-mouth respiration administrator can usefully change places as necessary. In children the force required to achieve a satisfactory circulation will be less than in adults and in infants massage can be easily accomplished with one hand on the back and one over the sternum. The position of the palm or heel of the hand must be correct or there is a distinct danger of causing major damage to the rib cage or to the soft organs beneath, such as the liver. Though peripheral circulation may be poor, the output from cardiac massage satisfies the demands of highly susceptible tissue, such as the brain and major organs.

The criteria of successful resuscitation are a conscious patient, spontaneous respiration and a stable circulation. Such criteria may not be reached for some time and, after the initial phases of resuscitation, a more prolonged regime may be required to overcome some degree of cerebral damage or to achieve a stable circulation. Pupillary signs are unreliable, but fixed dilated pupils for longer than fifteen minutes with deep unconsciousness, absent spontaneous ventilation and a circulation requiring full support are poor prognostic signs.

Drug therapy. Once the first phase of resuscitation has been established, specific drug therapy will be required and an intravenous infusion must be established to effect this. Some drugs, such as adrenaline or calcium chloride, may be given by intracardiac injection in the initial phases (see Table 6.5).

Table 6.5 *Resuscitation drugs*

Drug	*Container*	*Concentration*	*Dose*	*Remarks*
Myocardial stimulants:				
adrenaline	1 ml ampoule	1 in 1000	2–5 ml of 1 in 10 000	Always given i.v. or intracardiac in emergencies May also be used as an i.v. infusion 2–5 ampoules of 1 in 1000 in 500 ml
calcium chloride	10 ml ampoule	10% or 20%	5–10 ml (0·5–1 g)	
calcium gluconate	10 ml ampoule	10%	5–10 ml (0·5–1 g)	

Drug	*Container*	*Concentration*	*Dose*	*Remarks*
isoprenaline (Suscardia)	ampoules	2 mg in 2 ml	0·5 ml of 1 in 20 000	Used similarly to adrenaline Suscardia used for i.v. infusions 1–2 ampoules in 500 ml dextrose
Dysrhythmia control:				
digoxin (Lanoxin)	2 ml ampoule	0·5 mg in 2 ml	ml (0·25 mg)	Dose may be doubled or repeated to achieve digitalization
lanatoside C (Cedilanid)	2 ml ampoule	0·4 mg in 2 ml	0·2–0·4 mg i.v.	
lignocaine (Xylocaine)	500 ml flask 10 ml ampoule 2 ml. ampoule	0·1% 1% 2%	50 mg i.v. followed by i.v. infusion of 1 mg/kg/h	Can be strengthened for slower drip rate
procaine amide (Pronestyl)	10 ml ampoule	10%	25–100 mg/min i.v. maximum 600 mg	Lignocaine causes less myocardial depression
practolol (Eraldin)	5 ml ampoule	0·2%	2 mg repeated at 2 minute intervals to a maximum of 10 mg	
Muscle relaxants:				
pancuronium bromide (Pavulon)	2 ml ampoule	0·2%	2–4 ml (4–8 mg)	Duration of action 45 min. Minimal effect on systemic blood pressure as compared with *d*-tubocurarine
suxamethonium chloride (Anectine)	2 ml ampoule	5%	1 ml (50 mg)	Action lasts 3–5 min
	(may be used to control convulsions):			
Anticonvulsants:				
diazepam (Valium)	2 ml ampoule	0·5%	2–4 ml (10–20 mg)	
thiopentone sodium (Pentothal)	0·5 g ampoules and 20 ml ampoule of water	made up to 2·5% solution	4–20 ml (100–500 mg)	
Dehydrating agents:				
frusemide (Lasix)	2 ml ampoule	1%	2–4 ml (20–40 mg)	
mannitol	500 ml flasks	20%	1–1·5 g/kg	

Drug	*Container*	*Concentration*	*Dose*	*Remarks*
Metabolic acidosis treatment:				
sodium bicarbonate	500 ml flask 100 ml bottle	4·2%, 5% or 8·4%	50–200 mEq (1 ml of 8·4% contains 1 mEq)	Higher concentrations involve less fluid load. Dose may be increased or supplemented if bicarbonate level low on estimation
trisaminol (Tham)	25 ml	0·3 M 3·66%	500 mg/kg	In not less than 1h

Condition	*Drug*	*Container*	*Concentration*	*Dose*
Miscellaneous conditions:				
adrenal cortical hypofunction	hydrocortisone sodium succinate*	100 mg ampoule and 2 ml water	5%	(2–4 ml) 100–200 mg
allergic reactions	chlorpheniramine maleate (Piriton)	1 ml ampoule	1%	(0·5–1 ml) 5–10 mg†
bradycardia‡	atropine sulphate	1 ml ampoule	0·06%	(1 ml) 0·6 mg
bronchospasm	aminophylline	10 ml ampoule	2·5%	(10–20 ml) 250–500 mg
cerebral depression	nikethamide (Coramine)	2 ml ampoule	25%	(2–4 ml) 0·5–1 g
cerebral oedema	fructose	500 ml	10 or 20%	90 g i.v.
coronary ischaemia	amyl nitrate	0·2 ml vitrellae		0·2 ml inhaled
hypoglycaemia	glucose	50 ml ampoule	50%	20–50 ml (40–100 g)**
hypotension	methylamphetamine	1·5 ml ampoules	30 mg/1·5 ml	15–30 mg i.v.
	noradrenaline (Levophed)	2 and 4 ml ampoules	1 mg/1 ml	2 ml diluted in 500 ml
		2 ml ampoule	0·1 mg/ml	1–2 ml intracardiac
opiate overdosage	levallorphan (Lorfan)	1 ml ampoule	0·1%	1–2 ml (1–2 mg)
opiate overdosage	nalorphine (Lethidrone)	1 ml ampoule	10 mg/1 ml	5–10 mg i.v.

* Large doses of 0·5–1 g may be used for cerebral oedema.
† May be given as an infusion 10 mg in 500 ml.
‡ Bradycardia may be a warning of severe myocardial depression or hypoxia.
** Dosage dictated by patient response.

Correction of metabolic acidosis: myocardial contractility is greatly reduced in the presence of metabolic acidosis. Immediate correction of this is vital, for it will render attempts at electrical defibrillation and the action of adrenaline to improve myocardial tone ineffective.

Metabolic acidosis is treated by the administration of sodium bicarbonate intravenously or, less commonly, THAM. The amount of bicarbonate to be given can be roughly assessed from the patient's weight and the duration of arrest: in an adult this would amount to approximately 50–70 mEq per minute of arrest or 1 mEq/kg/min. A more accurate measurement can be obtained from an analysis of arterial blood for bicarbonate content, though the time factor for such analysis should not detract from starting bicarbonate infusions. An 8.4% solution of sodium bicarbonate contains 1 mEq per ml while a 5% solution contains 12 mEq in 20 ml.

Myocardial contractility: cardiac arrest, of any duration, is associated with poor myocardial tone, either in the asystolic or the fibrillating state. Evidence of poor myocardial activity will be seen by a failure to respond to external massage following adequate bicarbonate infusions or by failure to defibrillate. With the chest open the myocardial tone can be felt on massage. Adrenaline or calcium chloride are the drugs commonly used either by intracardiac injection or into a free flowing intravenous infusion to improve tone:

calcium chloride: 5–10 ml of 10% calcium chloride or calcium gluconate

adrenaline: 2–5 ml of a 1 in 10 000 solution, obtained from the standard 1 in 1000 ampoule diluted from 1 ml to 10 ml

These doses may be repeated if no response is obtained or if the response is short-lived

isoprenaline: 0.5–2 ml of a 1 in 20 000 solution may be used in preference to adrenaline. Less peripheral vasoconstriction will occur, but isoprenaline may not be so freely available as adrenaline, unless standard drug sets are prepared for resuscitation trolleys

Other drugs should also be available for the treatment of specific conditions. Dysrhythmias may be treated with procaine or lignocaine, digoxin and β-adrenergic blockers, such as practolol (see Table 6.5); muscle relaxants and anticonvulsants are used for control of convulsions.

Defibrillation. Once external massage and effective alveolar ventilation have been established, the exact nature of the cardiac rhythm should be ascertained by electrocardiographic monitoring. No delay in its procurement should prejudice the patient's recovery if massage is already adequate. In the presence of ventricular fibrillation, or less commonly ventricular tachycardia, artificial defibrillation should be attempted. The electrical impulse can be supplied by an a.c. (alternating current) or a d.c. (direct current) apparatus.

An a.c. defibrillator will supply a current for 0.1 or 0.2 s at a voltage of 50–900 V. A range of 50–300 V is available for internal defibrillation, with the electrodes applied directly to the heart surface and 300–900 V for external defibrillation, with electrodes applied to the chest wall. Larger voltages are required for external defibrillation, due to the added resistance of the chest wall.

A d.c. fibrillator is more effective than an a.c. defibrillator, since the electrical energy being discharged is 25–400 watt seconds or joules. As in the a.c. defibrillator, lower ranges are for internal use and higher ranges for external; the design of the equipment incorporates safety switches, preventing the wrong range of electrical energy to be used at any time.

Method of defibrillation: adhere strictly to instructions given with each defibrillator. Ideally, two people should be holding the electrodes by the insulated handles and they should be insulated from earth. There must be no direct contact between the patient and any person during the defibrillating shock. A setting is selected on the apparatus for voltage (or for joules) depending on the size of the patient, and one discharge shock given. If defibrillation does not occur, the discharge should be repeated or increased in strength.

Attention must be paid to the metabolic state. The use of β-adrenergic blockers may be valuable where fibrillation does not respond to repeated efforts at defibrillation. In the presence of asystole, or bradycardia, the use of artificial pacing of the heart should be considered. This may be by an internal electrode, commonly introduced into the right side of the heart from a large peripheral vein such as the antebrachial vein, or by an external electrode on the chest wall.

Summary of management of cardiac arrest

Cardiac arrest: immediate treatment

Diagnosis

(a) Absent pulse in major artery (carotid or femoral)
(b) Pallor; may be cyanosis

You have only THREE minutes – note the time

Treatment

1. Raise the legs
2. Thump the precordium with fist – if no response in five seconds –
3. External cardiac massage
4. Clear the airway and institute mouth-to-mouth ventilation
5. Send someone else for: (a) assistance; (b) resuscitation equipment

External cardiac massage

1. Lay the patient on firm surface (floor) or insert large board between mattress and springs of the bed
2. Compress lower third of sternum with both hands, one on top of the other
   (a) sternum should move 3–4 cm
   (b) 60 compressions per minute
3. Concurrent artificial ventilation – timed so that compression and inflation do not coincide. If only one person is present both can be done by one person – at eight heart beats to one breath
4. Check the response of
   (a) palpable pulse
   (b) constricting pupils
   (c) capillary filling
5. Inject sodium bicarbonate – 1 mEq/kg body wt/min of cardiac arrest into a major vein or by intracardiac injection.
6. Establish intravenous infusion. If response is satisfactory, continue treatment until resuscitation trolley arrives, or more sophisticated aid arrives.

   If no satisfactory response, review the technique or proceed to internal cardiac massage.

Internal cardiac massage

1. Positive pressure ventilation is necessary
2. Incise 4th to 6th intercostal space from one inch lateral to border of sternum, extending well into axilla on the left side
3. Separate ribs forcibly
4. Place one hand beneath the heart and compress heart between hand and sternum
5. If no immediate response, incise the pericardium anterior to phrenic nerve, then compress heart between the palmar surfaces of the *bases* of the fingers (*not* with the tips of fingers)

   Compress heart 60 times per minute.

Proceed as for:

(a) drugs for asystole

or

(b) internal defibrillation

Restoration of the heart beat

Connect patient to ECG oscilloscope

Diagnose

1. Cardiac asystole
2. Ventricular fibrillation. Coarse/fine

If asystole or fine fibrillation:

1. Calcium chloride 10 ml of 10% solution.
2. Adrenaline 1/10 000 solution 2–5 ml
   (these drugs improve cardiac tone, and convert 'fine' fibrillation to 'coarse')

Treatment

Metabolic acidosis – repeat treatment with $NaHCO_3$ as necessary (see page 182).

Cerebral oedema – 20% mannitol (1.5 g/kg body wt.). Large doses of steroids may be used and hyperventilation may be instituted. After the use of dehydrating agents, urinary catheterization should be carried out.

Hypotension: methylamphetamine up to 30 mg i.v.
adrenaline 2–4 mg/500 ml
isoprenaline 2–4 mg/500 ml } as an infusion
noradrenaline 2 mg/500 ml

If ventricular fibrillation, convert 'fine' fibrillation into 'coarse' and then proceed to defibrillate.

Defibrillation

External defibrillation

1. Produce 'coarse' fibrillation by the administration of calcium chloride
2. Wear rubber gloves if available
3. Each electrode should be held by a separate person
4. Cover electrodes with electrode jelly or soak pads in saline solution
5. Apply at base and apex of heart
6. Apply 100–400 joule (d.c.) or 300–900 V (a.c.) for maximum of 0.2 s; increase if necessary *or* give multiple shocks, with a.c. defibrillator
7. Continue pulmonary ventilation

Internal defibrillation

1. Produce 'coarse' fibrillation
2. Wear rubber gloves if available
3. Hold electrodes as above
4. Soak gauze-covered electrodes in normal saline or Ringer's solution
5. Place one electrode underneath, and one on top of the heart
6. Apply 150–300 V for 0.1 s (a.c.) or 30–100 joule (d.c.)
7. Continue cardiac massage and pulmonary ventilation, as necessary

Respiratory arrest

Expired air resuscitation

1. Clear airway by swabbing or suction
2. Keep head tilted back
3. Check, visually, that chest inflates with each breath

Mouth-to-mouth ventilation

Hold patient's chin well up, head tilted well back, pinch the recipient's nostrils with the free hand. Take a big breath and breathe into the patient's mouth. After chest has risen remove your mouth to let patient's lungs deflate. Repeat every four seconds.

Mouth-to-nose ventilation

As an alternative method the resuscitator may apply his mouth to the patient's nose during inspiration if the nasal airway is patent, holding the jaw forward and the mouth closed.

Mouth-to-airway ventilation

Place one end of the airway in patient's mouth over the tongue, close mouth, tilt head back, pinch nostrils, then breathe down airway. When patient's chest rises take your mouth off the airway and let the patient's lungs deflate.

Manual ventilation with bag and mask

Tilt patient's head well back, apply mask tightly to patient's face, hold chin well up and squeeze the rubber bag. When chest rises on inflation, release hold on bag to allow patient to breathe out, then repeat process every four seconds.

Intubation

With an endotracheal tube and intermittent positive pressure, ventilation can be established as equipment becomes available.

In any established hospital, some form of resuscitation policy should exist. The location and extent of the equipment will, of course, depend on the type of hospital and the extent of its use. In an acute general hospital, resuscitation should depend on first line resuscitation at ward level and second line aid by more sophisticated, expensive equipment and expert staff, shared by the hospital or unit as a whole.

Emergency treatment ward equipment

Every ward should have:

Mouth to mouth airway
Laryngoscope

Endotracheal tubes and connectors
A method of manual ventilation, e.g. Ambu Bag (or Water's circuit if an oxygen supply is immediately available)
Oxygen.

Each hospital should have at least one emergency trolley containing the following items:

Laryngoscopes
Endotracheal tubes and connectors
Manual ventilation apparatus
Oxygen
Bronchoscopes
Electrocardioscope with leads
Internal/external defibrillator with leads:
  modern equipment is battery operated and can be used anywhere
Pacemaker
Suction equipment
Tracheostomy set
Thoracotomy set
Full range of syringes and suction catheters
Transfusion sets and intravenous fluids including sodium bicarbonate, mannitol,
  5% dextrose, 0.9% saline
Suitable selection of extension leads and electrical adaptors
Comprehensive collections of drugs must be available as such a trolley may be required outside the ward atmosphere where many resuscitation drugs will be available routinely

7 *The Respiratory System*

Among the factors which must be considered by the anaesthetist are the uptake of oxygen and the elimination of carbon dioxide.

An adequate inspired concentration of oxygen is essential. This should be at least 30% and approaching 50% in subjects with respiratory, cardiac or oligaemic conditions. Inadequate concentrations of oxygen in the inspired mixture may arise because of lack of vigilance on the part of the anaesthetist, leading to failure of the oxygen supply. Warning systems have been devised to minimize this risk but most are not wholly reliable. Cyanosis should at all times be avoided and, indeed, never be relied upon to warn the anaesthetist of oxygen lack. The patient may be anaemic, in which case he may have insufficient haemoglobin to allow cyanosis to take place (at least 5 g per 100 ml of blood must be present before this becomes apparent): in the second place the warning will come too late; thirdly, clinical recognition of cyanosis is open to many variables, such as colour blindness, artificial lighting, and skin and mucous membrane blood flow.

Alveolar ventilation must be adequate to permit interchange of oxygen and carbon dioxide. The following relationships are basic to the understanding of the mechanisms involved:

$$\text{alveolar ventilation (ml/min)} = (\text{tidal volume (ml)} - \text{dead space (ml)}) \times \text{breathing frequency}$$

$$\text{alveolar ventilation (ml/min)} \propto \frac{\text{carbon dioxide production (ml/min)}}{\text{arterial carbon dioxide tension mmHg}}$$

$$\text{minute volume (ml/min)} = \text{tidal volume (ml)} \times \text{breathing frequency/min}$$

It will be appreciated that if there is a reduction in tidal volume arising from tachypnoea, (trichloroethylene and halothane), central respiratory depression and/or peripheral neuromuscular blockade, alveolar ventilation will tend to fall, with consequent carbon dioxide accumulation within the body. However, when breathing 21% oxygen, the alveolar ventilation will need to fall from approximately 5 l/min to 2.5 l/min to produce a significant fall in oxygen saturation of the blood. This effect tends to be masked if higher concentrations of oxygen are employed.

The dead space can be considered to be made up of three components: apparatus, anatomical and alveolar. The sum of all three has been defined as the 'functional dead space' whereas the sum of anatomical and alveolar dead space is what is known as the 'physiological dead space'.

Apparatus dead space should be kept to the minimum. The anatomical dead space is increased by bronchodilators, e.g. diethyl ether, halothane, etc., and is reduced by approximately half by endotracheal intubation. In old age and chest disease, in association with general anaesthesia, increased tidal volumes, hypothermia, hypotension and oligaemic states, some of the gas entering the alveoli either does not participate in gaseous exchange or is in excess of that required to 'arterialize' the blood. This gas is termed 'alveolar dead space'. During general anaesthesia the physiological dead space/tidal volume ratio is of the order of 0.3 in the normal patient with healthy lungs. In other words 30% of each breath is wasted.

It must be appreciated that under certain circumstances blood bathes underventilated parts of the lung, which can give rise to hypoxaemia. Such venous admixture, arising from underventilation in relation to perfusion, can usually be corrected by the administration of oxygen concentrations in excess of 30%. Further, hypoxaemia can arise by blood completely by-passing the lungs – a condition often found in congenital heart disease, bronchial obstruction, and alveolar collapse. If there is an imbalance between the amount of oxygen reaching the tissues and that being extracted, the effect of these 'shunts' is to aggravate hypoxaemia. Such a situation is likely to arise with a fall of cardiac output, anaemia, and excessive extraction of oxygen at the periphery, e.g. post-operative shivering. It is important to maintain stores of oxygen in the body as near to capacity as possible. Breathing 21% oxygen, these stores amount to approximately 1.5 litres, 50–60% of which are in combination with haemoglobin. One way to increase these stores is to wash out pulmonary nitrogen by administering 100% oxygen – the extra store being largely in the lung. Because of the shape of the oxygen dissociation curve for haemoglobin, no further oxygen can be added to the haemoglobin unless it is previously desaturated. By maintaining body oxygen stores as near to the normal as possible, some reserve of oxygen is offered to the patient, should momentary respiratory depression or obstruction occur. If mixtures of oxygen below 30% are offered to subjects under anaesthesia, this reserve diminishes and severe hypoxia may quickly arise. Cyanosis must never be allowed to occur as it represents approximately 75% saturation with an oxygen tension of about 50 mmHg: grave oxygen deficit can quickly arise in this situation. Progressive falls in oxygen tension have been reported during anaesthesia, and it is possible that the collapse of smaller air passages and alveoli may occur during the course of an anaesthetic, particularly in subjects with lung disease. The absence of the normal 'sigh' mechanism may partly account for this phenomenon, so the periodic hyperinflation of the lung, a mechanical sighing device, or ventilation with greater than normal tidal volumes with an added apparatus dead space may improve arterial oxygenation, by opening up collapsed air passages. (The added dead space is to counter the lowering of the carbon dioxide tension resulting from large tidal volumes.)

Under general anaesthesia, carbon dioxide production is diminished by about 15%. There is, however, an increase in dead space which tends to counter the expected fall in arterial carbon dioxide tension. The amount of alveolar ventilation necessary to maintain normal arterial carbon dioxide tension should, where possible, be estimated by either using the Radford nomogram or the Nunn blood/gas predictor. Such prediction depends upon the knowledge of the patient's weight and sex, correction being made for reduction of dead space by endotracheal intubation. Measurement of ventilatory volumes is full of inaccuracies, but the Wright anemometer, or Drager volume meter are adequate for clinical purposes. Clearly the only accurate way of estimating the efficiency of alveolar ventilation is to monitor either alveolar carbon dioxide concentration, or to measure the arterial carbon dioxide tension. At the moment, these methods of measurement are outside the bounds of normal clinical practice, and prediction, as outlined above, is satisfactory for routine purposes.

Tissue oxygenation

It is important for the anaesthetist to bear in mind constantly the factors responsible for the transport of oxygen from the lungs to the tissues which are given in Table 7.1.

Table 7.1 *Factors in transport of oxygen from lungs to tissue (normal resting values)*

available oxygen (ml/min)		cardiac output (ml/min)		haemoglobin concentration (g/100 ml)		oxygen saturation (%)		1·34 (mlO_2/gHb)
1000	=	5000	×	15	×	95/100	×	1·34

The normal demands for oxygen by the body, in the conscious resting state, amount to approximately 300 ml/min, in the fit adult male. A reduction by $\frac{1}{3}$ in each of cardiac output, haemoglobin and oxygen saturation may bring the patient perilously near to gross oxygen deprivation, but it is well to realize that such reductions individually can pass unnoticed, particularly in association with blood loss.

Pulmonary evaluation of surgical patients

Apart from being called upon to help in the management of a case of respiratory disorder requiring supportive therapy, such as artificial ventilation, the anaesthetist may require to administer anaesthesia in patients suffering from respiratory disease concurrent with an unrelated condition requiring surgery.

He should direct his attention to any evidence, which suggests that disease has given, or is giving, symptoms and signs of respiratory decompensation. Evidence of breathlessness is of particular value. Cyanosis may or may not be present; certainly it should not be relied upon in the assessment of the patient. The presence or absence of sputum is of importance, as this will influence the management of the patient under general anaesthesia and also the post-operative recovery and convalescence.

The common cold may not infrequently be found at the pre-operative assessment. It must be remembered that coryza sometimes precedes a much more serious illness. Antibiotic cover should be considered. As a general rule, if the patient will not suffer by postponing the operation, it is in his best interests to do so. When the operation cannot be postponed, conduction anaesthesia should be employed wherever possible.

A few tests of pulmonary function can be helpful to the surgeon and anaesthetist in the selection of patients for operation, and may indicate the need for pre-operative and post-operative measures. The following are of value:

peak expiratory flow rate (PEFR).
forced expiratory volume per unit time ($FEV_{1\cdot0}$)
rebreathing method for the determination of carbon dioxide tension
single breath nitrogen washout

Peak expiratory flow rate: this measurement may be carried out in a number of ways. The Wright peak flow meter is often used and is very handy at the bedside as it is readily portable: the peak expiratory flow rate correlates closely with the forced expiratory volume in one second ($FEV_{1\cdot0}$). (See below).

The Snider match test. This most useful test can be applied at the bedside without having to use complicated or cumbersome equipment. The patient is asked to extinguish a lighted match held at a distance of three inches (7.5 cm) from the widely opened mouth. This test correlates well with the maximum breathing capacity. Patients who are unable to extinguish a lighted match generally have a maximum breathing capacity less than 40 l/min, or 50% of predicted normal. Patients who can extinguish a lighted match at a distance of six inches (15 cm) from the open mouth can usually maintain adequate ventilation after thoracic or abdominal surgery. A patient who cannot extinguish a lighted match held at a distance of 3 inches should be submitted to quantitative tests before a decision is reached whether to operate or not.

The de Bono whistle. De Bono has described a whistle, of value in measuring peak expiratory flow rates up to 300 l/min. The advantage of this method of assessment is that the apparatus is inexpensive and readily portable.

The timed vital capacity. (Forced expiratory volume per unit time): this measurement requires slightly more sophisticated equipment which will enable the volumes of air forcibly expired to be measured in relation to time: the volume expired in one second is the figure most frequently measured. This value, the $FEV_{1\cdot0}$, normally constitutes 75% or more of the total volume that can be forcibly expired from the lungs (the forced vital capacity – FVC). It is reduced in conditions where there is either reversible or irreversible obstruction in the air passages. The $FEV_{1\cdot0}$ may, therefore, be taken as a simple measurement by which response to therapy may be quantitatively measured. The maximum breathing capacity (MBC) may be indirectly derived from a knowledge of the one second forced expiratory volume ($FEV_{1\cdot0}$):

$$\text{Indirect MBC (l/min)} = FEV_{1\cdot0} \times 35 \text{ (l/min)}$$

The maximum breathing capacity is measured in litres per minute and varies according to age, sex and body size. The normal value for the average adult male lies between 100 and 140 litres per minute. Patients with a maximum breathing capacity below 40 l/min are usually unable to maintain ventilation above resting levels as readily as those with MBC value above 40 l/min. Those with pulmonary emphysema and a MBC less than 40 l/min, will often have resting arterial oxygen saturation below 92% and a carbon dioxide tension in arterial blood in excess of 40 mmHg, particularly if chronic bronchitis is present too. Patients with a MBC above 40 l/min are unlikely to develop increasing respiratory acidosis during inhalation of 100% oxygen. Low levels of MBC are associated with degrees of breathlessness in grades 3–5 as below:

- Grade 1 Performance on walking and climbing hills and stairs as good as that of other persons of a similar age and build
- Grade 2 Normal performance on walking, but inability to keep up with others on hills and stairs
- Grade 3 Ability to walk a mile or more at own speed, but inability to keep up with others
- Grade 4 Inability to walk more than 100 yards without rest

Grade 5 Breathlessness on talking or undressing and inability to leave the house

Measurement of carbon dioxide tension by the re-breathing method. A measurement of the arterial carbon dioxide tension will give an accurate estimate of the efficiency of alveolar ventilation, but, unfortunately, this estimation carries with it the disadvantage of having to make an arterial puncture and the necessity of a sophisticated analysis of arterial blood. Campbell and Howell (1960) have devised a modification of the original technique. In this method the gas within the lungs is rebreathed, and the lungs are used as a 'tonometer' in which the blood bathing the lungs comes into equilibrium with the rebreathed gas. The subject is requested to rebreathe into a 1.5–2.0 litre bag containing 100% oxygen, for approximately $1\frac{1}{2}$ minutes. A period of 3 minutes is allowed for the patient to resume a steady state, and the bag reapplied, making sure that there are no leaks around the mouth and through the nose. Rebreathing is permitted for 20 seconds. The carbon dioxide concentration within the bag is then estimated, using either a modified Haldane gas analyser or other chemical method of analysis, or a carbon dioxide analyser working on physical principles. This method can be used for patients under general anaesthesia, but apparatus for analysis must be used which has been appropriately modified for the estimation of carbon dioxide in the presence of anaesthetic gases and vapours. Using this method the arterial carbon dioxide tension (mmHg) = carbon dioxide concentration × [(barometric pressure − 47) − 6mmHg].

Endotracheal intubation

Endotracheal intubation may be satisfactorily carried out either via the nose or mouth. The nasal route is of particular value for operations upon the mouth and teeth, but carries the disadvantage that foreign material may be passed down into the trachea. Nasal intubation may be difficult where there is nasal obstruction, e.g. by nasal polyps, deflected nasal septum or enlarged adenoids; nevertheless, the nasal route is often employed where prolonged intubation is required, as for treatment with artificial ventilation. The oral route carries with it the added advantages that, as a general rule, a larger tube may be passed: the nasal route requires a reduction in the size of the tube especially if a cuff is incorporated (see Table 7.2).

There are very many varieties of endotracheal tubes, some of which may be armoured to prevent kinking. Jackson-Rees has designed a nasal tube primarily for use with children. It should be borne in mind that in children, the narrowest part of the upper respiratory tract is at the level of the cricoid ring; a tube that will pass through the external nares will almost certainly pass satisfactorily into the trachea. Tunstall has designed a disposable pre-sterilized tube for neonatal resuscitation purposes. Recently a nasal tube with 'streamlined' cuff has been introduced.

Table 7.2 *British Standard (B.S. 3487: 1962) relating to endotracheal tubes*

Internal dimensions (mm)

Oral and cuffed	*Nasal*
2·5	2·5*
3·0	3·0*
3·5	3·5*
4·0	4·0*
4·5	4·5*
5·0	5·5
5·5	6·0
6·0	6·5
6·5	7·0
7·0	7·5
7·5	8·0
8·0	8·5
8·5	9·0
9·0	10·0
9·5	11·0
10·0	—
11·0	—
11·5	—

* available through 'Portex'

Technique for oro-tracheal intubation. Before endotracheal intubation it is mandatory to look through the tube against the light, by straightening it, to ensure that no foreign body is present in the lumen. The cuff should be checked by inflating it in a sterile glass tube of roughly the same diameter as the trachea, to ensure correct inflation of the cuff and the absence of leaks. The ability of the patient to open his jaw and the presence or absence of dental caries or bridges and crowns and the number of teeth, must also be noted.

In order to pass an endotracheal tube via the mouth, adequate relaxation of the mouth, jaws and laryngeal muscles must be achieved. Using inhalational agents this relaxation can be achieved with diethyl ether, cyclopropane, or halothane, provided the anaesthetist is prepared not to 'rush' the induction: with halothane and cyclopropane, relaxation of the jaws occurs before adequate depression of the laryngeal reflex. Prior to the passage of the laryngoscope the occiput should be supported by a shallow pillow. With a right-handed anaesthetist the laryngoscope is held in the left hand and passed backwards over the right-hand side of the tongue, a movement which can be facilitated by the prior lubrication of the laryngoscope blade. The left hand pulls the laryngoscope away from the upper teeth and gums (at no time should the teeth be used as a fulcrum for the laryngoscope). With this action the tip of the Macintosh laryngoscope is passed in front of the tip of the epiglottis into the vallecula and the laryngeal aperture visualized. With the Magill laryngoscope the tip of the blade is passed behind the epiglottis. Before passing the endotracheal tube into the trachea, many anaesthetists prefer to spray the vocal cords and upper trachea with topical anaesthetic solution. This is important in patients with heart and chest disease, and in neurosurgical operations and other procedures upon the head and neck, where movement of the head is likely to occur. Coughing and straining on the tube during surgery will be obviated in these circumstances. A well-lubricated tube (with local anaesthetic agent if desired) is then held in the right hand and passed between the vocal cords. The tip of the assistant's little finger can be used to give traction to the angle of the mouth to facilitate a good view. Where topical anaesthesia is applied to the larynx, it is particularly important to ensure that nothing should be given by mouth for at least four hours after application of the local anaesthetic solution – the nursing staff must receive clear written instructions which must be displayed for all to see at the patient's bedside.

Blind nasal intubation: the anaesthetist must use all his sensory perception to the full in this technique, practising the procedure regularly so that when confronted with a situation requiring it he will be capable of putting this experience to the test. After a sleep dose of thiopentone, the patient should be allowed to breathe either halothane, diethyl ether, or trichloroethylene and, once anaesthesia has been established, a small pillow is placed under the occiput and the head hyperextended. In order to achieve mucosal decongestion, the nose may be sprayed thoroughly through each nostril with no more than a total of 4 ml of 5% cocaine. A well prepared nasotracheal tube (with a curve approximating to that achieved by storage in a 10 inch diameter biscuit tin) is then passed gently through the nostril, using the right side for preference. The patient should be breathing adequately at this stage and may be encouraged to hyperventilate by the judicious addition of 5% carbon dioxide to the anaesthetic mixture. With the left hand keeping the patient's chin well forward, the neck flexed and the head hyperextended, the anaesthetist should watch the region of the larynx carefully, at the same time advancing the tube towards the midline and listening to the breathing through it. With careful observation the tube is pushed downwards at the commencement of an expiration: should this procedure fail, slight elevation of the occiput from the pillow may facilitate the passage of the tube. Reasonable care can avoid epistaxis and should this occur it is treated in the normal way by suction. It is essential to incorporate some means of making absolutely sure that the tube cannot under any circumstances slip down the air passages and become inaccessible.

With either method, it must be remembered that the trachea ends approximately 10 cm below the larynx in the adult. A tube inserted further than this distance will enter a bronchus – usually the right. Care must be taken to avoid this, and both sides of the chest should be observed and auscultated after intubation to ensure both lungs are being inflated.

Disturbance of cardiac action during endotracheal intubation: there is strong evidence that both intubation and extubation, particularly in patients with burns, cause cardiac dysrhythmias which are potentially dangerous. To reduce the incidence of cardiac involvement during intubation, muscle relaxants should be used, but in the case of burns, paraplegia, and severe trauma involving muscle injury, suxamethonium should never be used. The autonomic reflex can be further obtunded by premedication with atropine, and the application of a topical anaesthetic agent to the larynx, trachea and tube. (β-adrenergic blockade has been suggested as of possible value in preventing this autonomic reflex in cases with tetanus and in certain hypertensive patients.)

The avoidance of hypercarbia and hypoxaemia will help to reduce the incidence of dysrhythmias.

Lesions of the respiratory tract following endotracheal intubation. Trauma to the upper respiratory tract, larynx, and trachea may arise during direct laryngoscopy and insertion of the endotracheal tube. With the profound relaxation now made possible by using neuromuscular blocking agents, traumatic sequelae are far less common than when intubation was carried out under inhalational agents. Lesions may result from the presence of the tube in the larynx and trachea; these are particularly prone to occur if movement of the tube is allowed during the course of the operation, or when the tube is left down for any length of time. Glottic oedema may occur, particularly in young children, and may constitute a hazard after extubation, as respiratory obstruction may supervene. Prolonged intubation may lead to ulceration of the larynx and laryngeal stenosis, or to granulomata of the larynx, especially in those subjects where movement of the head has occurred (e.g. operations on the head and neck). Glottic oedema should be treated by oxygen therapy, with added helium if necessary, and efficient humidification: hydrocortisone powder applied locally to the vocal cords often has a dramatic effect. Antibiotics may be necessary in the case of tracheobronchitis.

Sore throat and anaesthesia. Sore throat is not an uncommon sequela to general anaesthesia and can be so distressing that it takes precedence over the discomfort from the site of operation. There is a high incidence after naso-gastric intubation and it also tends to occur after endotracheal intubation, but it should be borne in mind that it can also occur with an ordinary oro-pharyngeal airway. These factors must be considered, but should not take precedence over the maintenance of a clear airway.

Laryngeal spasm

Laryngeal spasm was not uncommon in the days before neuromuscular blocking agents. Attempts to induce and maintain anaesthesia with intravenous barbiturates would sometimes lead to laryngeal spasm, particularly if the patients were at a light level of anaesthesia. Although modern techniques have reduced the incidence, saliva and sputum coming into contact with the larynx can give rise to spasm. Operations on the mouth particularly, may lead to the inhalation of blood, pus or other debris and thus irritate the cords. Certain anaesthetic agents e.g. thiopentone and cyclopropane, are said to lead to laryngeal spasm, as can also diethyl ether, because of its irritant properties: conditions of the throat, particularly infectious conditions, can similarly predispose to excessive laryngeal irritability. Hypoxia can lead to laryngeal spasm and the spasm can intensify the hypoxia causing a vicious circle. Vomiting and regurgitation may likewise provoke spasm. Laryngeal spasm can be associated with bronchospasm.

The anaesthetist should learn to recognize such situations as are likely to irritate the larynx and lead to laryngeal spasm. Ludwig's angina, an acute infection of the floor of the mouth, producing marked swelling under the jaw and in the neck, is often associated with oedema of the larynx, respiratory obstruction and excessive laryngeal irritability: the use of general anaesthetic agents in these cases is fraught with dangers, of which laryngeal spasm is only one. Operations on the upper respiratory tract carry with them the danger of inhalation of material, and the anaesthetist must be absolutely certain that debris cannot be inhaled. This may be achieved by efficient packing as described in the section on dentistry, or by intubating and sealing off the trachea, either by cuff or packing. Insertion of an oropharyngeal airway under light anaesthesia may produce laryngeal spasm, so the patient must be sufficiently 'deep' for surgical stimuli to have no reflex effect on the laryngeal muscles. Dilatation of the anus or cervix may be an intense stimulus which also, must be countered either by adequate depth of anaesthesia, or by ablating the laryngeal reaction by intubation and/or the use of muscle relaxants. Excessive laryngeal irritability is sometimes associated with asthma and great care must be taken not to attempt intubation in a patient too lightly under general anaesthesia, for fear of triggering off laryngeal spasm and associated bronchospasm. Laryngeal spasm may sometimes be observed in patients during recovery of consciousness particularly following intubation.

Treatment of laryngeal spasm. The onset of laryngeal spasm is not only disturbing to the anaesthetist but also dangerous to the patient. Should it occur, the anaesthetist must quickly appraise the situation. Is the 'depth' of anaesthetic appropriate for the surgical stimulus? Is there any foreign material in the upper respiratory tract causing excessive laryngeal irritability such as saliva, blood, pus, tooth fragments or gastric contents? The anaesthetist, as he gains experience, will learn to detect the difference between laryngeal spasm and obstruction of the upper respiratory tract by the epiglottis, tongue, or soft tissues of the neck.

Having checked the airway and depth of anaesthesia, further steps must be taken to deal with the spasm should it persist. Light anaesthesia should be deepened cautiously, making sure that the subject is breathing an oxygen enriched mixture. Some anaesthetists deepen the anaesthetic and at the same time increase pressure in the circuit by tightening the expiratory valve, occasionally adding carbon dioxide for a brief period of time in order to stimulate ventilation. The anaesthetist should always have the appropriate drugs and equipment available, as it may be advisable to intubate the larynx and trachea under a muscle relaxant in these circumstances. Where relaxant drugs are not available, any intention to intubate should be considered in the light of the fact that instrumentation may tend to make the larynx more irritable. In an outpatient dental procedure the wisest precaution (failing the measures outlined) is to allow the patient to recover, ensuring adequate oxygenation, and to abandon the operative procedure. Where this is not possible oxygen should be delivered via the face mask, using positive pressure on the reservoir bag to inflate the lungs; it is essential to make sure that there is no obstruction above the level of the larynx. Care must also be taken to avoid inflating the stomach. Happily, laryngeal spasm is unusual today in well-conducted anaesthetic practice. Episodes of apnoea and straining under anaesthesia can be reduced by the application of topical 4% ignocaine spray to the larynx and trachea. The relative effectiveness of 4% lignocaine and 4% prilocaine as topical anaesthetic agents has been studied. It would appear that lignocaine is superior to prilocaine, and, provided the anaesthetist is prepared to wait five minutes after administration of the lignocaine, there is unlikely to be any response of the laryngeal reflex to direct stimulation. No more than 5 ml of 4% lignocaine or 10 ml of 4% prilocaine should be used for a fit 70 kg young adult. Atropine neither prevents nor abolishes laryngeal spasm.

Endotracheal suction

Excessive and careless suction within the trachea can lead to reduction in the lung volume and resulting hypoxia. Stimulation of the trachea has been known to produce sudden death and exaggerated autonomic reflexes particularly in cases of tetanus. Unless precise attention is paid to the application of asepsis to this procedure, infection of the tracheo-bronchial tree may result, with catastrophic consequences to the patient.

Suction catheters should be of transparent plastic material, so that the nature and quality of aspirate can be visualized. They should have a single orifice at the tip, be pre-sterilized and preferably disposable. In order to allow free ingress of air, there must be free communication between the outside of the suction catheter and the inner wall of the endotracheal tube, with the external diameter not more than half the internal diameter of the airway. So that the negative pressure can be intermittently applied by placing a finger over the side tube, the suction catheters should be connected to the suction line by means of a T tube. The maximum negative pressure required should not exceed 25 mmHg and the suction apparatus – B.S. 4199 applies – should have a free air flow of at least 30 1/min. At all times suction of the tracheo-bronchial tree should be carried out under full aseptic 'no touch' technique.

It is sometimes necessary to carry out frequent tracheo-bronchial toilet in patients not under general anaesthesia, where there is a tendency to retain secretions, but where tracheostomy is thought inadvisable. These patients may receive full topical anaesthesia to the upper respiratory tract with the blind passage of a naso-tracheal tube or alternatively a block of the superior laryngeal nerve may be carried out.

Superior laryngeal nerve block. With the patient either lying down or sitting up, the head is extended, using a small pillow to facilitate this manoeuvre and the patient is instructed neither to talk nor swallow. The landmarks are checked: these are the thyroid notch in the mid-line, and the greater hyoid cornu on each side. Using an aseptic technique an intradermal wheal is raised in the mid-line, the hyoid being held in the left hand, the thumb on one cornu and the index finger on the other. An 8 cm needle is inserted and 2–3 ml of 2% lignocaine injected in the region just below and anterior to the cornu, another 2 ml being injected on withdrawal: after 'cocainization' of the nasal mucosa, blind nasal intubation is carried out. The suction catheter can then be passed through the naso-tracheal tube into the tracheo-bronchial tree.

Respiratory obstruction

One of the greatest challenges facing the anaesthetist can be the management of a case of respiratory obstruction. The obstruction may vary in severity from difficulty in establishing and maintaining an airway to a case with severe respiratory decompensation.

Routine examination of all cases pre-operatively will enable the anaesthetist to determine whether there is mobility of the jaw and neck. Inability to move the neck may be associated with many conditions, including ankylosing spondylitis, injury to the neck, rheumatoid and osteo- arthritis. The jaw may have limitation of movement because the chin is on the chest as a result of deformity of the spine, or severe scarring from burns; alternatively, infection may make it impossible for the patient to open his mouth whilst conscious because of spasm of the masseters. It is well to remember that the temporo-mandibular joint may be involved in rheumatoid arthritis or, again, condylar hyperplasia may cause limitation of the movement of the jaw. Underdevelopment of the jaw such as occurs in Treacher-Collins syndrome may make intubation difficult if not hazardous: similarly, injuries to the jaw may seriously impair the anaesthetist's ability to intubate the patient with safety.

Particularly where limitation of movement of the jaw is associated with respiratory obstruction and the use of the accessory muscles of respiration, the obstruction must be relieved prior to the induction of anaesthesia. Even when movement of the jaw is free it is hazardous to induce anaesthesia in the presence of respiratory obstruction. Tracheostomy may be considered to be the safest way of overcoming an obstruction at the level of the larynx or above, and in most instances should be carried out under local anaesthesia. However, in certain circumstances, even this procedure may prove to be impossible because the chin is fixed on the sternum by virtue of deformity of the spine. Where the anterior aspect of the neck is accessible intubation can be carried out in patients suffering from deformities of the upper airway. After infiltration of the skin with local anaesthesia, a Tuohy needle is passed through the crico-thyroid membrane and 2 ml 4% lignocaine injected through it into the trachea. Following this a catheter is guided upwards between the vocal cords into the nasopharynx, the catheter rescued by means of a hook and a nasal or oro-tracheal tube can then be threaded over the catheter and passed into the trachea. This procedure can be carried out under light general anaesthesia in certain cases, but the advisability of doing so will depend on the circumstances and if there is any doubt the whole procedure should be carried out under topical anaesthesia. With lesser degrees of respiratory obstruction and with limitation of movement of the jaw, the passage of a nasal tube either into the pharynx or into the trachea must be considered, with hooks passed through the mouth to help on its passage.

Ludwig's angina is a condition associated with acute infection of the floor of the mouth, producing marked swelling under the jaw and in the neck. Trismus, or inability to open the jaw, is often present and oedema of the larynx and swelling of the aryteno-epiglottic folds may complicate the condition and place the patient's life in a very precarious state. Respiratory obstruction which is often present may lead to use of the accessory muscles of respiration. Whenever laryngeal oedema and/or respiratory obstruction is present, general anaesthesia must on no account be employed. External drainage may have to be performed under topical freezing with ethyl chloride spray.

Lesser degrees of infection are still a grave hazard to the patient, but usually general anaesthesia can be employed. If drainage is contemplated from the outside, in the absence of trismus and oedema of the larynx, general anaesthesia may proceed, with the passage of a naso-pharyngeal tube to maintain an airway. With trismus a mouth gag (with Ackland jaws) should be inserted gently between a gap in the teeth prior to the induction of anaesthesia. When anaesthesia is established the spasm of the muscles will become reduced and careful intubation can proceed. Any case requiring drainage from within the mouth will require endotracheal intubation and careful and gentle packing with swabs soaked in saline.

The use of general anaesthesia for tracheostomy in acute laryngeal obstruction has been advocated. The commonest form of acute inflammatory laryngeal obstruction in children is acute laryngo-tracheobronchitis, which is often of sudden onset, associated with rapidly increasing respiratory embarrassment, with inspiratory stridor, a harsh irritating cough, intercostal recession and cyanosis. The performance of tracheostomy in such a grave condition is an extremely hazardous procedure and may be associated with considerable struggling in a conscious child. Macintosh has stressed the dangers of general anaesthesia in patients with partial obstruction due to glottic oedema, advising intubation before induction, but this is clearly not always practicable in children. Whilst recognizing the hazards associated with general anaesthesia in such conditions, it is perhaps less hazardous for the patient than attempting to carry out tracheostomy whilst he is fully conscious.

Acute epiglottitis is another form of acute respiratory obstruction occurring in children. This condition is particularly prevalent in Sweden, and depending on the severity of the case, the patient may present in extremis. With good organisation and team work the mortality can be almost insignificant.

On admission to the hospital, the patient should receive 100% oxygen by mask at the point of reception, where intubation is also carried out. During the period of pre-oxygenation, intramuscular hydrocortisone is given, and an intravenous infusion established. Halothane is added to the oxygen, until relaxation of the jaws is adequate, and an endotracheal tube passed orally. A wide range of tubes of varying size must be to hand. As direct visualization of the cords is generally impossible, passage of the tube is facilitated by the use of a stylette. Once the patient's condition has been stablilized (usually within 5–10 minutes) the oral tube is replaced by a PVC naso-tracheal tube, whilst the child is still under the influence of anaesthesia. The tube is firmly secured and the patient allowed to regain consciousness, when sedative doses of diazepam are given intravenously. This sedation together with intensive antibiotic and steroid therapy and humidification, is maintained for up to 48 hours, by which time, in most instances, extubation can be carried out.

Treacher-Collin's syndrome: This condition results from defective growth of the first branchial arch and produces mandibulo-facial dysostosis. It is often associated with coloboma of the iris, oblique axis of the eyes, external or middle ear abnormality, underdevelopment of the maxillae and a high foreshortened palate. Many of these patients come to surgery for the correction of hare-lip or cleft palate or because of a poorly developed and receding chin and obtuse angle of the jaw; they often create extreme difficulty in intubation. On no account should neuromuscular blocking agents be given prior to intubation as, with relaxation, inflation of the lungs may be difficult without intubation. In order to pass an endotracheal tube is may be necessary to pass a gum elastic bougie blind and then thread the endotracheal tube over it.

Other similar conditions such as Pierre-Robin syndrome (micrognathia, glossoptosis and cleft palate), and Engelmann's disease (osteopathia sclerotisan multipax infantalis – associated with limited jaw and neck movement) also constitute problems in relation to the maintenance of a patent airway. With Pierre-Robin syndrome the tongue may have to be fixed with a Kirschner wire to overcome obstruction, giving rise to nasopharyngeal insufficiency. The glottis is extremely low in the neck and a long laryngoscope blade is helpful. By the age of 2–3 years, relatively little difficulty is experienced with the airway and, with the less severe case, nursing in the face-down position facilitates airway patency. In Engelmann's disease intubation may be helped by passing a catheter through the crico-thyroid membrane.

Tracheostomy

Tracheostomy is one of the procedures that may be performed to maintain unimpeded ventilation in the presence of obstruction in the upper respiratory tract. Because of the very real danger of general anaesthesia producing profound respiratory insufficiency in patients who already have a degree of respiratory decompensation, it may be necessary to perform tracheostomy prior to induction.

The operation is frequently performed when long term management of the unconscious patient is envisaged. Patients requiring prolonged artificial ventilation may also require tracheostomy. However, where it is thought that the need is of short duration, there is an increasing trend towards naso-tracheal or oro-tracheal intubation, particularly in children. A tracheostomy carries a high risk of complications, and if these can be avoided by oro-tracheal intubation it is clearly in the best interests of the patient. Some workers have relied upon prolonged intubation using the nasal route, minimizing glottic oedema by not using too large a tube. A mortality of 3.4% directly due to tracheostomy, and a complication rate of the order of 50% has been reported (McClelland, 1965): the latter included pulmonary infection, tracheitis, pneumothorax, haemorrhage, surgical emphysema, structural deformities, displaced and obstructed tube.

Tracheostomy or prolonged endotracheal intubation by-passes the upper respiratory tract, reducing dead space and facilitating both the work of breathing and tracheo-bronchial toilet. However, because the warming and humidifying mechanisms of the upper respiratory tract are by-passed, there is a great tendency towards the development of viscid secretions. Humidification of the inspired gas should therefore be efficient.

Where there is no contraindication to general anaesthesia, tracheostomy is best performed in an unhurried manner, with the patient unconscious and immobile. The procedure is facilitated, particularly in children, by the passage of a lighted bronchoscope down to the level of the incision. There are very many types of tube available, but red rubber tubes are best avoided on account of their irritant properties. Where there is difficulty in coughing and swallowing, a cuffed tracheostomy tube is desirable: as prolonged pressure of the inflated cuff on the mucosa can produce necrosis, regular intermittent deflation and inflation may be used. Various devices have been developed to enable the cuff to be inflated in phase with the ventilator.

Management of tracheostomy. Provided adequate humidification and warming of the inspired air is insisted upon, the accumulation and blocking of the air passages with thick viscid secretions can be largely eliminated. The instillation of saline has been advocated: a total of 10 ml of sterile saline per hour in divided doses will do no harm in an adult and will facilitate the aspiration of secretions. Heated nebulizers are of additional value. At all times a strict regime of aseptic suction must be adhered to with suction of the pharynx always carried out prior to the regular and frequent deflation of the cuff. It should be unnecessary to change the tubes more frequently than every 3–5 days if humidification has been efficient, but following extubation of the laryngeal route, it is advisable in children to apply hydrocortisone powder to the larynx, or, if preferred, systemic cortisone may be administered.

Acute chest disease

Acute chest disease is often a complication arising unrelated to the condition presenting for surgery. Patients with broncho-spasm and acute bronchitis have one feature in common, namely airway obstruction.

Pneumonia. Occasionally the anaesthetist will be confronted with a patient suffering from pneumonic consolidation of the lung. Such a patient may be pyrexial, toxic and have a productive cough. General anaesthesia should be designed to avoid using irritant agents such as diethyl ether. Cyclopropane, because of its broncho-constricting properties may also create difficulties for the anaesthetist. Although intravenous induction agents are used an inhalational induction, using halothane and oxygen, is to be preferred. It is worth bearing in mind that propanidid can lead to histamine release with resulting broncho-spasm, whilst the barbiturates can cause excessive irritability of the tracheo-bronchial tree. Pre-oxygenation is desirable and premedication should be limited to agents such as phenothiazine or benzodiazepine drugs. Atropine may increase the viscosity of the secretions. Intubation may be carried out under neuro-muscular blocking agents, such as pancuronium, alcuronium and gallamine which produce less histamine release than curare. Humidification of the inspired gas mixture is desirable. Prior to the termination of anaesthesia, gentle tracheo-bronchial aspiration should be carried out, if necessary via a bronchoscope. Finally, the patient should receive antibiotic therapy appropriate to the sensitivity of the particular organism causing the disturbance.

Asthma

The patient with a history of asthma may be presented to the anaesthetist, either for an operation requiring the giving of a general anaesthetic, or for the management of status asthmaticus. Sometimes these patients are debilitated and may exhibit excessive anxiety.

General anaesthesia carries an incidence of circulatory and respiratory complications, both during and after anaesthesia. The main difficulties arise as a result of broncho-spasm being provoked by the premedication, anaesthetic agents or instrumentation. Instrumentation of the respiratory tract, particularly under light anaesthesia, is perhaps the most potent cause of broncho-spasm developing in relation to general anaesthesia. The resultant broncho-spasm can seriously imperil the patient's well-being, being accompanied by straining, hypoxia and hypercarbia and the retention of secretions. Thiopentone and cyclopropane are said to be contraindicated in asthmatics because of their parasympatheticomimetic properties. Diethyl ether initially provokes broncho-spasm because of its irritant properties, but with deeper anaesthesia good broncho-dilatation is achieved; because of this it has been advocated for the treatment of broncho-spasm. Halothane is a potent broncho-dilator. Curare has the disadvantage of leading to histamine release.

Where possible conduction anaesthesia should be employed, but in making this recommendation it should be borne in mind that broncho-spasm may be precipitated in an over-anxious individual. Lack of awareness of the operation, even with its associated hazards, may be in the best interests of the patient, rather than local anaesthesia.

Preparation of the asthmatic patient for general anaesthesia. A careful enquiry will elicit a history of broncho-spasm and the possible relationship between attacks and precipitating factors; the frequency of attacks, their control by therapeutic agents, and the degree of respiratory compensation between the attacks, will give the anaesthetist an idea as to pre-operative therapy. Whilst no patient should receive a general anaesthetic without the anaesthetist ascertaining what drug therapy, if any, he has been receiving, this is especially important where asthmatics are concerned: for example, some asthmatics may receive therapy with 'steroids' and these drugs may impair adrenal cortical function. A thorough examination may reveal debility, anaemia and respiratory decompensation. Attention must also be paid to adequate hydration as under-hydration is often an associated factor of status asthmaticus.

Where the operation is not urgent and the anaesthetist feels that the patient may derive benefit from a period of drug therapy and breathing exercises, he should not hesitate to postpone surgery in order to allow therapy to take place. Where the operation cannot be postponed the patient should receive broncho-dilator therapy pre-operatively as shown in Table 7.3 where doses are for a fit adult man weighing 70 kg. Antibiotics may be given where indicated.

In order to allay his anxieties, the patient should be sedated as much as possible and particular attention paid to a personal approach. Barbiturates are best avoided as they are known to provoke an acute attack in certain individuals; in addition, the opiates and similar respiratory depressants are unsuitable for the majority of cases. The patient should already be receiving antispasmodics and the response to this therapy can, if necessary, be measured quantitatively, using the forced expiratory volume or the peak expiratory flow rate. Sedation is best achieved with the phenothiazine group of drugs or other ataractics; though atropine should be given, particularly when suxemethonium, diethyl either or halothane are to be used, it must be recognized that it can make secretions more viscid and difficult to void.

General anaesthesia: on arrival in the anaesthetic room, aminophylline 0.25–0.5 g in 10 ml water should be slowly administered intravenously. After three minutes of pre-oxygenation the induction of anaesthesia can be carried out using a non-barbiturate intravenous induction agent (e.g. Althesin) or alternatively nitrous oxide/oxygen/halothane. (Thiopentone and propanidid have the theoretical disadvantage of triggering an attack of broncho-spasm.) The patient should then breathe halothane and

Table 7.3 *Drugs for broncho-dilator therapy*

Drug	**Administration*	*Dose*	*Remarks*
isoprenaline	aerosol†	1%–2% (0·1–0·3 ml)	not more often than every 2 hours
ephedrine	oral	30–60 mg	6 hours between doses
	sub-lingual	10 mg	8 hourly
salbutamol (Ventolin)	metered aerosol	100 μg	said to produce less cardiac effects than isoprenaline (do not prescribe concurrently with - blocking agents)
	oral	4 mg	6 or 8 hourly
methoxyphenamine (Orthoxine)	oral	50 mg–100 mg	6 hourly
orciprenaline sulphate (Alupent)	oral	20 mg	6 hourly
	metered aerosol	20 mg	
Franol:			
theophylline	oral	120 mg	8 or 12 hourly
phenobarbitone	oral	8 mg	
ephedrine	oral	10 mg	
adrenaline	subcutaneous	0·5 ml	give over 5 minutes and repeat in not less than 30 minutes
iso-etharine (Numotac)	oral	10 mg	6 or 8 hourly a derivative of isoprenaline and ethyl noradrenaline said to be better than isoprenaline no increase in pulse
proxyphylline (Thean, Brontyl)	oral	300 mg	8 hourly
	i.v. slowly	300–400 mg	said to cause less pain at site of injection and less irritation on oral administration than aminophylline
	i.m.	300–400 mg	
aminophylline	i.v.	0·25 g in 10 ml	slowly
	rectal suppositories	0·7–1·0 g	daily
	i.m.	0·48 g	once or twice per day
	oral	0·2–0·4 g	8 hourly
choline theophyllinate (Choledyl)	oral	100–400 mg	8 hourly
deptropine citrate (Brontina)	aerosol	2 mg/ml	1–3 inhalations 8–12 hourly
	oral	1 mg	8 hourly
hydrocortisone‡ sodium succinate	i.v.	100 mg–200 mg	
prednisolone‡	oral	2·5–5·0 mg	

* cromoglycote (Intal) has been administered by inhalation in some patients with varying degrees of success

oxygen until the jaw is relaxed and an oro-pharyngeal airway carefully introduced without irritation to the upper air passages. Should intubation be required, after establishing spontaneous ventilation on oxygen and halothane, 50 mg of suxamethonium should be administered intravenously. The patient should be gently ventilated, the vocal cords and upper trachea sprayed with 4% lignocaine or prilocaine and a well-lubricated cuffed endotracheal tube placed in the larynx under direct vision.

Should intubation be carried out with an ultra-light induction agent and short acting relaxant sequence, coughing and straining are almost certain to arise as the relaxant wears off. Halothane and oxygen with or without further relaxants, should be used for the maintenance of anaesthesia (curare should be avoided because of its known effect of producing histamine release in certain subjects). Alcuronium (Alloferin) is said to produce less histamine release than curare and its use is suggested in patients with a history of broncho-spasm: pancuronium may also have a place. Halothane, being an effective antispasmodic, is in our opinion, the general anaesthetic agent of choice, but some anaesthetists prefer to employ diethyl ether, which also has marked broncho-dilator activity. Care should be taken with the induction if ether is used, as it may provoke broncho-spasm before dilatation, because of its irritant properties, under light anaesthesia.

With an endotracheal tube in place, ventilation should be carried out by means of a slow inspiratory phase, followed by a slow expiratory phase, as the obstruction to ventilation affects both inspiration and expiration. For this reason a volume-cycled ventilator should be used. Humidification of inspired gases is essential and high inflation pressures may be necessary to ensure adequate ventilation. Suction and removal of tracheal secretions can be carried out by passing a catheter down the endotracheal tube, but the greatest care must be taken not to irritate the tracheo-bronchial tree by anything but the gentlest suction. Surgery should not be permitted until the patient is at an appropriate depth of anaesthesia for the surgical stimulus, for if in too light anaesthesia, it might provoke severe broncho-spasm.

Should broncho-spasm develop during the course of general anaesthetic, it can be a most disturbing event: it may even prove impossible to

---

† A small number of sudden and unexplained deaths of asthmatic patients have been reported. In some cases the circumstances of death were strongly suggestive of overdosage from aerosols containing broncho-dilating drugs, in particular isoprenaline. Recent reports suggest a possible link between excessive use by patients of such aerosols and a recorded rise in the death rate from bronchial asthma

‡ dexamethasone can be administered in the form of an inhalation. Recent evidence suggests that adrenal cortical depression is less likely than with these preparations

inflate or deflate the patient's lungs. Attempts should be made to deepen the level of anaesthesia by increasing the concentration of inhalational anaesthetic agent. Oxygen alone should be used as the vehicle, and aminophylline given intravenously (0.25–0.5 g) as well as hydrocortisone 100 mg. Even massage of the lungs, with or without thoracotomy, has been employed.

Pulmonary embolism

Pulmonary embolism usually occurs 7-10 days post-operatively. It is more common in association with lower abdominal procedures, but can follow any form of surgery. It is a risk which is anticipated and where at all possible, steps should be taken to reduce the predisposing factors (see page 162). Nevertheless, it may still occur.

Severity varies from immediate death to mild embolic-pneumonia giving rise to minimal symptoms. There is a group of patients however, who, after a severe attack, survive for a few hours. It is these who are amenable to pulmonary arterial embolectomy (Trendelenberg's operation). As most of them are critically ill, with great increase in the alveolar dead space and decreased cardiac output, oxygen therapy is essential, and intermittent positive pressure ventilation desirable whilst awaiting operation. Surgeons are usually reluctant to operate until confirmatory evidence in the form of pulmonary angiograms and radio-active scanning of the lungs have been carried out. ECG usually produces a picture similar to a massive posterior infarct. Estimation of the physiological dead space is a further diagnostic aid. With ventilatory support already in hand, general anaesthesia is relatively easy to induce, many of the patients requiring minimal quantities of drugs. Most surgeons carry out this operation with an assisted circulation in the form of a cardio-pulmonary by-pass: with the development of emergency extracorporeal circulation facilities, operative results should improve. The importance of having disposable oxygenators readily available cannot be overstressed. The use of fibrinolytic enzymes such as streptokinase is gaining popularity in the treatment of pulmonary embolism.

Chronic chest disease

Chest deformities

Kyphoscoliosis. Severe kyphoscoliosis may reduce the total lung volume and the vital capacity to as little as a quarter of normal. However, in the young these small lungs are ventilated with an efficiency only a little less than normal; the mixing of inspired gases is seldom abnormal and usually airway obstruction is not present. As the spinal curvature increases so the lung volumes decrease, and the maximum breathing capacity may be reduced partly because of associated muscle weakness. Kyphoscoliosis arises from many causes and may be associated with neuromuscular disease, such as the after-effects of poliomyelitis, or in association with neurofibromatosis, syringomyelia, Frederich's ataxia and paraplegia; or it may be related to disease of the vertebrae such as tuberculosis, tumour, fracture, dislocation or osteomalacia. Sometimes it is associated with Marfan's disease and Klippel-Feil syndrome and with such thoracic disease as empyema and thoracoplasty. Finally, it may be congenital in origin or just arise apparently idiopathically.

In severe cases of kyphoscoliosis heart failure may occur in later life, probably due to the development of ventilation/perfusion imbalance in the lung. The clinical picture of heart failure closely resembles anoxic cor pulmonale, due to emphysema, and is associated with a reduction in the arterial oxygen saturation and increase in the arterial carbon dioxide tension. Patients suffering from kyphoscoliosis have a high oxygen consumption because of the mechanical disadvantage at which their respiratory muscles are working.

In children various types of operative procedure have been devised in attempts to correct the deformity.

The Harrington operation: this technique combines spinal fusion with internal metallic fixation and is designed to improve cardio-respiratory function – an extensive and formidable operation associated with much blood loss (which must be carefully replaced). Laryngeal intubation may be difficult in these cases and adequate controlled ventilation is essential. The patient must be carefully postured on the table, so that the vertebral column can be slightly flexed and adequately supported during operation. Hypotensives and local infiltration are employed by some, and prevention of venous engorgement and maintenance of a low mean intrathoracic pressure are necessary. Metabolic acidosis should be corrected, should this arise as a consequence of blood transfusion. The ECG should be monitored. Post-operative oozing from the site of the surgical procedure occurs and will require replacement, as said earlier. The children are often sent back to the ward on a plaster bed and this may necessitate extreme care to maintain a patent airway for the first hour or so.

In the adult it may be necessary to administer a general anaesthetic to a patient suffering from kyphoscoliosis, for some unrelated surgical procedure. A detailed pre-operative examination is essential, particular attention being paid to the presence or absence of heart failure and the presence of bronchitis. Appropriate therapy should be instituted immediately if any of these are present. It should be remembered that these patients, besides having a diminished ventilatory capacity, have disturbances in ventilation and perfusion within the lung: therefore they may well be hypoxaemic. Before induction of anaesthesia, particular attention should be paid to the possibility of difficult intubation. Limitation of the cervical spine and involvement of the temporo-mandibular joint may make intubation difficult if not hazardous. These patients should be pre-oxygenated and ventilation controlled throughout the course of anaesthesia. Even post-operatively ventilation may be inadequate, and if necessary should be supported artificially for as long as required.

Chronic bronchitis and emphysema

The selection for surgery of patients suffering with chronic bronchitis and/or emphysema is no easy task. Both these conditions have one feature in common, airway obstruction. However, although these two conditions are often linked together, it is important to realize that one or other of the conditions predominates. In heavily industrialized conurbations, atmospheric pollution is a very real problem, and this factor, together with tobacco smoking, is thought to contribute to the aetiology of chronic bronchitis. Chronic bronchitis is commonest in males over the age of forty years and carries risks for the patient both during the operative and post-operative periods. Apart from causing disturbances in blood gas homeostasis, the disordered physiology associated with chronic bronchitis and emphysema can influence the uptake and elimination of inhalational agents.

Patients with chronic bronchitis and emphysema presenting problems in relation to surgery and anaesthesia can be broadly divided into two groups. Firstly, the patient with mild to moderate emphysema, and secondly, the patient with severe emphysema with or without cor pulmonale. In the former group the problem consists of a patient with a 'compensated' ventilatory defect, with or without the additional hazard of sputum, oedema of the bronchial mucosa and the possibility of broncho-spasm. In these patients, general anaesthesia as a whole does not constitute an insurmountable problem, but there is very little latitude available for misjudgement of dosage, and induction must be smooth. Patients with frank cor pulmonale are a severe risk. Induction of anaesthesia may be prolonged if it is carried out with inhalational agents. The use of an anaesthetic agent of low potency, such as nitrous oxide, will especially give rise to a slow induction. Broncho-spasm, too, is a recognized hazard and is particularly likely to occur in patients suffering with chronic bronchitis, if intubation is carried out under imperfect relaxation, or light anaesthesia. Furthermore, the agents thiopentone and cyclopropane are said to be 'vagotonic' and broncho-spasm may be provoked by their administration.

As the emphysema becomes more and more severe the problem of the anaesthesia in these subjects becomes greater. There is no doubt that in the severely handicapped patient local anaesthesia should be employed wherever possible. Local field block in conjunction with abdominal surgery may be employed, particularly for operations involving the lower abdomen. Where the upper abdomen is concerned the problem is somewhat different, as the intra abdominal pressure is often increased and the abdominal contents are likely to be extruded and thereby increase the difficulty of the procedure. The use of general anaesthesia with spontaneous ventilation in this situation may not improve the operative conditions for the surgeon. In addition, if spontaneous ventilation is permitted, depression of ventilation may occur leading to further carbon dioxide retention. This tendency to underventilation may be aggravated by oxygen enrichment of the inspired mixture that is mandatory under general anaesthesia. Controlled ventilation under general anaesthesia is in our opinion the most suitable technique for upper abdominal surgery. Further problems may arise in establishing adequate ventilation in the post-operative period and there is also an increased likelihood of post-operative pulmonary complications.

Whenever possible, the surgical procedure should be carried out under conduction anaesthesia in subjects with severe respiratory decompensation. Where this is not possible, and for all operations upon the upper abdomen, general anaesthesia with controlled ventilation should be used. The anaesthetist and his team must be prepared to offer prolonged ventilatory support to such patients in the post-operative period as, in general, a patient with a pre-operative maximum breathing capacity below 35 litres/minute will be unlikely to survive an upper abdominal operation without post-operative supportive artificial ventilation. The tendency of the patient to excessive bronchial secretions will perhaps be the one factor which will mainly influence the anaesthetist; any procedure which may further impair the patient's already small capacity to shift air will inevitably lead to sputum retention. Gross deviation in pre-operative arterial oxygen and carbon dioxide tensions are often associated with problems during and after general anaesthesia. Some take the view that elective surgery may only be considered with an arterial carbon dioxide tension below 50 mmHg, but with post-operative IPPV this factor in itself should not be a contraindiction to surgery.

Pre-operative preparation: a full clinical and respiratory function assessment should be carried out. Where sputum is present this should be treated with antibiotic therapy, assisted by breathing exercises and postural drainage. Antispasmodics should be prescribed, and attempts made to make the sputum less viscid.

Premedication: opiates and other respiratory depressants are best avoided and atropine should not be given, as it has the tendency to increase the viscosity of the sputum. Other sedative drugs without respiratory depressant properties may be allowed.

Anaesthesia. If general anaesthesia is decided upon, induction is best carried out using propanidid or Althesin and intubation carried out using a neuromuscular blocking agent, after a thorough application of topical anaesthetic to the larynx and upper trachea. Anaesthesia should be maintained using nitrous oxide/oxygen with 0.5–1.0% halothane, the oxygen percentage being at least 35%. The humidification of inspired gases is essential. Gallamine is probably the neuromuscular blocking agent of choice, but pancuronium or alcuronium may be used. The ventilatory requirement of the patient should take into account the increased alveolar dead space associated with chronic respiratory disease, and should probably be about 150% of that predicted for a normal patient. At the termination of operation the tracheo-bronchial tree should be cleared of secretions using a suction catheter, and if need be a bronchoscope. Reversal of neuromuscular blocking action should be carried out in the normal manner, but if there is any evidence of ventilatory insufficiency, IPPV should be maintained, preferably for at least 48 hours in the case of an upper abdominal operation, or until the inhibitory action of pain upon ventilation ends (confirmed if possible by blood gas studies). The patient may be returned to the ward and sat up as soon as possible. Oxygen therapy may be necessary, but graded concentrations should be exhibited. Whenever possible pain relieving drugs with respiratory depressant properties should be avoided, and, if pain relief is essential, the use of continuous extradural block considered. Efficient physiotherapy, continued antibiotic therapy, the use of antispasmodics, and the humidification of the inspired atmosphere should continue well into the post-operative period.

Technique of anaesthesia for intrathoracic operations

As well as the routine evaluation of the patient it is important to note the amount of bronchial secretions being expectorated daily, and whether these are easily voided. The chest should be rendered as clear as possible by vigorous physiotherapy, antibiotic therapy considered, and breathing exercises instituted.

Many anaesthetists prefer to carry out a preliminary bronchoscopy prior to intubation in lung cases, thus enabling the exact site of the lesion to be determined, secretions to be aspirated, and the type of tube to be selected to avoid its impinging on the growth. Several points should be noted:

all spontaneous respiratory movements must be abolished by the use of neuromuscular blocking agents and/or central respiratory depressants

secretions must be regularly aspirated from the bronchial tree

as at least 30%, and possibly higher concentrations of oxygen (particularly when a blocker is employed) must be given in the inhaled mixture in order to maintain blood oxygenation, it is likely that nitrous oxide/oxygen anaesthesia on its own will be inadequate. It should be supplemented by, for example, 0.5–1.0% halothane or intravenous analgesics

Right lung to be collapsed			*Left lung to be collapsed*		
Single lumen tube	*Double lumen tube*	*Bronchus blocker*	*Single lumen tube*	*Double lumen tube*	*Bronchus blocker*
*Machray modification. Magill endobronchial tube in left main bronchus	Carlen's tube	†Vernon Thompson blocker right main bronchus + endotracheal tube.		‡Carlen's tube	†Vernon Thompson blocker left main bronchus + endotracheal tube
*Magill endobronchial tube in the left main bronchus	‡Bryce-Smith/Salt tube into right main bronchus	†Magill bronchus occluder + endotracheal tube	*Magill right tube with wire coil	Bryce-Smith/Salt tube into right main bronchus allows vent right upper lobe	Magill bronchus occluder + endotracheal tube
MacIntosh-Leatherdale left endobroncheal tube	Bryce-Smith tube into left main bronchus		MacIntosh/Leatherdale left bronchus blocker & combined endotracheal tube	‡Bryce-Smith tube into left main bronchus	
Brompton-Pallister left sided with one cuff on tracheal tube and two on bronchial	Left sided Robertshaw tube		Gordon/Green right sided tube (allows ventilation right upper lobe)	Right sided Robertshaw tube	
	‡White right-sided (carinal hook)			White right-sided permits ventilation right upper lobe (carinal hook)	

For right upper lobectomy:
1 Magill bronchus occluder plus endotracheal tube
2 Vellacott right sided tube } allowing ventilation right middle and
3 Green right-sided tube } lower lobes and left lung

† must be introduced through bronchoscope
* must be introduced over bronchoscope
‡ although can be used for this purpose – best avoided for pneumonectomy

the collapsed parts of the lung (see Table 7.4) should whenever possible be inflated at regular intervals; it is sometimes surprising how much pressure is necessary to accomplish this

because there is a tendency, when the chest is open, for the mediastinum to shift away from the side of operation, it is important to either maintain a slightly raised end-expiratory pressure, or to intermittently increase the inflation pressure of the ventilated lung. This is best achieved by manual compression of the reservoir bag

all portions of the lung remaining must be fully inflated before final closure of the pleura, and establishment of underwater drainage

Post-operative points:

an intrapleural drainage tube with underwater seal will be in place, and must be checked to see that there is free movement of fluid up and down the tube with ventilation

if there is any doubt as to the adequacy of ventilation, this should be supported by employing artificial ventilation

routine oxygen administration by mask is recommended

pain is, on the whole, less distressing with a thoracotomy wound than an upper abdominal. Pain should, however, be so controlled as to facilitate coughing without depressing ventilation

early institution of deep breathing, postural drainage and assisted expectoration is important

Broncho-pleural Fistula

Communication between a bronchus or bronchiole and the pleural cavity – which may contain gas or fluid or both – constitutes a very real hazard. The communication may be valvular and allow movement in only one direction. Should positive endotracheal pressure be applied, tension pneumothorax may result or pus, blood or serous fluid flood the bronchial tree. Broncho-pleural fistula may result from breakdown of a bronchial stump suture following an operation upon the lung or it may arise from rupture of bullae, or of a lung abscess. Traumatic injuries to the chest may also give rise to a communication between the air-containing parts of the lungs and the pleural cavity.

Once the diagnosis of broncho-pleural fistula has been established, it is essential to drain the pleural cavity by means of a thoracotomy tube and underwater seal, prior to induction of anaesthesia. Some anaesthetists would advise intubation under spontaneous ventilation, either employing general anaesthesia or topical anaesthesia. In all cases it is essential to ascertain that the water level in the thoracotomy bottle swings freely with respiration and the tube is left unclamped.

Induction of anaesthesia is best carried out with the patient in a head up position. Most authorities would recommend the passage of a bronchus blocker, or selective intubation (Table 7.4) so that the affected side may be isolated and the leak of air or pus prevented from communicating with the whole tracheo-bronchial tree. Some prefer to intubate their patients with an endo-bronchial tube or blocker, following bronchoscopy under topical anaesthesia. Crichothyoid puncture with the insertion of 2 ml 4% lignocaine, may be followed by induction of anaesthesia and intubation with the patient breathing spontaneously under general aaesthesia.

Thoracoplasty

Though once an essential operation for the management of pulmonary tuberculosis in the pre-antibiotic era, this operation is seldom performed today. However, the operation of thoracoplasty is very occasionally carried out in a patient who is suffering from tuberculosis with a resistant strain or cavity formation in the lung, as it would be dangerous to attempt lobectomy, pneumonectomy or localized excision of the lung where there is a real danger of the suture line being broken down by resistant organisms. In addition it is sometimes employed after pneumonectomy. Because of the danger of the spread of infected material from one part of the lung to another, surgeons preferred to carry out this operation under local anaesthesia with sedation and preservation of the cough reflex. Today, however, when this operation is performed, it is usually conducted under general anaesthesia with controlled ventilation, incorporating blockage where necessary.

Local anaesthesia: this is a very distressing procedure for the conscious subject and it is doubtful whether local anaesthesia has any place, particularly in view of the modern advances in general anaesthesia. Should the method be employed, however, adequate sedation of the patient is essential. In order to cover the operative field, brachial plexus block, posterior intercostal block, and infiltration in the anterior end of each intercostal space is necessary.

Post-operative chest complications

Patients with a history of respiratory disease are particularly liable to develop post-operative pulmonary complications. The pre-operative presence of chronic productive cough predisposes to the post-operative development of sputum retention, particularly if the patient experiences pain on coughing. Measurement of the capacity of the patient to shift air (peak expiratory flow rate and forced vital capacity) will be helpful to the surgeon and anaesthetist in the assessment for operation and indicate the need for pre-operative prophylactic measures. Probably because *Haemophilus influenzae* is the most commonly encountered pathogen in the bronchial tree of the bronchitic patient and is not sensitive to penicillin, a course of penicillin before operation and five days after operation does not necessarily reduce the incidence or severity of post-operative chest infections. A five days' course of penicillin with streptomycin (Crystamycin) continued over the time of the operation does, however, significantly reduce the incidence of post-operative chest complications. Such chest infections are more frequent in the male than the female, and after upper abdominal operations rather than lower abdominal operations.

Atelectasis. Routine suction of the tracheo-bronchial tree, provided that it is carried out under aseptic conditions, can reduce the incidence of trouble. There appears to be no difference in the incidence of atelectasis, whether or not the patient has been ventilated with air or the more soluble oxygen for ten minutes at the termination of anaesthesia. Routine intermittent positive pressure ventilation combined with broncho-dilators and detergents does not prevent the occurrence of post-operative atelectasis nor accelerate clearance of patients with a normal bronchial tree, though the latter is of some value to patients with chronic respiratory disease. The routine administration of 5% carbon dioxide in oxygen by nasal catheter for 10 minutes hourly in the immediate 24 hours following operation reduces respiratory complications from about 65% to 22% (Enderby, 1947). Another method of producing the same effect is the use of a rebreathing tube of 100 ml capacity.

Pain: there is no doubt that pain may cause restriction of active respiratory movement and can seriously impede the patient's post-operative progress by leading to atelectasis. Pain relief must be adequate but opiates should not be exhibited to such a degree that the cough reflex is obtunded or depression of the respiration produced. (A cough belt has been advocated and may be of some help.) Rapid post-operative recovery of reflexes with early ambulation will help to reduce pulmonary complications.

Some writers have been unable to establish any statistically significant difference in the incidence of respiratory sequelae in relation to whether or not the patients have been intubated. Laryngeal incompetence does occur post-operatively in a significant proportion of patients in either case. It might, therefore, be advisable to avoid anything by mouth including sips of water, for the first 4 hours post-operatively. Postural drainage and/or breathing exercises, supervized by a physiotherapist in the post-operative period, can be of general help in reducing pulmonary complications. The inhalation of aerosols containing antispasmodic and mucolytic agents may also be used and are shown in Table 7.5.

Table 7.5 *Antispasmodic and mucolytic agents*

Drug	*Administration*
isoprenaline hydrochloride	controlled nebulizer
acetylcysteine 20% (Airbron)	by instillation or nebulizer
tyloxapol (Alevaire)	nebulizer
orciprenaline (Alupent)	metered aerosol
ascorbic acid + copper sulphate* (Ascoxal)	nebulizer

These agents should be avoided in the asthmatic patient

* active only for 15 min after mixing

Post-operative hypoxaemia

For many years it has been recognized that patients recovering after anaesthesia have been prone to post-operative hypoxaemia. It was generally accepted that this hypoxaemia was a result of alveolar hypoventilation, resulting from residual depression and the inability to breathe adequately, on account of pain from the operative wound. However, Fink (1955) drew attention to an additional factor, the diffusion of anaesthetic gases into the alveoli at the termination of anaesthesia, leading to dilution of the inspired oxygen. It has recently been shown that hypoventilation in the post-operative period may arise following prolonged hyperventilation during operation. The reduction of arterial oxygen tension during air breathing for at least 24 hours after anaesthesia and surgery with no evidence of carbon dioxide retention, led to the conclusion that the hypoxaemia has arisen because of small airway collapse and reduced FRC leading to disturbed ventilation/perfusion relationships within the lungs. It has been calculated that a shunt equivalent to 25% of the pulmonary blood flow would cause the degree of post-operative desaturation experienced in some patients. This venous admixture effect may be further accentuated by the low mixed venous oxygen content consequent upon increased oxygen extraction at the periphery (post-operative pain with increased muscle tone and shivering), and a low cardiac output associated with blood loss. The fact that this hypoxaemia is least marked in the young, fit subject and most marked with advance in age, length of operation, and pre-existing cardio-pulmonary disease, suggests that areas of pulmonary collapse may be a cause of increased venous admixture.

To summarize: periodic inflation of the lung and tracheo-bronchial toilet during anaesthesia and oxygen administration, maintenance of blood volume, adequate pain relief, and the prevention of hypothermia post-operatively, will reduce the tendency to hypoxaemia.

Oxygen therapy

Where arterial hypoxaemia is entirely due to alveolar hypoventilation, caused by failure of reversal of central respiratory depressants, or of reversal of peripheral neuro-muscular blockade, correction will occur by using air, provided that alveolar ventilation is made adequate by immediate artificial ventilation. Under certain circumstances, however, it is necessary to increase the concentration of oxygen in the inspired gas mixture. Underventilation of perfused alveoli may occur in association with general anaesthesia; this phenomenon gives rise to venous admixture which can usually be corrected by the administration 30–35% oxygen. A normal arterial oxygen saturation can thus be restored under such circumstances by a mixture moderately enriched with oxygen. At an atmospheric pressure of 760 mmHg it is possible to raise the alveolar oxygen tension to nearly 680 mmHg by breathing 100% oxygen (provided alveolar ventilation is maintained at a level adequate to produce normal levels of carbon dioxide elimination). When alveolar hypoventilation is present, carbon dioxide will be retained in the body and reduce the effective tension of oxygen at alveolar level; this becomes progressively more important as lower concentrations of oxygen are inhaled. When oxygen therapy raises the alveolar tension to 600 mmHg, as much as 1.5–1.7 ml of additional oxygen are taken up in solution in each 100 ml of plasma. The addition of blood which has completely by-passed collapsed alveoli, to blood which has been fully oxygenated by ventilated alveoli, produces a state of hypoxaemia if the venous admixture or shunt is significant. Such situations arise in pneumonic consolidation and bronchial obstruction. If such areas of totally collapsed alveoli are present, pulmonary arterial blood will be 'shunted' through these areas of collapse and will mix with blood from ventilated alveoli; this, in turn, will give up the extra dissolved oxygen and oxygenate some of the blood coming from the collapsed alveoli. Provided the mixed venous blood is moderately well saturated, this mechanism can compensate for a shunt of approximately 33% of the total pulmonary blood flow when 100% oxygen is breathed. Larger shunts will be accompanied by persistant hypoxaemia, in spite of 100% oxygen. Where pure anatomical shunts exist, as in congenital defects in the cardiovascular system, the effect of oxygen enrichment will depend upon the degree of shunt. A further indication for oxygen enrichment of the inspired gases is the presence of a diffusion defect. Increasing the oxygen tension gradient across the diseased alveolar membrane will encourage the transference of oxygen into the blood.

The arterial hypoxaemia which is present in oligaemic states associated with haemorrhage, may partly result from alveolar hypoventilation, due to an increase in physiological dead space and the reduction of tidal volume by agents such as morphine, and also to the venous admixture through normal shunts of grossly desaturated blood returning to the lung from poorly perfused tissues. Such a situation is improved by the maintenance of adequate ventilation and oxygen enrichment.

Signs and symptoms of oxygen deficiency: minor hypoxaemia is difficult to recognize and one cannot rely upon signs and symptoms. It is well known that cyanosis may be difficult to recognize under certain lighting conditions and indeed may be absent in anaemic states. A slight fall of arterial oxygen saturation represents a considerable fall of the arterial oxygen tension, even before cyanosis. The presence of cyanosis indicates that the oxygen saturation has fallen to approximately 75%, corresponding to a tension of 40 mmHg. Furthermore the arterial oxygen saturation is no longer on the plateau on the top of the oxygen dissociation curve, but down on the steep part: any further reduction of oxygen tension, therefore, will bring a proportionate reduction of oxygen saturation.

Oxygen therapy in conditions associated with chronic elevation of the arterial carbon dioxide tension. The danger of carbon dioxide retention in patients suffering from chronic hypoxic lung disease while receiving oxygen was described as early as 1931. These patients rely upon hypoxic drive of the respiratory centre in order to maintain ventilation however inadequate. Investigation of the various modes of oxygen administration in these patients has shown that intermittent oxygen administration does not correct hypoxaemia for any appreciable length of time, indeed that hypoxaemia following such administration is often more pronounced than before therapy. Elevation of the arterial carbon dioxide tension tends to be accentuated in patients with hypoxic lung disease who are receiving intermittent administration of oxygen. Campbell (1960) has recognized this problem and has defined the relationship between oxygen concentration of the inspired gas and the arterial blood in these patients. Continuous administration permits the inspired concentration to be controlled within limits of ± 1.0% over the range 24–35% and Venturi masks have been developed which will deliver 24%, 28%, 35% and 40% oxygen and which can be changed to suit the patient (Campbell, 1963). Therapy should be started with 24% oxygen in patients suffering with chest disorders and the oxygen concentration increased as the patient's condition allows.

Leigh (1970) has classified the methods of giving oxygen therapy to spontaneously breathing conscious patients, these being shown in Table 7.6.

The Ventimask provides a constant controlled inspired oxygen tension without imposing functional apparatus dead space. With an oxygen flow rate of 2–4 l/min the total flow rate of oxygen plus entrained air is 40 l/min. Under these circumstances a constant concentration of inspired oxygen can be offered to the patient. On the other hand, with oxygen therapy systems other than anaesthetic equipment, the inspired concentration of oxygen varies with the flow rate and tidal volume of the patient. These other systems cannot satisfy the peak inspired demand of the patient (40 l/min) and therefore air is inevitably entrained with dilution of the inspired oxygen. Simple nasal catheters have been designed but the danger of rupture of the stomach by nasal catheters delivering oxygen cannot be overstated. Particular care should be taken to ensure that the tip of the catheter does not pass down below the level of the tip of the epiglottis: for adults fixing a disc 12 cm from the tip prevents the catheter slipping down. In selecting a mask consideration must be given not only to its oxygen yield but also to its capacity to fit snugly to the face and resist twisting with resultant occlusion of flow.

Table 7.6 *Methods of giving oxygen therapy to spontaneously breathing patients*

Fixed performance systems:	
Characteristics:	Give a controlled oxygen concentration independent of patient's condition
Types:	High flow – Ventimasks
	Low flow – semi-closed anaesthetic circuits
Variable performance systems:	
Characteristics:	These are mainly air/oxygen admixture systems in which oxygen is administered at a rate much less than the inspiratory flow rate. The performance is dependent upon the character of the patient's breathing
Types:	No-capacity systems: oxygen catheters or nasal cannulae at low oxygen flows
	Capacity systems:
	Small capacity system: for oxygen only – catheters or cannulae at high oxygen flows
	For both oxygen and carbon dioxide (i.e. with rebreathing) – M.C. & Edinburgh masks
	Large capacity system: for both oxygen and carbon dioxide (i.e. with rebreathing) – pneumask, polymask, oxyaire, BLB, portogen, oxygen tent and incubator

With the MC, Edinburgh Polymask, Pneumask, and BLB masks the dead space is large. Because of the hazard of rebreathing it has been suggested that these masks should be used with caution in subjects liable to carbon dioxide narcosis.

Several oxygen head tents have been devised. The Venturi head tent has a dome 12in in diameter, a high air flow with oxygen enrichment – an inspired oxygen concentration which can be regulated up to 47% by using a throttle on the air intake to change the entrainment ratio of a Venturi tube. It is an efficient form of oxygen administration, particularly for confused patients who will not tolerate a face mask. The oxygen concentration in conventional tents has been investigated and concentrations of about 40% can usually be attained.

Intra-gastric oxygen. Several workers have investigated the efficiency of intra-gastric oxygen in the resuscitation of the newborn. The general opinion is that the method is valueless.

Humidification. Efficient humidification is essential for prolonged administration of oxygen: there are several humidifiers and nebulizers designed for this purpose (see page 31).

Further reading

Green, I. D. (1972) Methods of Administration of Oxygen. *Brit. J. Hosp. Med. Equip. Supplment.*, May, 33.

Hyperbaric oxygenation

According to Henry's Law, the solubility of the gases in the blood is directly proportional to the pressure of the gases in the alveoli. By increasing the partial pressure of the oxygen in the respired gas mixtures the whole body can, if necessary, be drenched with oxygen. Breathing 100% oxygen at 3 atmospheres pressure is equivalent to an arterial oxygen tension of approximately 2260 mmHg and an oxygen content of 27 vol per 100 ml. At this pressure approximately 20 vol per 100 ml will be carried in combination with haemoglobin, and the remaining 7 vol per 100 ml in solution with the plasma. With a cardiac output of the order of 5000 ml per minute, at least 350 ml of oxygen could be made available to the tissues per minute by the transport of oxygen in simple solution within the plasma; in fact the red cells could be disposed of at this pressure, and, in theory at least, oxygen transport would be satisfactory.

Hyperbaric oxygen therapy is used for increasing the sensitivity of neoplastic cells to radiotherapy. Its use has also been applied to the treatment and management of a multiplicity of conditions, including occlusive vascular disease, carbon monoxide poisoning, infections associated with *Cl. welchii, Cl. tetani,* and *staphylococcus,* haemorrhagic shock, cardiovascular surgery, neurosurgery, and plastic surgery.

The problems of anaesthesia within the hyperbaric chamber (McDowall, 1964) and the problem of anaesthesia for the patient receiving radiotherapy under hyperbaric oxygen conditions (Sanger *et al.*, 1955) have been detailed in the literature.

Hyperbaric anaesthesia. The 'depth' of anaesthesia is a function of the partial pressure of the anaesthetic agents within the blood. By increasing the partial pressure of nitrous oxide, as a result of increase in the ambient pressure, increased depth of anaesthesia can be obtained; however, this carries the risk of bubble formation in the tissues when decompression occurs. If the same effect as 100% oxygen at 3 atmospheres is required, while breathing 80% nitrous oxide and 20% oxygen, then the ambient pressure will have to be greatly increased, with all the attendant increased risks on the staff within the chamber. Nitrous oxide must never be used as a vehicle for halothane under hyperbaric conditions, because it widens the inflammability range of halothane. Halothane in clinical concentrations at 4 atmospheres pressure can be ignited by diathermy, but, provided that it is vaporized in 100% oxygen, it is safe at pressures below 4 atmospheres. Methoxyflurane may be safer at all pressures likely to be used for clinical work. If possible, volatile anaesthetic agents should be avoided altogether and intravenous agents used.

General anaesthesia. Before the induction of anaesthesia, myringotomy must be performed, as damage to the tympanic membrane will result from the inability to swallow and equalize pressures across the ear drums. Flowmeters will not display an accurate and true value under hyperbaric conditions, because the density and viscosity of gases will be altered. McDowall (1964) has calculated the true values of flow from these meters.

The Wright respirometer will over-read at hyperbaric pressures. The performance of vaporizers will also vary: the concentration of a vapour above a liquid is independent of pressure but dependent on ambient temperature, so the doubling of the atmospheric pressure will result in the vapour being diluted in twice the volume of carrier gas, with a resultant halving in concentration. However, as the atmospheric pressure has been doubled and the concentration halved, the partial pressure of the vapour will remain the same. Air at high pressure conducts slightly more heat – therefore the heat to vaporize liquids is more easily supplied. The administration of general anaesthesia under hyperbaric conditions calls for efficient and reliable monitoring equipment.

Pre-oxygenation

This is a valuable procedure and can lead to an increase of the body oxygen stores by as much as 2000 ml. Pre-oxygenation is particularly valuable if a reserve of oxygen is required, e.g. if intubation is thought likely to be difficult and delay may occur in the re-institution of adequate ventilation; it will remove from the lungs appreciable quantities of the diluent nitrogen, and facilitate induction with inhalational agents; it is of use in electro-convulsive therapy, after the administration of the relaxant and prior to the shock. Pre-oxygenation is an essential component of the technique called oxygen diffusion apnoea, which is sometimes employed in the examination of the upper respiratory tract and in bronchoscopy. If it is used, the subject should breathe oxygen on a non-rebreathing system for at least three minutes–longer in the emphysematous patient. The employment of pre-oxygenation is essential in the management of anaesthesia for subjects likely to void stomach contents (e.g. obstetric cases and acute abdomen), and patients with cardiovascular disease, and may be employed in other circumstances.

Oxygen diffusion apnoea

Deliberate apnoea is sometimes employed to facilitate operations on and investigations of the respiratory tract. After a period of pre-oxygenation, and following intravenous induction, a neuromuscular blocking agent is used to produce apnoea. Further oxygen is supplied to the respiratory tract to replace that which is taken up by the pulmonary blood flow. The additional supply of oxygen is usually fed into the tracheo-bronchial tree at the level of the carina, using a gum elastic catheter connected to a source of oxygen, with a flow rate of at least 300 ml/min. Flows of oxygen should not be excessive, because of the drying action and possible damage from high pressure. The amount of carbon dioxide elimination will depend to a certain extent on the flow of the gas. With a fresh gas flow of 10 l/min the mean quantity of carbon dioxide elimination is approximately 20 ml/min (i.e. 13% of carbon dioxide production): in apnoeic cases that receive no insufflation the mean rate of carbon dioxide elimination is approximately 6 ml/min. The extent of the respiratory acidosis is thus directly related to the duration of the apnoea and the amount of fresh gas flow insufflated. There is no doubt that the heart beat will tend to flush some carbon dioxide out of the alveoli, which may reach the carina and stand the chance of elimination from the lungs. Even in the presence of high flow rates of gas, considerable elevation of the arterial carbon dioxide tension is inevitable with this technique, rising as high as 250 mmHg in one hour. However, provided that the method is employed for only a short period of time the level of carbon dioxide retention achieved will not seriously embarrass the patient's own ability to compensate for this change. If the technique is used for a prolonged period of time correction of the pH may be possible with the use of THAM. 0.3 M THAM (36.6 g/l) is given rapidly intravenously in the dose of 0.2–0.3 ml/kg/min. The side effects from the THAM are minimal, particularly if the dose is kept well below 55 mg/kg.

The arterial oxygen tension during apnoeic oxygenation in men has been studied and values in excess of 400 mmHg have been found, even after five miutes of apnoea when oxygen has been replaced from above. However, when air was allowed to diffuse down from above there was a rapid fall of arterial oxygen tension.

Bronchoscopy

This procedure is called for in order to examine the tracheo-bronchial tree for diagnostic or therapeutic purposes and to remove foreign bodies or aspirate bronchial secretions. Many of the patients will be suffering from varying degrees of respiratory decompensation and some will have disability from infective or neoplastic processes. Where general anaesthesia is concerned, the anaesthetist may temporarily have to transfer the care and supervision of the airway to the surgeon.

General anaesthesia. Premedication with effective sedation is advisable. Induction agents with a very short duration of action are not advised and anaesthesia is induced with 2.5% thiopentone followed by 50 mg suxamethonium or a non-depolarizing blocker; after inflation of the lungs with 100% oxygen, the cords and upper trachea are sprayed with either lignocaine or prilocaine. The bronchoscope is introduced into the trachea, and ventilation immediately recommenced by fitting a Magill endotracheal tube into it and rhythmically squeezing the reservoir bag. This tube is removed for such periods of time as are required by the surgeon, but replaced periodically if apnoea is still present, to maintain adequate oxygenation. Complete co-operation between anaesthetist and surgeon is obviously required here. Further intermittent injections of thiopentone are given and suxamethonium may be re-administered if the patient does not settle to quiet breathing on the bronchoscope, or if the surgeon requires an apnoeic patient where a prolonged procedure is anticipated. In order to ensure unconsciousness, the patient may be given a continuous intravenous infusion of thiopentone. Alternatively, halothane 0.5% is blown down the side tube of the bronchoscope, or through a catheter which has been passed down to the level of the carina, prior to the passage of the bronchoscope. The technique of oxygen diffusion apnoea may be preferred and is described on page 223. There have been many modifications of bronchoscopes in order that ventilation may be assured during observations, possibly the best being one which operates on a venturi principle, allowing the surgeon free access to the tracheo-bronchial tree. Inflatable cuirasses have been employed to ensure adequate ventilation, and the passage of a 5.5, 6.0 or 6.5 mm endotracheal tube alongside the bronchoscope with artificial ventilation carried out through it has also been suggested. As there is a very real risk of the patient being aware of what is happening, talking must be forbidden throughout the procedure. Patients with bronchogenic carcinoma may be sensitive to both non-depolarizing and depolarizing blocking agents and care should, therefore, be taken when using these drugs.

Local anaesthesia. An increasing number of surgeons now employ general anaesthesia for bronchoscopy, but there is still a tendency for physicians to carry out diagnostic bronchoscopy under a local anaesthetic. Therapeutic bronchoscopy for aspiration of retained secretions is often carried out in extremely ill patients, and under these circumstances bronchoscopy is frequently managed under topical anaesthesia.

Procedure. The nature of the procedure must be explained where possible to the patient. Adequate sedation should be achieved, bearing in mind the patient's age, temperament and physical status. Intravenous diazepam in divided doses up to 20 mg for an adult is an excellent adjunct, and opiates are best avoided. On arrival in the anaesthetic room the patient should sit and be invited to retain in the mouth, without swallowing, flavoured lignocaine gel 2%. After swilling the mouth the gel should be spat out. The patient should then be made comfortable, with a nurse standing on his left side, supporting his back. The anaesthetist should draw up not more than 10 ml 4% prilocaine, basing the dose on age, weight and physical status – a fit 70 kg individual should receive no more than the above quantities. Holding the patient's tongue between gauze held in the left hand, his throat is thoroughly sprayed. With the patient's mouth wide open and his head extended a Krause's forceps holding a swab soaked in 4% prilocaine solution is placed deliberately and firmly into each pyriform fossa in succession. Each swab is held in position for two minutes, while the patient is instructed to breathe deeply. He may then lie down. After a period of about two minutes, a laryngoscope is gently passed, the glottis visualised and thoroughly sprayed, the jet being passed down between the cords to the level of the carina. The patient must now be made as comfortable as possible. Bronchoscopy may then proceed, and further quantities of solution sprayed down the bronchoscope with the aid of a long-nosed spray. At no time should the maximum safe dose for the particular patient be exceeded.

Some authorities have advocated the injection of anaesthetic solution through the crico-thyroid membrane.

Insufflation anaesthesia

Boulton *et al.* (1965) have pointed out that modern methods of 'insufflation' for bronchography and bronchoscopy are not comparable with the method which was so widely used in the past. In the earlier descriptions of the use of endotracheal insufflation in major surgery, flow rates of 16 to 30 litres were used and muscle relaxants were not employed. Boulton *et al.* (1965) found high flow oxygen/nitrous oxide/ether insufflation a clinically acceptable technique, demonstrating that hypercapnoea did not normally occur when this technique was employed for abdominal surgery. Apnoea was only rarely achieved when very high flow rates were employed, the respiratory minute volumes usually being sufficient to eliminate excess carbon dioxide.

Bronchography

This procedure calls for the sharing of the patient's air passages with the operator. The majority of patients requiring this investigation will be suffering from pulmonary disease and may have varying degrees of impairment of pulmonary function. In addition, as many of the patients have sputum retention, the presence of large quantities may seriously impede the establishment of a quiescent patient.

Local anaesthesia: repeated bronchoscopy and bronchography under topical anaesthesia tend to make patients uncooperative. In order to fill completely the sections of the lung under investigation, it is important to have full topical anaesthesia of the area being observed. It is sometimes difficult to obtain the total co-operation of the patient and so general anaesthesia is often called for. Also the presence of sputum interferes with the achievement of effective anaesthesia.

General anaesthesia: absolute control of pulmonary ventilation is essential. The patient must be quiescent and unable to cough, yet intermittent positive pressure ventilation tends to push the contrast medium into the alveoli and spoils the detail of the X-ray picture: similarly, insufflation with oxygen at high flow rates will interfere with the introduction of the radio-opaque medium. The procedure may be carried out in the darkness of the X-ray department, and there is the ever present danger of explosions if flammable anaesthetic agents are used. All patients should be prepared by postural drainage and where necessary antibiotic therapy administered for several days prior to the procedure. Most physicians and surgeons prefer to aspirate as much pus and secretion as possible before the introduction of the dye, therefore bronchoscopy is regarded by many operators as essential immediately prior to the investigation.

Local anaesthesia. The patient should be prepared as for bronchoscopy under local anaesthesia. His co-operation can be facilitated by the use of intravenous diazepam up to 20 mg in an adult. This method has little to recommend it. Following the introduction of the bronchoscope and the removal of secretions by suction, further topical anaesthesia is achieved by spraying, with a long nozzled spray, down the bronchoscope those parts of the tracheo-bronchial tree that are likely to be involved by the introduction of dye. Great care must be taken to see that the maximum safe dose of the topical agent is not exceeded. Alternatively, a catheter can be passed through the crico-thyroid membrane, using local infiltration, and after injection of a topical solution through the catheter this can then be followed by the contrast medium if necessary.

General anaesthesia. It is probably best to investigate children under general anaesthesia, following sedation perhaps achieved with the appropriate doses of omnopon and scopolamine. However, in our view, opiates should be omitted from the premedication in order not to obtund the cough reflex, as efficient coughing in the post-operative period is essential. A Gordh, Mitchell or similar type needle is placed in a vein, and, following a sleep dose of intravenous thiopentone, relaxation is achieved with suxamethonium: the lungs are inflated with 100% oxygen, tracheo-bronchial aspiration is performed through a bronchoscope and a cuffed endotracheal tube is now put in place. Anaesthesia is maintained with nitrous oxide/oxygen and trichloroethylene or halothane. The contrast medium is introduced through a catheter which has been passed down the endotracheal tube with the patient postured to allow the dye to run down into the area under observation. At the termination of the procedure, a thorough aspiration of the tracheobronchial tree is carried out.

Alternatively, a somewhat similar procedure is used initially, but, following the bronchoscopy, an endotracheal tube is positioned in the trachea and apnoea maintained with intermittent doses of suxamethonium and sleep with intermittent doses of thiopentone; the patient is oxygenated by allowing a flow of oxygen to pass down an independent catheter to the region of the carina. Radio-opaque medium is injected down the tube through another small catheter. The permitted period of apnoea should be judged by the patient's condition: some prefer to complete the bronchogram within three minutes of induction, endeavouring, if possible, to carry out the bronchoscopy and bronchogram on the initial dose of suxamethonium. Clearly, there are advantages in this technique which aims for full and vigorous recovery of cough reflexes within a few minutes of recovery of consciousness. However, it can only be achieved through close and efficient co-operation between the anaesthetist and the operator. In our opinion there is no place for the employment of diethyl ether for this procedure.

Physiotherapy

The anaesthetist is concerned mainly with that branch of physiotherapy that is aimed at the achievement of optimum function of the respiratory system. As a result of pain, there is usually reluctance to expand the lungs fully after abdominal operations, but the pre-operative demonstration of breathing exercises is an excellent insurance against post-operative chest complications and these exercises should be re-instituted as soon as possible post-operatively. Respiratory complications occur because of unwillingness to breathe deeply and to cough; they are often the result of accumulated bronchial secretions.

If physiotherapy is important in patients with no pre-existing respiratory disease, it will be obvious that it is of paramount importance where such disease exists. Prior to an operation, several days of active physiotherapy are often necessary, consisting of instructions in correct breathing and postural drainage, and of encouragement in coughing and expectoration. This latter may be assisted by hard percussion of the chest while the patient coughs, or better still vibrations, with or without pressure. A more recent development is the employment of continuous manual pressure to the chest wall, with over-pressure at maximal expiration.

Post-operatively, these manoeuvres during coughing are of enormous value in voiding bronchial secretions, but it may be necessary to administer an analgesic about 30 minutes beforehand. Trichloroethylene/air, methoxyflurane/air, or nitrous oxide/oxygen may be employed to assist pain relief during this period. Active deep breathing exercises should be encouraged hourly, whilst the patient is awake.

In some cases of collapse of a segment of lung, this may be re-expanded by lying the patient on the sound side, placing the palm of the hand over the collapsed area, and then thumping over this hand with the fist while the patient coughs. Vibrations or rib springing may be employed instead of this. It may be necessary to do this two or three times.

In order to make secretions easier to void during physiotherapy, humidification of inspired air, mucolytics and anti-spasmodics in the form of aerosols, may be prescribed. Inhalations of carbon dioxide may facilitate the expansion of the lungs.

It is also necessary to encourage active leg movements post-operatively in all cases where this is not definitely contraindicated. This helps to prevent venous thrombosis in the legs, with subsequent risk of pulmonary embolism.

8 *Anaesthesia for Abdominal Surgery*

Vomiting and regurgitation

Reports on deaths associated with anaesthesia have focused attention on the fact that vomiting and regurgitation are one of the most important causes of death associated with anaesthesia. With the introduction of muscle relaxants the problem has become more acute since, with these agents, gastric contents may reach the larynx when the protective reflexes are in abeyance. Delayed emptying of the stomach is a well-recognized feature also associated with excessive nervousness, trauma, shock and pregnancy. Intestinal obstruction likewise gives rise to retention of gastric contents with increased risk of regurgitation and vomiting.

The sequelae from contamination of the respiratory tract with gastro-intestinal contents are well recognised. They may vary from acute respiratory obstruction, pulmonary collapse and lung abscess, to the extreme case, usually associated with pregnancy, where the patient succumbs to an acute fulminating pneumonitis, Mendelson's syndrome.

Management. The management of these cases starts with recognition of the type of patient who is likely to vomit and the institution of adequate precautions to prevent the inhalation of stomach contents, should vomiting or regurgitation occur. A patient who has recently ingested a large meal, the patient in shock and the woman in labour are particularly at risk. Some anaesthetists prefer to pass a large-bore stomach tube in the belief that this will ensure that the stomach is fully emptied. It must be stressed that this in no way guarantees that vomiting and regurgitation will be avoided. We feel that it is legitimate to pass a large-bore tube in order to provoke vomiting prior to induction of anaesthesia, where there is evidence that the stomach contains quantities of largely undigested food. Actual aspiration via the tube will not, of course, remove this material. It must be borne in mind, however, that the passage of a tube is extremely unpleasant for the patient, and should only be reserved for the patient who clearly has a full stomach. In all other cases it is probably better not to attempt to pass a stomach tube, but, nevertheless, to assume that the stomach is full. No patient whether there is evidence of a full stomach or not, should be subjected to general anaesthesia, without equipment being available for adequately dealing with the emergency of vomiting or regurgitation should it occur. This equipment should comprise suction apparatus, an endotracheal tube with cuff, a means of inflating the patient and a table on which the patient can be placed for induction of anaesthesia, with facilities for the head of the patient to be raised or lowered above or below the horizontal.

Oesophageal tubes. Cuffed oesophageal tubes have been described, and even advocated for passing under local anaesthesia, prior to induction of general anaesthesia. These tubes are by no means reliable and carry the potential hazard that, if inflated too much, they may rupture the oesophagus. Most anaesthetists would prefer to intubate the trachea, with a cuffed endotracheal tube.

Induction of general anaesthesia. Prior to induction of general anaesthesia the anaesthetist should check that all the equipment is available and working. The suction apparatus should be turned on, the endotracheal tube checked, the cuff tested and a syringe filled with air attached to the tube for immediate inflation of the cuff. In order to ensure that intubation can be carried out with rapidity, the teeth and jaw movements should be checked. The patient should be placed in whatever position the anaesthetist normally prefers for intubation; some anaesthetists prefer the lateral position but the head-up position is probably best. The induction of anaesthesia may be with intravenous agents or with an inhalational agent, bearing in mind that, if intravenous agents are to be used, relaxation of the cardiac sphincter will occur not only with neuromuscular blocking agents, but also anaesthetic agents such as thiopentone. Some anaesthetists mix the neuro-muscular blocking agent with the thiopentone in the same syringe in order to cut down the time from the induction of sleep to full muscle relaxation. Quite apart from the difficulties of miscibility of agents such as thiopentone and suxamethonium, we are against the practice of giving agents mixed together as this does not allow a fair judgement to be made of the patient's true response to each drug individually. Other anaesthetists give intravenous curare, gallamine or pancuronium prior to induction of sleep, but this again carries the hazard that should the needle inadvertently come out of the vein, the patient may remain paralysed but conscious. To obviate some of these risks, a secure venepuncture should be obtained prior to induction of anaesthesia by placing a Mitchell, Gordh or similar indwelling needle in the vein. Where possible the anaesthetist should have an assistant during the period of induction, as the assistant can be of great help in exerting backward pressure on the cricoid cartilage, thus reducing the risk of regurgitation of stomach contents. He can also hold the endotracheal tube in readiness so that the cuff can be immediately inflated once the tube is passed into the larynx. Some anaesthetists prefer to induce anaesthesia with inhalational agents, though such an induction will carry the risk of vomiting if induction is prolonged: agents such as halothane and cyclopropane are more suitable for this purpose than diethyl ether. The deliberate accumulation of carbon dioxide will encourage the patient to breathe deeply and reduce the chances of vomiting – but this technique should not be relied upon entirely to prevent the inhalation of gastro-intestinal contents. For details on induction of general anaesthesia see page 251.

Mendelson's syndrome (acid pulmonary aspiration syndrome). Animal investigations have shown that there exists a critical pH associated with significant pathological changes following aspiration of fluid into the lungs. The critical level of pH appears to be 2.5, and 42.3% of emergency obstetric patients were found to have gastric contents below this critical level (Taylor and Pryce-Davis, 1966). Oral administration of aluminium hydroxide or magnesium trisilicate mixture before induction of general anaesthesia neutralized the gastric contents and maintained the gastric pH above the critical level in the majority of patients. Magnesium trisilicate was the more effective antacid. Recently a mixture of both substances has been claimed to have better neutralizing capacity.

Management of a case of inhaled vomitus: Should inhalation of gastric contents occur, immediate bronchoscopy and tracheo-bronchial toilet should be carried out. Gentle lavage of the tracheo-bronchial tree with normal saline or sodium bicarbonate may be of assistance in reducing the degree of residual damage. Hydro-cortisone may be administered systemically and should always be given when inhalation occurs in association with pregnancy.

Vomiting on recovery from anaesthesia: we recommend the adoption of the lateral or semiprone position at times of extubation or immediately anaesthesia is discontinued, in order to minimize the risk of aspiration of stomach contents.

Post-operative vomiting

Certain operations carry with them a high incidence of nausea and vomiting. Eye operations, ear operations, orthopaedic operations and the operation for dilatation and curettage or evacuation of the uterus in particular are commonly associated with a high incidence of post-operative nausea and vomiting. In the case of eye operations, nausea and vomiting can seriously imperil the success of the procedure. There are many pre-disposing conditions, amongst which are the sex, age and bodily structure of the individual.

A careful history will elicit a tendency to motion sickness and vomiting in relation to previous general anaesthetics, but care must be taken not to create in the patient's mind the fact that he will necessarily vomit post-operatively. Where a history of vomiting in relation to general anaesthesia has been elicited, it is important to find out, where possible, if any agents such as opiates or diethyl ether can be implicated. Clearly, where a particular agent or group of agents can be held responsible, these should not be given to the patient. In situations where post-operative nausea and vomiting could seriously imperil the success of the surgery, agents which are known to predispose to this should be avoided at all costs. Stewart (1963) has reviewed the pharmacological background to vomiting, and those interested in the subject are recommended to this article.

The current trend is to abandon the use of morphine or pethidine before an operation; this may reduce the incidence of vomiting but will probably increase post-operative restlessness. Atropine has anti-emetic properties but the incidence of emetic sequelae following a constant form of general anaesthesia was found to be greater with pethidine 50 mg and atropine 0.6 mg than with atropine alone, whilst morphine 10 mg resulted in even more symptoms than pethidine.

Certain general anaesthetic agents predispose to post-operative nausea and vomiting. Chloroform and diethyl ether carry a high incidence, and to a lesser degree trichloroethylene and cyclopropane. Halothane has been shown to reduce the frequency of post-operative vomiting during the first hour after operation, following premedication with morphine. The incidence of vomiting following methoxyflurane is probably even less. Hypoxaemia and hypotension during general anaesthesia carry with them a high incidence of post-operative nausea and vomiting, particularly in the outpatient.

In all cases of vomiting the anaesthetist must satisfy himself that it has not arisen because of some serious post-operative surgical or medical complications. An obstruction to the bowel or paralytic ileus may be masked by the administration of anti-emetic agents and may seriously hazard the patient's subsequent recovery.

Management of post-operative vomiting

No patients should receive anything by mouth for the first hour post-operatively. Then depending on the surgical contraindications, they may be allowed to take sips of sweetened fruit juice. They should be kept as still as possible, as movement will increase the ocular, vestibular and cerebellar stimuli, and enhance nausea and vomiting: early ambulation should therefore be avoided. Nursing in the prone position reduces the incidence of vomiting. Should it persist, despite the administration of an anti-emetic, all oral intake should be abolished and an intravenous infusion set up. Children are rarely a problem.

Anti-emetic agents. Very many anti-emetic agents are available and some of them are listed in Table 8.1. They may be given prophylactically in the premedication or at the termination of general anaesthesia, or during the post-operative period. Promethazine, atropine or hyoscine may be given in the premedication either alone or in combination with other agents. Haloperidol 5 mg i.v. in early anaesthesia has been suggested, as has perphenazine (Fentazin) 0.07 mg/kg i.m. at the termination of general anaesthesia.

The relative effectiveness of anti-emetic agents has been the subject of much study, some of which is summarized in Table 8.1.

Table 8.1 *Anti-emetic agents*

Approved name	*Proprietary name*	*Dose*
promethazine chlorotheophyllinate	Avomine	25–50 mg oral†
cyclizine	Marzine	50 mg i.m. or oral†
promethazine	Phenergan	25–50 mg i.m. or oral†
dimenhydrinate	Dramamine	50 mg i.m. or oral†
diphenhydramine	Benadryl	50 mg i.m. or oral†
prochlorperazine	Stemetil	12·5 mg i.m. or 5–10 mg oral†
perphenazine	Fentazine	5·0 mg i.m. or 2 mg oral†
thiethylperazine-di-hydrogen-malcate	Torecan	10 mg i.m. or oral†
triflupromazine	Vespral	20 mg i.m. or 10–25 mg oral†
trimethoxybenzamide	Tigan	200–400 mg i.m. or oral†
haloperidol	Serenace	5 mg i.v. or 1·5–3·0 mg oral†
chlorpromazine	Largactil	25–50 mg i.m. or oral†
propriomazine	Indorm	20 mg oral†
trifluoperazine	Stelazine	2–4 mg/day oral†
trimeprazine	Vallergan	0·6–0·9 mg/kg i.m.*
		3·0–4 mg/kg (syrup 6 mg/ml) oral*
metclopramide	Maxolon	10 mg/8h oral†
		10–30 mg/day i.m.†

* children – premed † adults

Oesophagoscopy

The procedure of oesophagoscopy is generally carried for diagnostic purposes and usually under general anaesthesia, though some operators prefer to perform the investigation under topical anaesthesia. The underlying condition giving rise to the investigation may be a neoplastic condition of the oesophagus, oesophageal varices, or hiatus hernia. The patient may be cachetic and there is a very real danger of regurgitation of oesophageal and stomach contents.

Patients requiring general anaesthesia will need to be intubated. This is preferably performed in the sitting or semi-upright posture, the risk of regurgitation being further minimized by an assistant providing cricoid pressure. A cuffed endotracheal tube one or two sizes smaller than that which would be normally passed for the individual, should be passed so that it lies on the left of the tongue and in the left corner of the mouth. Immediately the tube is in position, the cuff should be inflated, though the passage of the oesophagoscope past the cricoid area can be facilitated by momentarily allowing the cuff to deflate, and at the same time producing full relaxation with a dose of suxamethonium: care should be taken, however, to guard against regurgitation. In view of this danger, particularly in the debilitated patient, topical anaesthesia to the larynx must be avoided. The patient should receive careful suction to the pharynx prior to extubation.

Anaesthesia for intra-abdominal operations

The main surgical and anaesthetic requirement for intra-abdominal surgery is relaxation of the anterior abdominal wall. This is best achieved by the use of neuromuscular blocking agents, with or without supplementation and potentiation by narcotic agents. In certain situations the activity of reflexes may produce adverse cardio-vascular effects on the patient; for instance traction on the oesophagus during vagotomy may produce bradycardia, vasoconstriction and sweating. The use of inhalational agents such as halothane, in addition to the neuromuscular blocking agents, reduces to a certain extent the degree of response to the noxious stimuli.

Lower abdominal operations, in particular the repair of inguinal hernia, may not need relaxation, and the patient may therefore be permitted to breathe spontaneously. Where, however, neuro-muscular blocking agents are employed, full control of ventilation must be taken either manually or mechanically in order to ensure that alveolar ventilation is adequate.

Extensive abdominal and pelvic operations, such as abdominoperineal resection of the rectum, are often associated with considerable blood loss and neurogenic shock. Although not necessary as a routine, hypotensive anaesthesia should be considered where blood loss is expected to be severe: spinal subarachnoid or epidural block is extremely effective in reducing bleeding and 'neurogenic' shock. Blood loss should be carefully measured in all these operations and adequately replaced, using the central venous pressure as one of the guides.

Anaesthesia and liver disease

Patients with liver disease may suffer impairment of processes that are responsible for the detoxication of agents used in general anaesthesia; for example, decreased sensitivity to non-depolarizing neuromuscular blocking agents, such as D-tubocurarine, has been noted. Liver damage may also lead to a reduction of plasma cholinesterase and create difficulties when depolarizing neuro-muscular blocking agents are used. Thiopentone is almost entirely destroyed in the body, mainly in the liver, and, in view of this, great caution must be taken when administering this agent to patients with severe liver damage. Even short administrations of chloroform may have serious toxic effects on the liver and depression of function always occurs: it should never be administered to a patient with a history of liver damage either past or present. Furthermore, chloroform is contra-indicated in diabetes mellitus, and in all cases associated with starvation and malnutrition, or when prolonged vomiting is associated with dehydration and electrolyte imbalance. The use of halothane is discussed on pages 45 and 52. Hypofibrinogenaemia may occur in association with cirrhosis of the liver, and give rise to uncontrollable haemorrhage. Pre-operative laboratory tests to ascertain the degree of depression of the plasma fibrinogen level (normal 200–400 mg/100 ml) should be carried out. The critical level at which increased bleeding appears is about 100 mg/100 ml, so 4 g of human fibrinogen should be administered intravenously to those patients suffering from a deficit.

The liver is the site of detoxication of citrate. As impaired detoxication of citrate occurs particularly in association with hypothermia, great care must be taken when transfusing massive quantities of stored citrated blood to the hypothermic patient.

Anaesthesia for patients suffering from disease of the liver

The exploration and removal of stones and obstruction from the biliary ducts, and the combating of haemorrhage from oesophageal varices are the two most common operations. Cholecystectomy and its associated operations require good upper abdominal relaxation. The anaesthetist may be called upon to co-operate with the radiologist during X-ray examination of the biliary tree, as complete cessation of respiratory movement is required during actual exposure of the X-ray film. Operations for the control of haemorrhage vary in detail but it should be borne in mind that these patients usually have severe impairment of liver function and care should be taken over the administration of anaesthetic agents (see above). In addition the patient may be anaemic and exsanguinated and will require careful management of blood replacement.

Cirrhosis of the liver and oesophageal varices

The operation of porto-caval anastomosis is undertaken for the relief of portal hypertension. Patients presenting for such a procedure often have a history of haematemesis and progressive liver failure. Various procedures have been devised for the alleviation of this condition. Porto-caval anastomosis is the procedure commonly employed, but difficulties of access and veins deep in the abdomen may add to the difficulty of the operation. Lieno-renal anastomosis is sometimes employed and on occasion the inferior mesenteric artery has been anastomosed to the inferior vena cava. Hepatic artery ligature ('Reinhoff's operation') may sometimes have a place. Resection of the proximal part of the stomach, to interrupt the venous flow to the oesophageal varices, may be combined with porto-caval anaestomosis if haemorrhage is uncontrollable. A transthoracic approach is often employed. These operations may be of long duration, the patients could be anaemic, have a reduced circulating blood volume on account of haemorrhage and varying degrees of impairment of hepatic function. Because of liver damage they may have a tendency to bleed, plasma pseudocholinesterase may be low, and there may be an increased sensitivity to thiopentone. They may also exhibit an increased tolerance to D-tubocurarine.

Adequate volumes of warmed blood should be available for transfusion. Thiopentone and suxamethonium are to be used with caution, though a grossly prolonged response to suxamethonium is unlikely. Pre-operative Vitamin K and controlled ventilation are necessary; cessation of respiratory movement may be required if the venous system is to be visualized radiographically using the injection of a radio-opaque dye. Care must be taken to avoid undue and unheralded respiratory movement during the period of anastomosis. Halothane should be avoided in these cases.

Some patients with gross liver disease have associated ventilation perfusion abnormalities in the lung that may lead to problems associated with adequate oxygenation during and after operation. Particular attention should be paid to this factor and controlled ventilation may be necessary post-operatively.

Post-operative jaundice

Post-operative jaundice may arise from a variety of causes; it may result from infection, from provoked or coincidental viral infection, from acute septicaemia and post-operative pancreatitis. Hypoxia, hypercapnia, hypothermia and hypotension can also damage the liver. Drugs may provoke a reaction: Phenothiazines can be responsible for an allergic reaction in a hypersensitive person and some patients receiving chlorpromazine become jaundiced. General anaesthetic agents are known to act on the liver, and chloroform, in particular, can give rise to a progressive jaundice as a result of necrosis of centrizonal cells.

Recently there have been reports of jaundice appearing post-operatively in patients who have received halothane anaesthesia. The reaction is said to be characterized in some instances by leucopenia, eosinophilia, drug fever and rash. It must be remembered that viral hepatitis and drug hypersensitivity have similar features, both having a fever, rash, leucopenia, arthralgia and cholestatic jaundice. The time of apperance varies from less than seven days to more than three months. In view of this, the transmission of viral hepatitis by transfusion, venepuncture or any other way, cannot be excluded. An association between hepato-cellular necrosis and halothane has been postulated. Retrospective studies have concluded that halothane is no more toxic to the liver than other anaesthetics. There is no evidence of increased liver damage in patients who have received halothane and who are already suffering from diseases of the biliary tract. Indeed, if there is any connection between halothane and liver damage it must be exceedingly infrequent. There is however, the possibility that there may be some relationship between the use of halothane on more than one occasion for the same patient, with subsequent development of jaundice. But so low must be the incidence of this occurrence, that halothane should not be contraindicated on these grounds. It might be better not to use halothane more than once in a period of four weeks. However, if there is a history of unexplained fever and jaundice after halothane, this should contraindicate its subsequent use for that particular patient.

Burst abdomen

Patients with 'burst abdomen' are usually very ill and often poorly prepared; they may be suffering from paralytic ileus and have a full stomach, and electrolyte and water imbalance may add to the anaesthetist's difficulties. The electrolyte picture should be determined and corrected as far as possible by the intravenous administration of suitable solutions. Full precautions should be adopted to avoid the inhalation of intestinal contents.

These are always major operations and should never be approached with the idea that the procedure will be short and simple. Even when only a small amount of peritoneum appears to have given way, the whole of the incision very often has to be resutured, as the defect is far more extensive than appearances would suggest. The major problem from the point of view of the surgical procedure is to effectively close the abdomen in the minimum time.

In view of the possibility of electrolyte imbalance and increased sensitivity to non-depolarizing neuro-muscular blocking agents, those such as suxamethonium may be employed, but in reduced quantity. Relaxation is particularly important during closure of the abdomen, where distended intestines will tend to make the task of the surgeon extremely difficult.

Intestinal obstruction

Intestinal obstruction, if it has been established for some time, may be associated with acid-base disturbance as well as electrolyte and water deficiency, while reduction of circulating blood volume may arise from strangulation and hyperaemia of the bowel. Such patients are often extremely ill and debilitated, may be sensitive to general anaesthetic agents and have a prolonged response to neuro-muscular blocking agents. Respiratory embarrassment may be caused by intestinal distension.

Time should be allowed for adequate pre-operative preparation of the patient, particular attention being paid to the replacement of water and electrolyte deficiency. They are often in a state of shock, and gastro-intestinal decompression by continuous suction, together with replacement of water and electrolytes, will greatly improve this condition. There is much to be said in favour of delay in operating, so that the shock can be adequately dealt with. Care must be taken, however, to ensure that there is not actual strangulation of the bowel.

Anaesthesia for intestinal obstruction. Apart from the disturbance to electrolyte and water balance, these patients present an additional hazard to the anaesthetist on account of the danger of regurgitation and vomiting. Gastric suction will not ensure against this hazard. Efficient and reliable suction must be at hand and the anaesthetic administration handled in such a way as to overcome this problem immediately by suction should it arise, and to reduce the possibility as much as possible. The patient should be placed on the operating table and anaesthesia induced either in the upright or head-down position according to the preference of the anaesthetist. Following pre-oxygenation, induction of anaesthesia may be carried out using intravenous agents and a short acting relaxant such as suxamethonium. General anaesthesia should be employed for, despite the grave condition of the patient, conduction block is often unsuitable on account of the distension of the bowel. Until the bowel has been decompressed, the surgeon will require full relaxation of the anterior abdominal wall. Evisceration may be necessary and this will at times be disturbing for the patient and may result in a temporary fall in blood pressure. The surgeon also experiences difficulties in approximating the abdominal wall at the termination of the operation. The volume of gas within the lumen of the bowel may increase 75–100% in two hours during the administration of nitrous oxide, and increase 100–200% in four hours. (A similar problem is experienced in association with a pneumothorax, where the volume can double in 10 minutes, triple in 45 minutes and quadruple in 2 hours and also exists in relation to general anaesthesia associated with pneumoencephalography). No such changes occur with oxygen and halothane. Faced with these difficulties of closure, the anaesthetist is often tempted to give an extra dose of relaxant. A short acting depolarizing agent such as suxamethonium should never follow the administration of a non-depolarizing agent. Indeed, we doubt the wisdom of using additional doses of relaxants for this purpose and suggest that any further relaxation required can be obtained by deepening anaesthesia with halothane or cyclopropane. In view of the likelihood of electrolyte disturbances, relaxants, particularly non-depolarizing agents, should be kept to the minimum, and relaxation obtained by the employment of the synergistic action of small quantities of relaxant together with an inhalational agent such as halothane, cyclopropane, or ether. The withdrawal of the inhalational agent towards the end of anaesthesia usually allows the return of spontaneous breathing, with only a small degree of neuro-muscular blockade which can be readily reversed with neostigmine. Post-operative ventilatory support should be employed, if there is any suggestion that ventilation is likely to be inadequate.

9 *Obstetrics and Gynaecology*

Pain relief in obstetrics

When considering pain relief in obstetrics, it should be remembered that at least two lives are involved. Pain relief should be as effective as possible, and should in no way conflict with the well-being of mother and child. In particular, uterine activity should not be impaired, prolonging the course of labour and hazarding the life of the child; the mother should not be made excessively drowsy or unco-operative; there should be no respiratory or cardiovascular depression of mother or child. If general anaesthesia is employed, particular care should be taken to guard against the well recognized hazards of vomiting or regurgitation of stomach contents. It is, in fact, impossible to satisfy any of these criteria to the full with present day methods. All agents at present used to sedate and relieve pain in labour cross the placenta to a varying degree and thus the baby is liable to be influenced by the substances.

Management of pain relief in labour

It cannot be overstressed that the management of pain relief commences in the antenatal period. The sympathetic and understanding midwife or doctor can do much to relieve the anxieties of the expectant mother. A thorough explanation of the physiology of child-birth in simple terms is essential. The antenatal instruction should include a talk on how it is possible, with the mother's co-operation, to minimize pain, pointing out that drugs and techniques are readily available to assist her; and further, that she will be able to administer and control some of these agents herself, if she so wishes. At the same time, care must be taken to avoid creating in her mind particularly if a primigravida, that pain is necessarily a major feature of childbirth. It must be stressed that she herself, by co-operating with the obstetrician, midwife and anaesthetist, can do much to help in bringing about effective relief. Antenatal exercises, particularly those which train the women to relax mentally and physically, have a very distinct place in the preparation for childbirth. Some anaesthetists attach more importance to these than others, but there is no doubt that a mother who has had adequate and correct antenatal instruction will benefit.

With the advent of intensive care facilities and the ability to monitor not only maternal but also foetal cardiovascular and acid-base status, there has been an increasing trend towards the deliberate induction and control of labour. Linked closely with this management has been the resurgence of the epidural method of pain control.

Nutrition. Clearly it is neither in the interest of the mother, nor the baby, for fluid and calorie intake to be limited, particularly as labour may be unpredictably long and arduous. Whilst recognizing the very real dangers associated with the inhalation of acid gastric contents in the parturient woman it must be assumed that the stomach is likely to contain material whether the patient has had oral nutrition or not. Feeding must be directed in such a way as to avoid the ingestion of solids, and a sieved diet is to be preferred. Liquids containing isotonic glucose may be permitted, with the proviso that adequate facilities and equipment are available to the anaesthetist should general anaesthesia subsequently become necessary. Mist. magnesium trisilicate, 10–20 ml, should be given routinely 2 hourly during labour in order to reduce gastric acidity and keep the pH above the critical level of 2.5. This is in case general anaesthesia, with the attendant hazard of reflex and aspiration, should become necessary. A further dose must be given immediately prior to induction of anaesthesia. Alternatively Andursil (aluminium hydroxide magnesium hydroxide mixture) may be given in a dose of 5–10 ml 6-hourly.

Use of drugs

The individuals responsible for pain relief have a wide variety of combinations of drugs available. There is as yet no standard form of medication universally accepted, and each hospital tends to develop its own particular pharmacological permutation. In the early part of labour there is likely to be general discomfort with backache; here the application of warmth and massage to the back will establish the correct relationship between the mother and the person managing the labour. In primigravidae in particular, the use of hypnotic agents at this stage is of value in encouraging sleep, and this, together with oral fluids and carbohydrate, will conserve the patient's strength for what lies ahead. Powerful analgesics are usually avoided at this stage, unless it is thought that labour is likely to progress rapidly.

Sedatives and analgesics. (See Table 9.1). The barbiturates at one time enjoyed popularity as hypnotics in the early part of labour, but as they are foetal respiratory depressants they should not be used in large doses, particularly if delivery is likely within a few hours. They are probably better avoided altogether, except for perhaps the case where labour fails after a short start and it is necessary to give a good night's sleep. In any

Table 9.1 *Some drugs used to relieve pain in labour*

Drug	*Dose*	*Route*	*Hypnosis*	*Analgesia*
chloral hydrate	1·2–2 g	oral	++	0
chloral hydrate syrup	5–20 ml	oral	++	0
dichloralphenazone (Welldorm)	2–3 tabs	oral	++	0
triclofos (Tricloryl)	0·59–1·0 g tabs. or syrup	oral	++	0
paraldehyde	2–8 ml	oral	++	0
	2–8 ml	i.m.		
barbiturates				
amylobarbitone sodium (Sodium Amytal)	0·1–0·2 g	oral	++	0
pentobarbitone (Nembutal)	0·1–0·2 g	oral	++	0
butobarbitone (Soneryl)	0·1–0·2 g	oral	++	0
quinalbarbitone (Seconal)	0·1–0·2 g	oral	++	0
*aspirin	0·3–1 g	oral	+	+
*codeine	10–60 mg	oral	+	+
DF118	30–60 mg	oral	++	++
	20–30 mg	i.m.		
scopolamine	0·4 mg	oral or i.m.	+	0
†phenothiazines				
chlorpromazine (Largactil)	25–50 mg†	oral or i.m.	+	0
promazine (Sparine)	25–50 mg†	oral or i.m.	+	0
promethazine (Phenergan)	25–50 mg†	oral or i.m.	+	0
*tinct. opii	0·25–2·0 ml	oral	++	+++
morphine	8–20 mg	oral or i.m.	++	+++
omnopon	8–20 mg	oral or i.m.	++	+++
diamorphine (Heroin)‡	5–10 mg	oral or i.m.	++	+++
*pentazocine (Fortral)	30–45 mg	oral or i.m.	+	+++
*pethidine	100–150 mg	oral or i.m.	+	+++
*pethilorfan	100–150 mg	oral or i.m.	+	+++

* These analgesics are at the disposal of the midwife

† Phenothiazines can be given with opiates or pethidine: for example, sparine 25 mg, pethidine 50 mg (always use reduced doses when together)

Better not to exceed 100 mg total dose

‡ Said to produce less respiratory depression, in the baby, than morphine

case, the longer acting barbiturates (e.g. phenobarbitone) should not be given at all and the shorter acting agents not given if delivery is anticipated within six hours. They tend to produce restlessness, particularly if the patient is in pain. On the whole, it is better to give drugs which are more rapidly excreted. Chloral hydrate is still commonly used by midwives. It is a good sedative in large doses, if pain is not a major feature; unfortunately, with large doses it is an irritant to the gastric mucosa, so that some prefer to use the less irritating derivatives, dichloral phenazone (Welldorm) or triclofos (Tricloryl). Tinct. opii is permitted by the Central Midwives Board to be given to mothers in labour and it is often useful when severe pain is becoming a feature. Paraldyde, largely because of its unpleasant smell, has fallen out of favour; methylpentynol (Oblivon) can be given in 250 mg doses by mouth. Hyoscine, together with morphine, was widely used in the early part of this century, the so-called 'Twilight Sleep'. Its claim to fame arose from the belief that amnesia occurred in many of the patients. It would appear that this was true, but this advantage was outweighed by the serious depression of the baby and the production of an unco-operative mother. Intramuscular hyoscine and pethidine have also been used during the first stage of labour: keeping the total dose of pethidine to 150 mg and the dose of hyoscine not more than 0.6 mg, and administering nitrous oxide/oxygen when required, the risk of depressing the baby has proved to be small. Mild analgesics such as codeine phosphate 10–60 mg have been administered in the early part of labour, as also the more powerful dihydrocodeine bitartrate (DF 118) 20–30 mg. Unfortunately, the powerful analgesics such as morphine, papaveretum, pethidine, diamorphine and pentazocine are all powerful depressants of the respiratory centre. In an attempt to overcome this depressant effect, these agents have been combined with analeptics and also, in reduced dose, with the phenothiazines. Morphine, Omnopon and diamorphine may all be given in doses of 10 mg; diamorphine is said by some to be more reliable in its action.

Levallorphan tartrate 1.25 mg in combination with 100 mg of pethidine, is known as Pethilorphan, and is said to be less depressing to the respiratory centre than pethidine: this combination is probably better not used, however, because of the unreliability of its action as an analgesic. The mixture of 100 mg pethidine and 5 mg nalorphine has been claimed to reduce the respiratory depressant effects of pethidine by about half. The analgesic effect of this mixture is probably at least as good as pethidine alone, labour is said not to be prolonged and there is no increase in the necessity for operative interference. The combination of morphine and tetrahydroaminacrine is also said to be satisfactory, but care must be taken if general anaesthesia is being contemplated in a patient who has received tetrahydroaminacrine, as the latter is known to potentiate the action of suxamethonium.

Pethidine alone, or in combination with other agents, may be given once labour is established. Opinions vary concerning how much should be given in any one labour, or how late in labour such agents should be employed. On average not more than 300–400 mg should be given in twenty-four hours, starting with a big dose (150 mg), 'topping up' with progressively smaller doses and ceasing within 3–4 hours of anticipated delivery. Clearly many factors must be borne in mind by the person responsible for the analgesia, i.e. the state of the mother, the progress of labour, the condition of the foetus, the total quantity of drugs given, whether any other agents such as phenothiazines have been employed and the time of the anticipated delivery of the baby.

Another way of overcoming the respiratory depressant effect of these agents is to reduce the dosage and combine the drug with a phenothiazine derivative. Many combinations of drugs have been employed, but perphenazine (Fentazine), chlorpromazine (Largactil) or promazine (Sparine) combined with pethidine are perhaps most commonly used. Chlorpromazine also sedates the patient, but has the disadvantage of tending to cause vasomotor instability. Chlorpromazine and pethidine have also been used in labour on a wide scale, while promethazine seems to have achieved considerable popularity, using doses of 25–50 mg of either chlorpromazine, promethazine or promazine in conjunction with 50–100 mg pethidine. Methotrimeprazine 15 mg and pethidine 75 mg or 3 mg haloperidol (Serenace) with pethidine 100 mg intramuscularly, may be given for pain relief. Droperidol (Droleptan), diazepam (Valium) and nitrazepam (Mogadon) have all been employed in obstetric practice. Phencyclidine (Sernyl) was claimed to produce adequate analgesia for most obstetric interventions and have no adverse effect on the baby: unfortunately, most patients developed catatonic stupor with bizarre hallucinations, but, if the psychotropic effect could be controlled or eliminated by simple means, then it would be a very useful drug. Recent evidence suggests that another 'dissociative agent' ketamine (Ketalar) may be more promising. Gamma-hydroxy-butyric acid and chlormethiazone (Heminevrin) may also have a place. As a general rule, if the progress of labour is satisfactory, it is wiser to supplement the basal analgesic effect of these powerful agents with volatile and gaseous agents, or conduction anaesthesia. The conduction agents are not, however, as rapidly eliminated from the body as the gaseous and volatile and there is some risk of affecting the baby. The two inhalational agents commonly employed today are nitrous oxide and trichloroethylene, though methoxyflurane is increasing in popularity. All these substances can be administered by midwives, provided certain criteria are satisfied (C.M.B. rules).

Inhalational agents

Nitrous oxide. Nitrous oxide and air was first introduced into obstetric practice by S. Klikovitch in 1880. For many years the Minnit gas/air machine and other gas/air machines were used for pain relief in labour. The Minnit gas/air machine was specified to deliver 50%/50% gas/air for tidal volumes up to 500 ml with a respiratory rate of 12 to 18 per minute. Furthermore, it was specified by the Central Midwives Board (C.M.B.) that the oxygen concentration should not fall below 10.4%, because breathing these mixtures, patients would be subjected to hypoxia. Studies of patients in labour have shown tidal volumes of 350–2250 ml with rates of 12 to 72 per minute, and minute volumes varying from 7–90 litres. However, gas/air machines have been shown to deliver 12%

oxygen within the range 5–9 l/min, but when subjected to minute volumes of 40–50 l/min the oxygen percentage falls to the region of 8%. Further studies of gas/air machines have revealed that the majority of machines violated C.M.B. rules and some appliances were potentially dangerous, depressing the arterial oxygen saturation in the mother. In an effort to ensure more adequate oxygen for the mother, without sacrificing pain relief, the Lucy Baldwin machine was introduced. This machine allows mixtures of nitrous oxide and oxygen, containing no more than 70% nitrous oxide, and automatically cuts off the nitrous oxide, if the oxygen source fails. It was found that 70/30 nitrous oxide/oxygen gives optimum analgesia with retention of co-operation of the mother: there was no advantage to be found in using concentrations higher than 70%.

In 1945 the use of premixed gases was suggested, and in 1961 the British Oxygen Company introduced cylinders of premixed nitrous oxide 50% and oxygen 50% (Entonox). In certain parts of the world cooling will occur, particularly if storage is out of doors or the cylinders are used in domicillary work. It was soon realized that cooling could cause phase separation below −7°, but this risk could be overcome by warming the cylinders, inverting three times and then keeping them in the horizontal position. If phase separation occurs with cooling, the cylinders will deliver an oxygen-rich mixture early in life and a nitrous oxide-rich mixture later on. Ideally nitrous oxide/oxygen cylinders should be stored in an environment where the temperature does not fall below 10°C.

There is no doubt that nitrous oxide/oxygen correctly self-administered can bring considerable benefit to the patient, provided that she learns to inhale the mixture prior to the onset of pain. By careful timing and observation, inhalations can commence so that appreciable blood levels of nitrous oxide are attained before pain reaches its peak. The theoretical and yet unproven possibility that the Fink effect might occur in the baby after delivery, bears consideration.

Trichloroethylene. Trichloroethylene and air have been used since 1943. The Tecota inhaler and Emotril inhaler will deliver 0.5% and 0.35% trichloroethylene in air, regardless of ambient temperature, as they have a temperature compensator incorporated within them. Care should be taken with the Emotril inhaler, however, when using it under hyperbaric conditions or at high altitude. Patients receiving a general anaesthetic, who have had trichloroethylene administered to them during the course of labour should not be allowed to have a closed circuit anaesthetic for fear of the exhaled trichloroethylene reacting with soda lime. Although trichloroethylene is a cheap, effective analgesic (and the equipment readily portable) prolonged administration leads to drowsiness and lack of co-operation on the part of the mother.

Methoxyflurane. The use of methoxyflurane in obstetric work has been reported. 0.35% methoxyflurane is significantly better than trichloroethylene as far as pain relief, restlessness and effect on the course of labour are concerned. There is no evidence that methoxyflurane administered in this concentration is nephrotoxic.

Evidence available at the time of writing suggests that oxygen enrichment of the inspired mixture may be beneficial to the foetus, and therefore present opinion favours the use of unaugmented nitrous oxide/oxygen mixtures which, in addition, allow a rapid recovery. Throughout the administration of the inhalational mixtures it is essential to maintain the mother's co-operation, so that intermittent administration is advisable unless a suitable concentration can be found; this may be achieved by using the Entonox or the Lucy Baldwin machine, which allows continuous administration and, at the same time, maintains adequate analgesia.

Placental transmission

The important factors which govern the selection of drugs for placental transmission are well known. It may be safely assumed that the majority of agents employed in obstetric analgesia and anaesthesia will traverse the placenta to a varying degree. Whether the agent is harmful to the foetus is dependent on the nature of the substance and the amount transferred, as any substance found in the maternal or foetal blood will be able to penetrate the placenta to some extent, unless it is destroyed or altered during passage. However, a very low degree of permeability may slow the entry to a rate which renders a drug physiologically inactive and pharmacologically undetectable. All membranes allow the transfer of non-ionized drugs more readily than those which are ionized: passage is favoured by pH in the direction which increases the concentration of the undissociated form, so non-ionized drugs with a high fat solubility are transferred rapidly, whereas lipoid insoluble agents penetrate poorly. Other factors influence placental transfer, such as the concentration, gradient, distribution, protein binding, and metabolism and excretion by mother and infant, as well as factors which influence the permeability of the placenta (such as disease, circulatory upset and asphyxia.)

Relaxants. Drugs containing the quaternary nitrogen group are highly ionized and possess a low degree of fat solubility. Suxamethonium and tubocurarine are examples of these and, therefore, they tend to cross the placenta more slowly. In clinical doses of D-tubocurarine and pancuronium only traces are found in the foetus, and, despite the alleged sensitivity of the newborn to non-depolarizing neuro-muscular blocking agents, there appears to be no detrimental effect upon the baby. It has been found that suxamethonium does not cross the placenta in demonstrable quantities in the usual clinical dose. Decamethonium iodide in 3 mg doses has been administered with no apparent ill effect on the baby, but gallamine is found in foetal serum in readily detectable and probably significant amounts after administration to the mother; therefore it should not be used.

Thiopentone. It was at one time thought that there was a partial delay in thiopentone transmission through the placenta for up to ten minutes, and after that time the concentration increased in the foetus for a further ten minutes or so. Recent work has disproved this, and present evidence suggests that the barbiturate content of the foetal blood is a variable fraction of the maternal content, irrespective of time. Thiopentone produces anaesthesia in the mother by a high plasma concentration, quickly binding itself in the maternal circulation to plasma protein and entering muscle. It is only if intermittent injection is performed that the thiopentone accumulates in the foetus and produces harmful effects. In normal induction doses thiopentone is unlikely to depress the baby.

Methohexitone. Methohexitone rapidly crosses the placenta with peak umbilical venous concentration occurring 2–3 minutes after the maternal injection. However, there seems to be no reason why methohexitone should not be used in obstetric work.

Propanidid. Because of its rapid distribution and breakdown, propanidid may have a place in obstetrical anaesthesia. It should probably not be given to the unpremedicated Caesarean section because of fear of consciousness during the operation, if reliance for the maintenance of unconsciousness is placed upon nitrous oxide/oxygen alone.

Althesin. Because of its short duration of action this drug may lend itself as an induction agent in obstetric anaesthesia. Awareness in anaesthesia may however be a problem, unless an adjunct to nitrous oxide is used.

Pethidine. When pethidine is given intravenously to a pregnant patient, it begins to reach the foetus in measurable quantities within two minutes. Significantly more pethidine reaches the foetus after intravenous than intramuscular injection as, following the intramuscular administration of pethidine to a pregnant patient at term, slightly less than 10% of the dose reaches the foetus during the subsequent few hours. If given intravenously pethidine should be administered just before the start of a uterine contraction, to minimize placental transfer. Pregnant women and neonates preferentially excrete pethidine (in urine) in the unchanged state.

Promazine. Results of urine analyses suggest that approximately 0.5% of the amount of promazine given intravenously to the mother reaches the foetus. A small amount of promazine is retained in the placental tissue. Studies of the pattern of urinary excretion of pethidine, promazine, and a selection of their metabolites, suggest that the metabolism of these agents is rendered somewhat deficient during pregnancy.

Local anaesthetics

In the past, local anaesthetic techniques have been employed in many cases because it was thought that these were less harmful than general anaesthetics to the babies, but recent work suggests that local anaesthetic agents also traverse the placenta and affect the baby. Methaemoglobinaemia induced by prilocaine administered as a continuous epidural block may occur in the foetus as well as the mother. The presence of methaemoglobin may produce cyanosis in the baby and lead to difficulties in diagnosis.

Hyperventilation occurs during well established labour. As foetal asphyxia has been reported in subjects where low levels of arterial carbon dioxide tension have been found in the mother during labour, it is probable that prolonged hyperventilation may be harmful to the baby, possibly because of reduction of the mother's cardiac output. Where induction/delivery time is short, hyperventilation is probably not harmful, but it would appear to be unwise to rely upon the hyperventilation technique for obstetric anaesthesia, not only because of the remote chance of harm to the baby, but also because of the danger of consciousness. Present evidence suggests that it is probably of value to maintain maternal normocapnia during general anaesthesia.

Effect of drugs upon the uterus

Adrenaline. Although a single intravenous injection of noradrenaline to the mother produces a transient bradycardia in the foetus, this is less common with adrenaline. It is suggested that the bradycardia is due to uterine vasoconstriction with subsequent foetal hypoxia: consequently many believe that, by virtue of their potentially deleterious effect on the foetal environment, vasopressor agents are contraindicated during pregnancy, unless essential for maternal survival. However, adrenaline may be employed to balance the absorption of local anaesthetic solution which in itself is harmful to the foetus.

Inhalational anaesthetic agents. Trichloroethylene and 'light' cyclopropane have no effect upon uterine contraction, but 'deep' cyclopropane decreases muscle tone and produces some inhibition of contractions.

Nitrous oxide has no effect on uterine contraction, whilst diethyl ether and chloroform inhibit according to depth, due to direct action.

Halothane causes a dose dependent uterine relaxation and can give rise to alarming bleeding during, and after, delivery, which may fail to respond to oxytocic drugs. The specific action in relaxing the uterus is, however, sometimes of value, as in external cephalic version, and operative delivery when manipulations are hindered by uterine hypertonicity, and occasionally in manual removal of the placenta and acute inversion of the uterus. Halothane is not recommended by us for obstetrical anaesthesia except when uterine relaxation is needed. Some highly skilled anaesthetists hold contrary views and commonly use 'light' halothane anaesthesia at the same time administering oxytocic drugs.

Suxamethonium. There is no evidence that suxamethonium has any direct action on uterine musculature.

Vomiting. It has been recognized for some time now that there are very real dangers in the vomiting and regurgitation of acid gastric contents associated with general anaesthesia in obstetric patients. Inhalation of gastric contents in the parturient woman may lead to a fulminating pneumonitis, terminating in death in a proportion of patients. It must be fully appreciated that delayed emptying of the stomach may occur despite the absence of recent feeding, so it is safer to assume that the stomach is full. Some authorities advocate the passage into the stomach of a tube and the supposed emptying of the stomach : in our opinion, besides being distressing for the patient, this procedure in no way ensures that the stomach is empty. Others advocate the use of apomorphine induced vomiting: again, we feel that there is no justification for the use of this unpleasant technique. It is wiser to ensure that only fluids and alkalis have been taken by mouth and to anticipate that the patient may well vomit or regurgitate on induction.

Therefore, before commencing anaesthesia, the patient must be placed on a bed or table which will enable the head to be lowered or raised according to the anaesthetist's wishes. A thoroughly reliable suction apparatus must be available at the patient's head, checked and working, and a selection of cuffed endotracheal tubes chosen, the cuffs of which have been tested for leaks and with an inflating syringe attached ready to inflate the cuff. A malleable introducer should be at hand. It is absolutely essential to have an assistant present prior to, and during, induction of anaesthesia. The degree of opening of the mouth and characteristics of the teeth should always be determined prior to induction of anaesthesia.

Posture of patient. Anaesthetists differ as to the position in which anaesthesia is induced; the sitting position is advocated by some. Using the head-up position, intubation is best facilitated by the use of suxamethonium. Others advocate the lateral position for the induction of anaesthesia but, whatever position is employed, cuffed endotracheal intubation must be carried out. Cricoid pressure by the assistant should always be used to reduce the chances of regurgitation of stomach contents. It should be borne in mind that in some patients the adoption of the supine position results in hypotension arising from compression on the inferior vena cava by the gravid uterus, and for this reason a rubber wedge has been developed for tilting the patient laterally. The use of the lateral position for general anaesthesia and intubation will depend on the skill of the anaesthetist, and the co-operation of the obstetrician. One grave disadvantage of the use of local techniques such as pudendal block is that, should the technique fail or the obstetrician subsequently require general anaesthesia, the anaesthetist will be confronted with a patient in the lithotomy position with the obstetrician urgently requiring an unconscious patient. *Under no circumstances should anaesthesia be induced in the lithotomy position.* For choice the anaesthetic technique most familiar to the anaesthetist should be the one employed, remembering that induction with any agent may be associated with regurgitation.

Mendelson's syndrome. Should the inhalation of stomach contents occur, immediate therapy is needed. Gentle bronchoscopy, suction and lavage of the tracheo-bronchial tree with normal saline or 5% sodium bicarbonate solution should be carried out: careless bronchoscopy might well aggravate the condition. Hydrocortisone 100 mg should be given intravenously and the patient maintained on further doses of intramuscular cortisone and, in addition, ventilation with 100% humidified oxygen through an endotracheal tube may be indicated. The prophylatic administration of antacids in all obstetric patients should be standard practice; the oral administration of colloidal aluminium hydroxide, or better still, magnesium trisilicate, 15–30 minutes before the commencement of the operation, reduces the gastric acidity significantly in obstetric patients. A combination of these two substances known as Andursil has good buffering properties.

General anaesthesia

The movement of the jaws and the characteristics of the teeth must be ascertained before the induction of anaesthesia. The patient is placed in the position to which the anaesthetist is most accustomed. A vein should be sought and an intravenous cannula, such as Gordh or Mitchell needle established within the vein.

Premedication. Atropine 0.6 mg or hyoscine 0.4 mg intravenously should be administered prior to the induction of anaesthesia or promethazine 50 mg intra-muscularly may be given one hour pre-operatively. Pre-oxygenation with 100% oxygen is then carried out for at least three minutes.

Induction. A sleep dose of 2.5% thiopentone is given slowly. With shorter acting agents such as propanidid there is a very real danger of consciousness during anaesthesia. 100 mg of suxamethonium is then given; this produces optimal conditions for uncomplicated intubation. (Manual inflation of the lungs before intubation should not follow as this may provoke regurgitation.) Cuffed endotracheal intubation is now carried out using the procedure outlined on page 194.

Maintenance. Anaesthesia is maintained with nitrous oxide/oxygen 70/30. In order that adequate oxygen may be given, and hyperventilation avoided, cyclopropane, light ether, or trichloroethylene can be used to avoid the risk of consciousness. Soda lime should not be used when employing trichloroethylene. As soon as spontaneous ventilation recommences D-tubocurarine 30 mg or pancuronium 4–6 mg is given and controlled ventilation maintained. Some anaesthetists prefer to give intermittent suxamethonium, or to use a 'drip' of suxamethonium, tetrahydroaminacrine (Tacrine) may be used to potentiate the suxamethonium. Initially 20 mg tetrahydroaminacrine and 25 mg suxamethonium are given intravenously – this usually produces paralysis lasting about 14 minutes, and continued relaxation is achieved by further doses of suxamethonium (the average total dose of suxamethonium being about 60 mg). There are no serious side effects in the mother and child. Tetrahydroaminacrine crosses the placenta and is a powerful morphine antagonist. It should be remembered that there is an incidence of severe muscle pain in about 16% of cases following the use of suxamethonium for Caesarean section. Owing to the risk of dual block non-depolarizing neuromuscular blocking agents may be preferred. Thought should be given as to whether hyperventilation is admissible, as evidence is collecting which suggests that this may lead to a reduction of placental blood flow and resultant foetal acidosis.

Ergometrine or oxytocin are used to encourage uterine contraction. It should be remembered that ergometrine constricts alpha and beta blood vessel receptors giving rise to hypertension and sometimes pulmonary oedema. Oxytocin, on the other hand, causes transient dilatation of alpha and beta vessels and may cause hypotension (alpha vessels are those supplying kidney, skin, splanchnic and meningeal regions whereas beta vessels supply skeletal muscle).

Oxytocin: the posterior pituitary hormone, oxytocin, which may contain vasopressor contaminant vasopressin, has been held responsible for the occurrence of ventricular fibrillation in a parturient patient receiving cyclopropane. As cardio-vascular shock has been reported in a patient receiving an intravenous dose of oxytocin under the influence of halothane, it would appear to be unwise to exhibit oxytocin in the presence of trichloroethylene, halothane or cyclopropane. It has been suggested that oxytocin when administered by continuous infusion, may modify the response of the motor end plate to suxamethonium so that the action of the latter may present features of a non-depolarizing block. This fact, however, has not really been substantiated.

When the baby is about to be delivered, or just after, the intravenous injection of ergometrine is often required, though this can cause a rise in blood pressure or pulmonary oedema, particularly in toxaemic women. Syntometrine, which does not contain natural oxytocin, but is a mixture of synthetic Syntocinon (which is free from vasopressor activity) and ergometrine, is sometimes used instead of pure ergometrine and is effective, but it is regarded as a potential hazard by some.

Following the delivery of the baby by Caesarean section, it is unnecessary to give further relaxants, as no difficulty will be experienced by the obsetrician in closing the flaccid abdominal wall. Some authorities maintain anaesthesia with intravenous pethidine, or cyclopropane, from this stage until the end of the operation. Ventilation is assisted where necessary and neuromuscular blockade reversed at the termination of the operation.

Anaesthesia for forceps delivery. Undoubtedly pudendal block is of great value for forceps delivery, but should difficulties arise in delivering the baby under pudendal block, the subsequent administration of general anaesthesia, which is called for in a hurry, poses problems for the anaesthetist. The use of epidural (single dose) or 'saddle block' spinal subarachnoid anaesthesia may be of value here.

Anaesthesia for external version. The ability of general anaesthesia to reduce uterine tone is sometimes used in the antenatal period, when there is a reasonable prospect of turning the baby with a relaxed uterus. The procedure is optimally performed around the 36th to 37th week of pregnancy. Obstetric contraindications are hypertension, toxaemia, a small baby with lack of liquor, any evidence of placental insufficiency, or any history of bleeding or previous Caesarean section. Deep halothane anaesthesia is generally suitable.

Heart failure in obstetric practice. Patients with cardio-vascular disease may develop cardiac failure during the latter few weeks of pregnancy, when the blood volume increases. If the patient can be tided over the delivery there is often a dramatic improvement in her condition. Anaesthesia should take into account the fact that incipient pulmonary oedema may be present, so a quick acting diuretic such as i.v. frusemide (20 mg) should be administered two hours pre-operatively. Digitalis, or other agents to control cardiac dysrhythmias, may be required. Patients should receive induction of anaesthesia with head up and lying towards the left side, in order to obviate the supine hypotensive syndrome. Preoxygenation, the administration of intravenous aminophylline and the application of venous tourniquets should be considered.

Intravenous induction agents are best avoided; however cyclopropane is an effective agent for induction, followed by suxamethonium and endotracheal intubation. Ergometrine should be avoided because of its alpha-adrenergic stimulating effect.

Pre-eclamptic toxaemia. In the past eclampsia has carried a mortality as high as 10% and is still the third most important cause of maternal death in the U.S.A. Rapid stabilization of blood pressure is essential, with control of muscular irritability and/or convulsions: rising blood pressure and increasing oedema may, indeed, require induction of labour and possible forceps delivery or Caesarean section. The knowledge that the pathogenesis of this disease is associated with peripheral arteriolar vasoconstriction enables establishment of treatment methods indicated below, and in all these cases management requires sedation and a quiet atmosphere.

Chlorpromazine, promethazine, pethidine, diazepam, bromethol, and chlormethiazole have been employed along with other sedatives. (100 ml of 0.8% of i.v. chlormethiazole given in 5 minutes produces deep sleep.) Epidural anaesthesia or ganglion blockade has also been used. Reserpine safely and effectively reduces vasoconstriction and hypertension and 5–10 mg may be given i.m. 6 hourly. Alternatively, hydralazine, a potent vasodepressor which may also cause tachycardia with a resultant increase in cardiac output and renal blood flow, may be given: 10 mg of hydralazine intravenously is recommended. Reserpine may be used before hydralazine, since this drug neutralizes the rapid heart action associated with hydralazine. It should be remembered that reserpine causes bradycardia and nasal congestion both in the baby and mother, so respiratory difficulty may arise from consequent nasal obstruction in the neonate.

To control convulsions 4–6 g magnesium sulphate may be given intravenously as a primary dose followed by an intramuscular dose of 4–10 g with subsequent doses of 5 g 6-hourly, or, as an alternatives, 1.0 g may be given i.v. hourly. Deep tendon reflexes should be carefully looked for as these reflexes disappear before respiratory paralysis appears. It should be remembered that patients in receipt of magnesium sulphate require smaller doses of neuromuscular blocking agents (both depolarizing and non-depolarizing), if these are employed subsequently for anaesthesia. Both muscular relaxation and intermittent positive pressure ventilation have been employed for the control of convulsions. The only certain cure is delivery of the foetus, although fits may occur up to 48 hours after delivery. Ergometrine should not be used.

Hypofibrinogenaemia. This condition is not uncommon in obstetric practice, particularly in association with accidental haemorrhage. There is a need for a rapid estimation of fibrinogen in such cases. Serial estimations are of considerable value in the management of cases. Epsilon-amino-caproic acid may have a place in the treatment of hypofibrinogenaemia; alternatively, fibrinogen or triple-strength plasma transfusions may be given. Caution should be observed in the rate of administration of the latter because of its high potassium content.

Domiciliary midwifery. Some centres employ 'flying squads' to bring expert help to the mother in her home in an emergency. The role of the anaesthetist in such a squad may vary from a purely resuscitative role, of mother or baby, to the administration of general anaesthesia in far from ideal circumstances. The mother may be ill prepared, probably with a full stomach, possibly in a state of shock. There may be an open fire in the room and the patient will be on a bed which is impossible to tilt. Chloroform, though in many ways an apparently ideal agent for such purposes, (potency, simplicity, non-inflammability and cheapness), poses very distinct problems associated with its administration in inexperienced hands. Some prefer to use a portable anaesthetic machine (and aspirator), inducing anaesthesia in the upright posture, passing a cuffed endotracheal tube under suxamethonium and maintaining ventilation with an Oxford bellows or similar machine.

Epidural and subarachnoid anaesthesia

Provided that labour is well established, neither spinal subarachnoid nor spinal epidural anaesthesia is likely to abolish uterine contractions, as long as the blood pressure is maintained within normal limits and small doses are used. If blood pressure falls, not only may uterine contractions be impeded but foetal bradycardia may result. Factors associated with the sensation of pain, bearing down, and increased muscle tone, which may enhance or inhibit uterine contractility, may be modified by subarachnoid or epidural anaesthesia. Intrinsic uterine work is preserved. Acute hypotension, however, causes decreased uterine contractions, but any attempt to correct acute hypotension with vasopressor agents may cause tetanic uterine contractions and severe foetal distress. It is best treated by rapid restoration of the circulating blood volume with the infusion of plasma expanders and posturing. If pressor agents are used, it is even more important to monitor the foetal heart rate, the uterine contraction and the maternal haemodynamics.

Epidural anaesthesia (see page 366).

Continuous. With the patient in the lateral or sitting position and using full aseptic precautions, the epidural space is entered at L2–L3 using a graduated Tuohy needle with the bevel pointing cephalad. (L4–L5 may be used particularly if the non-selective technique is used.) A polyethylene catheter is passed into the needle and is further advancd for 3–5 cm beyond the tip. Holding the catheter stationary the needle is withdrawn and the catheter strapped to the back – the patient is laid on her back making sure she is not inclined to one side.Using the sitting position for puncture, L4–L5 level is probably better than a higher injection site, for the dura may bulge and there is a greater risk of puncturing it. Use of the lateral position for puncture obviates this risk. 2–3 ml of 0.5% lignocaine without adrenaline are injected. The patient should then be observed for signs of a spinal tap (movement of the legs should be unimpaired, blood pressure and pulse should be noted). After waiting at least five minutes, 10–15 ml of 1.5% lignocaine solution or 6–8 ml of 0.25% bupivacaine solution are slowly injected and the patient's blood pressure and pulse and the foetal heart rate checked at 5 minute intervals for 15–20 minutes. The patient should be nursed either in the lateral position or with a pillow under the buttocks. The height of the block should then be tested; within five minutes the patient should be having painless contractions and she should receive further injections as soon as she experiences a return of painful sensation. The only exception to this rule is when epidural block is being used for the management of toxaemia, and under these circumstances a further injection may be given when the blood pressure begins to rise, before there is a return of pain. No more than 10 ml bupivacaine should be given and usually less in a single top-up dose. Great care should be taken to check the blood pressure when the mother forcibly pushes as this has the effect of the Valsalva manoeuvre, and the lack of compensatory vasoconstriction may lead to a fall in blood pressure, with a fall in the foetal heart rate.

In primigravidae, when the voluntary forces of expulsion are removed, epidural block may tip the balance towards forceps delivery, where, under normal circumstances, forceps delivery might be unnecessary. However, with the multigravida, the baby can often be actively expelled. In occipitoposterior deliveries experiencing much pain, and in patients who are selected because of abnormal factors, the forceps rate tends to be high.

Tachyphylaxis is less common with bupivacaine, but if tachyphylaxis occurs with lignocaine (10–15 ml being required every 3/4 hour) one must start thinking of changing to bupivacaine or supplementing the effect with pethidine to avoid toxic effects of the local anaesthetic on the mother and baby. 2% lignocaine should not be used in patients who are pregnant, as a greater volume of solution is required to produce an effective block than in the non-pregnant patient.

Epidural anaesthesia for Caesarean section should be reserved for those who want to remain awake, those who have bad chests or oral deformities, etc. A catheter should be passed at L2–L3 level and left in for topping-up purposes, should this be required during the course of operation. Spinal subarachnoid anaesthesia (see page 362) is far more suitable for Caesarean section, particularly in under-developed countries.

Selective epidural. It is argued that selective epidural block of T10–L12 produces adequate pain relief, but allows crowning and rotation of the head with a very low incidence of forceps delivery. Much less local anaesthetic agent tends to be required but, undoubtedly, the effect of the drugs spreads downwards and, in certain cases, backache persists. Epidural anaesthesia has received widespread acceptance in North America. It is part of the technique of 'controlled delivery' using in many instances an oxytocic intravenous infusion and culminating in some cases with a forceps delivery. However, labour usually outlasts the effects of a single injection and the continuous method is now employed.

Caudal anaesthesia (see page 369) abolishes efferent pain impulses from the perineal area. There is often delay of the presenting part on the perineum with the result that there tends to be a high incidence of forceps delivery with this technique, unless the caudal injection is delayed until labour is fully established. The time to administer the caudal block is when the cervix is at least 4–6 cm dilated, and if any doubt exists it is best to wait until the cervix is 6–8 cm dilated. It is important to have made sure that the patient has not suffered any damage to the coccyx and is not suffering from any neurological or skin disease. The left lateral position is usually suitable for the insertion of the needle but, in the obese subject, the knee-elbow position makes insertion of the needle easier.

The procedure is often painful and on occasion the anatomy is not easy to identify. Using the Oxford malleable needle, if bone is not encountered at a depth of ½ cm the needle should be slightly withdrawn, for there is a very real danger of piercing the baby's head: once in the sacral canal the hub should be depressed and the needle advanced 3–4 cm. If the patient is in the knee elbow position, additional care should be taken not to penetrate the subarachnoid space. The needle should be aspirated; if blood and CSF are absent; then, with a syringe containing 10 ml of air attached to the needle and the other hand pressed firmly over the lower part of the back, a small amount of air should be injected and loss of resistance ascertained. Pressure on the subcutaneous tissue will detect crepitus if air has been injected in the wrong space: if there is loss of resistance and no crepitus, the catheter can be threaded up the needle; if there is bleeding, the catheter or needle can be flushed with normal saline and the tip of the needle moved slightly. The patient is then placed on her back after firmly securing the catheter, 5 ml of local anaesthetic solution as used for epidural blocks is injected and the movement of the legs, blood pressure and pulse rate noted. After 5 minutes, 15 ml of 0.5% bupivacaine solution are injected. If the blood pressure falls the patient should be placed on her left side with the head down and plasma expanders given intravenously, with injection of local anaesthetic given in between contractions because excessive spread is less likely. The foetal head usually comes well down and rotates.

The disadvantage of caudal anaesthesia is motor weakness of the legs, which can be trying if labour takes a long time, together with more marked loss of perineal sensation and difficulty in always getting spread up to T10; with the lumbar route smaller doses are usually required, with less loss of motor power of the legs. There is a lower incidence of success with caudal as compared with spinal epidural anaesthesia.

Spinal subarachnoid anaesthesia. (see page 362) Spinal subarachnoid block has been employed for normal labour, mid and low forceps and Caesarean section. The patient is conscious and co-operative, and therefore not likely to inhale stomach contents should she vomit or regurgitate, and, in theory, the drugs have no depressant effect on the baby. It carries the disadvantage that a severe drop in blood pressure with depression of ventilation may occur should the subarachnoid block involve the lower dorsal segments. Nausea and vomiting are often present and the procedure can itself be somewhat frightening for the patient.

Anaesthesia to the level of at least T10 is necessary for Caesarean section and this level of anaesthesia, together with splinting of the diaphragm by the gravid uterus, may well lead to respiratory inadequacy. Hypotension may be worsened by the supine position. Compression of the inferior vena cava may often be diagnosed pre-operatively, but should a spinal subarachnoid block be administered inadvisedly to someone suffering from the supine hypotensive syndrome, a catatrophic fall in blood pressure may occur. Many workers have advised the use of pressor agents to correct the hypotension which may arise in association with spinal anaesthesia in obstetrics, but this practice is to be condemned as pressor agents undoubtedly reduce placental blood flow. An intravenous infusion of Hartmann's solution or plasma expander may be employed to correct venous return. Straining to expel the baby should be avoided as this causes the blood pressure to fall, because the response to the Valsalva manoeuvre is impaired following the lack of vasoconstrictor response. It also increases the possibility of post partum headache.

In a comparative study of spinal anaesthesia and general anaesthesia for elective Caesarean section (Crawford, 1966), it was found that children born after general anaesthesia (thiopentone/suxamethonium/nitrous oxide/oxygen) were less asphyxiated than those delivered under spinal anaesthesia. It was suggested that the relatively greater asphyxia under spinal anaesthesia was a result of the obligatory use of vasopressors and their action on the uterine blood flow.

Procedure for inducing spinal anaesthesia: it should first be determined whether the patient suffers from the supine hypotensive syndrome. If not, lumbar puncture at the L4–L5 interspace is carried out with the patient in the left lateral position, with slight head-up tilt, or actually sitting up. 1.5–1.7 ml of heavy spinal solution is administered for Caesarean section, and 0.9 ml for vaginal delivery using a saddle block. Pressor agents should be avoided as far as possible, until the delivery of the child has taken place. As soon as the solution has been injected, the patient is placed supine, with the head and shoulders slightly raised, and is maintained thus until the anaesthetic agent is 'fixed' – about 5 minutes. After this time a head down tilt may be employed if it is desired.

Paracervical block. Paracervical block is particularly valuable in cases of incomplete abortion, where difficulties may arise in obtaining an anaesthetist. It has the advantage that no agent is being used which affects uterine activity, and is considerably safer than general anaesthesia in the unprepared patient. It is of use for facilitating dilation and curettage in day cases. It is extremely effective in controlling the pain of the first stage of labour. There are several disadvantages; some patients develop a parametritis, particularly if the block has been maintained by continuous administration, and it should not be used in the presence of sepsis. Another disadvantage is the high level of local anaesthetic circulating in the foetus.

Method: Cooper (1963) uses a 15 cm long needle sheathed in a rigid guard tube with the tip projecting 7 mm and recommends that each lateral fornix be pierced at the '3 o'clock' and '9 o'clock' position. He injects 10 ml of 1% lignocaine with 1:200 000 adrenaline on each side. It is claimed that relief of pain in the first stage of labour from one or two hours is achieved; completely in 71% cases and partially in 25%. Crawford (1963) suggests that it is unwise to use adrenaline, as vasoconstriction of the placental site may occur.

Tatjeen *et al.* (1966), using a pre-curved Teflon catheter (20 gauge – 36 cm long), threaded over a specially designed stylet marked at 22.5 cm and 24 cm, introduce the catheter through a 13 gauge thin-wall stainless steel needle, 20 cm long, into each lateral fornix, to a depth of 1.5 cm. Following an aspiration test, 3 ml of 1% mepivacaine (Carbocaine) may be injected and further quantities of 5 ml mepivacaine are given according to the patient's needs. Using this continuous technique they claim elimination of discomfort from the first stage of labour.

Kuah and Yates (1967) have used 20 ml 0.5% bupivacaine with 1 : 200 000 adrenaline claiming that it lasts 3–4 hours.

Pudendal nerve block. Pudendal block can be employed in normal delivery, both at the time of presentation of the head at the vulva and for repair of episiotomies and tears. It can also be employed for the application of the Ventouse extractor in the first stage of labour, but if the block is completed too early in labour delay may occur. A carefully applied pudendal block produces efficient pain relief for all mid and low forceps, except some of those requiring manual rotation.

The pudendal nerve should be surrounded by local anaesthetic solution at the point where it enters the pudendal canal at the level of the ischial spine – it should be remembered in performing these blocks that the anterior part of the vulva derives its nerve supply from the ilio-inguinal nerve and therefore a separate block should be carried out to involve these nerves. Two routes are available, the transvaginal and the transperineal.

Transvaginal approach: with a forefinger placed in the vagina, the ischial spine is located and a 12 cm needle guided along the forefinger and directed into the region of the ischial spine. To facilitate this manoeuvre various guides have been devised to avoid piercing the vagina at the wrong point, the finger, or the foetal scalp. 4–20 ml of 0.5% lignocaine without adrenaline, or prilocaine without adrenaline, are injected just posterior to the tip of the spine. The procedure is repeated again on the other side. The ilio-inguinal nerves are also infiltrated in the region of the symphysis pubis.

Transperineal approach: with the forefinger placed in the vagina a small bleb is raised in the skin midway between the anus and ischial tuberosity. A 12 cm needle is then guided into position using the finger in the vagina to facilitate this. No more than 200 mg lignocaine without adrenaline or 400 mg prilocaine without adrenaline should be used, for the complete procedure.

Failed forceps. The difficult forceps may still call for general anaesthesia. Herein lies a very real hazard, for if general anaesthesia is required for a patient who has had a failed forceps under local anaesthesia there is a great temptation to induce general anaesthesia with the patient lying on her back in the lithotomy position – a potentially dangerous situation should she regurgitate. Induction of general anaesthesia should never be allowed with the patient in this position. Full facilities to deal with vomiting and regurgitation should be available. General anaesthesia should proceed along the lines suggested in Caesarean section. A very real dilemma presents itself to the anaesthetist when called in to give a general anaesthetic in a breech delivery when the after coming head is arrested. Here it may be best to temporarily lower the legs and have them held by an attendant at each side. As soon as the patient is safely intubated the legs are again suspended and extraction of the head immediately commenced. It should be stressed that any woman possibly requiring such an anaesthetic should be delivered on a 'bed' that can be positioned head or feet up. In addition, because general anaesthesia was not anticipated it is possible that the usual precautions for ensuring against a full stomach have been omitted. The anaesthetist should satisfy himself that antacid has been administered. The passage of a tube into the stomach is not always practicable in this situation.

Neonatal resuscitation

Provided careful management has been present throughout labour, depression of the foetal respiratory and circulatory systems will be minimized. The establishment of rapport between the mother and her attendant, the use of hypnosis, 'natural child-birth', and regional anaesthesia, will all lead to a reduction of the need for potent analgesics.

Monitoring of the foetal blood acid-base status, the presence of foetal bradycardia, and meconium-stained liquor will warn the attendant that the baby is likely to be distressed. With adequate warning, arrangements can be set in motion for skilled resuscitation. The various physical signs of foetal depression are conveniently summarized in the Apgar score (Apgar, 1953) (see page 453). A baby with an Apgar score of 7 to 10 usually requires little help except prevention of airway obstruction, but children with scores of less than 7 will require varying degrees of assistance. A correlation has been found between the heart rate, pH of blood obtained from the caput, and the Apgar score, so amnioscopy and the determination of the foetal acid-base picture are investigations which may help in subsequent management. It should be remembered that apnoeic attacks (lasting more than 60 s) are particularly common in premature babies (1000–1750 g): a very high proportion of such cases terminate fatally unless the recurrent apnoeic attacks are treated energetically.

All children at birth should be wrapped in a warm towel to minimize cooling and laid upon a firm surface with the head slightly lowered, a pad under the shoulders and the body in the semi-lateral position. Gentle suction must be applied to the mouth and nasopharynx in order to clear the upper respiratory tract of mucus – this stimulus will generally provoke breathing. The stomach may also be emptied.

If the baby fails to breathe adequately, i.e. fails to become pink on air after 1 minute or is apnoeic for this period of time, the following regimen is embarked upon:

(1) Aspirate pharynx and larynx under direct laryngoscopy with a soft sterile catheter (breathing may be initiated by this manoeuvre).

(2) If the baby does not respond to this stimulus by breathing adequately, intubation should be carried out, the stimulus itself provoking vigorous 'crying' in some instances. A fine catheter is then passed down the endotracheal tube and with weak suction, carried out in short periods, any debris is cleared from the tracheobronchial tree; if help is still necessary intermittent ventilation of the lungs is then instituted using humidified oxygen: pressures of 30–60 cmH_2O may be necessary to inflate the lungs initially. Short puffs of oxygen at a pressure of 25–35 cmH_2O for a fraction of a second should be applied in order to expand the lungs, and this should be followed by pressures of 5–10 cmH_2O. Once expansion has occurred, ventilation of each lung should be checked by listening with a stethoscope. IPPV may be carried out for long periods of time.

(3) If spontaneous ventilation is sluggish the inspired air may be enriched with oxygen and delivered to the face with a mask. If for any reason intubation is not possible (lack of skill on the part of the resuscitator or lack of equipment), IPPV should be carried out using mouth to mouth ventilation or a face mask with a gentle pressure on the reservoir bag. Great care must be taken to avoid inflation of the stomach: this can generally be avoided by correct positioning of the head and the avoidance of too high inflation pressure.

(4) Where there is definite evidence that cardiac activity ceased just prior to delivery, there is justification in applying cardiac massage. This should be carried out using the tips of the forefinger and middle finger and pressing them firmly but gently over the midpoint of the sternum. The massage should continue in a rhythmical manner at approximately 60 beats per minute. Oxygen therapy with positive pressure ventilation of the lungs should be carried out concurrently.

Drugs. There has been considerable debate in recent years over the role of drugs in neonatal resuscitation. It is now felt that attention should be paid, primarily, to the correction of the inevitable metabolic acidosis which occurs in association with neonatal cardio-pulmonary depression.

Correction of metabolic acidosis. Provided adequate artificial ventilation is being carried out with oxygen, sodium bicarbonate may be given intravenously as a 0.6 M (1.4%) solution in a dose of 7.7 ml/kg. Trihydroxymethylaminomethane buffer (THAM) may also be considered, but it has the disadvantage that it lowers the carbon dioxide tension, thereby possibly reducing respiratory drive. It is also highly irritant to the tissues if deposited outside a vein. The intravenous administration of glucose may well be a more rational approach to this problem of metabolic acidosis associated with the newborn.

Analeptics. Specific antagonists are rarely indicated, but where there is definite evidence that the mother has received one predominant drug in large dosage there may occasionally be a case for exhibiting an analeptic. If large doses of pethidine or morphine have been given to the mother, levallorphan or nalorphine may be administered into the umbilical vein of the baby in a dose of 0.25 mg or 0.2 mg respectively. The drug nalorphine can be administered to the mother in a 10 mg dose before delivery of the baby if the mother has received morphine or pethidine. Naloxone (Doxopram) has also a place as an opiate antagonist. There is no conclusive evidence that other analeptics are of value. The use of deliberate 'back-slapping' and sublingual analeptics are, in our view, neither valid nor useful forms of therapy; indeed, they waste valuable time.

Oxygen. Intragastric oxygen has been shown to be of no value whatsoever, but intra-rectal oxygen has been recommended, particularly for breech deliveries. Though it is claimed that a significant increase in the levels of oxygen in the umbilical vein is achieved, further evaluation is necessary before this technique can be recommended. Hyperbaric oxygen has also been advocated, but it is certainly of no value in the totally apnoeic child. In our view it has nothing to recommend it and resuscitation should be directed towards establishing effective ventilation by intubation and artificial ventilation. Prolonged ventilatory insufficiency and recurrent neonatal apnoea should be treated by intermittent positive pressure ventilation. IPPV may also be of value in small premature infants at high risk: the timing and technique are of particular importance, in that situation.

Respiratory distress syndrome

Whatever the reason for its absence, lack of pulmonary surfactant is fundamental to the development of the respiratory distress syndrome of the newborn. Respiratory distress syndrome (RDS), or hyaline membrane disease, affects premature babies, causing the death of three to four per cent, but is rare in full term babies except those of diabetic mothers. At, or immediately after birth, the respiratory rate increases from about 30 up to 100 per minute. Breathing is laboured with retraction of the lower chest wall, grunting and expiratory whimper. Apnoeic periods intervene and increasing cyanosis appears, resistant to oxygen therapy; lung compliance is decreased and the work of breathing is up at four times that normally required. Metabolic acidosis from anoxia, with fall in blood pressure, body temperature and cardiac output causes a fatal outcome in about 50% or more affected. Treatment should include IPPV, oxygen therapy with humidification and the correction of metabolic acidosis. Recently the maintenance of an end-expiratory positive pressure under spontaneous ventilation has had some popularity in the treatment (Gregory Box).

Gynaecology

Patients presenting for gynaecological operations in many instances come to their doctor on account of abnormal or excessive blood loss. They are frequently anaemic and particular attention should be paid to this factor when first seen. In many cases treatment of the anaemia can commence as an outpatient whilst awaiting admission for surgery, thus saving considerable time and bed accommodation. In view of the problems of transfusion of blood in patients of child-bearing age, attempts to raise the haemoglobin content of blood by transfusion are best avoided and iron therapy used where possible. Many of these patients receive tranquillizing drugs of some form or another, and great care should be taken to ensure that the nature of these drugs is known. In some instances, blood loss may be both acute and severe and the result of this will be very different from the result of chronic blood loss. Both a ruptured ectopic pregnancy and an incomplete abortion may result in reduction of the circulating blood volume. There should be no undue delay in procuring the arrest of the haemorrhage, and, within reason, restoration of blood volume by transfusion should await the control of haemorrhage. An intravenous drip should, however, be secured before induction of anaesthesia. It must be remembered that patients suffering from acute haemorrhage will have an increased sensitivity to general anaesthetic agents, and intravenous agents in particular. Minimal quantities of agents should therefore be exhibited. In the case of a severe ruptured ectopic pregnancy, induction and maintenance of general anaesthesia with nitrous oxide/oxygen together with relaxants may be all that is required. Once the haemorrhage has been controlled, the patient may be rapidly transfused with warm blood. Certain perineal operations and the operation of pelvic exenteration are associated with troublesome and excessive bleeding and the surgeon may wish to have some reduction of this loss by deliberate hypotension.

In order to carry out certain gynaecological procedures the surgeon may wish to be assisted by posturing the patient. The Trendelenberg, lithotomy and knee-elbow position carry with them problems from the point of view of potential nerve and tissue damage and impairment of the circulatory and respiratory systems. Finally, the presence of a large abdominal tumour may produce hypotension when the supine position is adopted. To reduce this problem, the patient may be turned slightly to one side whilst the abdomen is being opened and the tumour mobilized.

Meig's syndrome. This is a condition in which an ovarian tumour is associated with a pleural effusion, the latter possibly causing severe ventilatory distress and consequent cardiovascular decompensation. As the pleural and peritoneal effusions collect rapidly after drainage, the cavities must be tapped immediately prior to operation. Many of the patients are under-nourished, emaciated and cachectic, with anaemia and electrolyte imbalance.

Blood loss during vaginal surgery. The blood loss has been variously reported as averaging between 200 ml and 750 ml during vaginal hysterectomy without adrenaline. The use of a disposable plastic bag is advisable in that the blood lost can be contained and the loss measured. Following infiltration with pituitrin or adrenaline containing solutions the loss can be significantly decreased, and such infiltration will reduce the time of operation by maintaining a clearer operative field. However, although infiltration of the operative site and paracervical tissues with pituitrin has been found to be satisfactory in reducing blood loss, many still use adrenaline. It must on no account be employed where halothane, cyclopropane, trichloroethylene, or chloroform are being used as inhalational agents. Further reduction of blood loss can be obtained by deliberate hypotension, thus offering opportunity for better and more rapid surgery. This does not release the surgeon from the obligation of securing haemostasis. Such lessening of blood loss reduces the need for blood replacement. Spinal subarachnoid anaesthesia, or continuous epidural anaesthesia, also reduces blood loss, the latter being possibly more effective in this context.

Peritoneoscopy. This procedure may require the preliminary insufflation of large quantities of carbon dioxide into the peritoneal cavity. The subsequent embarrassment to ventilation is further aggravated by the adoption of the Trendelenberg position. Problems may also arise from the carbon dioxide being placed extraperitoneally.

Anaesthesia should be carried out with IPPV through a cuffed endotracheal tube. Because of inevitable absorption of carbon dioxide from the peritoneal cavity, ventilation should be in excess of the usual requirements. Regurgitation of stomach contents may occur. Gallamine is the relaxant of choice, because any residual effect lasting after neostigmine has been administered will be countered by carbon dioxide retention and fall in pH. In case of excessive absorption of carbon dioxide, halothane should not be used because of the danger of dysrhythmias.

10 *Anaesthesia and Eye, Ear, Nose and Throat Surgery. Plastic, Orthopaedic and Urological Surgery*

The eye

In order that the ophthalmic surgeon may carry out his work in a satisfactory manner, certain criteria must be satisfied:

he must have a quiescent patient who is either unconscious and immobile, or conscious and co-operative
the patient's eye must be immobile
there must be minimal bleeding
he must have some measure of control, either directly or indirectly over the intra-ocular pressure
a smooth post-operative recovery, with the minimum of restlessness, nausea and vomiting, must be ensured

General anaesthesia and local anaesthesia each have their protagonists and each method has its distinct advantages and disadvantages.

Local anaesthesia

A number of operations can be performed satisfactorily without general anaesthesia. Some writers advocate the use of local anaesthesia, together with heavy sedation, particularly for cataract operations. The advocates for local anaesthesia argue that:

early ambulation and feeding by mouth is possible
there is less nausea and vomiting
there is less bleeding
there is no risk of explosion
less post-operative care is required
the incidence of pulmonary complications, such as cough, is less
secretions are controlled more effectively

A mixture of chlorpromazine and pethidine may be used, or even heavier sedation employed. It is claimed that patients are well sedated but co-operative, the eye becoming white and soft, bleeding being reduced, and retrobulbar anaesthesia becoming unnecessary. After the heavier sedation the patient is quiet, often passing into sleep, but without depression of respiration. Few patients have any memory of the operation. A disadvantage of this technique is that a sudden fall in blood pressure, usually associated with bradycardia, commonly happens during traction on the ocular muscles; because of this phenomenon adequate and careful supervision is necessary. Another technique consists of the oral administration of promazine (Sparine) in a long acting preparation the night before operation, the dose being decided by age and blood pressure and general physical status. $1\frac{1}{2}$ hours prior to operation, promazine, promethazine (Phenergan), pethidine and atropine are administered intravenously, the dose once again being determined by age and blood pressure. On arrival in the operating theatre the blood pressure is checked and a further dose of intravenous pethidine and promazine is given, if sedation is not adequate and the blood pressure has not fallen. A somewhat similar technique, using phenazocine (Narphen) or pentazocine (Fortal) instead of pethidine at the time of the operation may be used. Here it is claimed that provided the patient is co-operative and refrains from making sudden movements, none of the problems associated with recovery from general anaesthesia are encountered. The main disadvantage of these techniques seems to be that very careful supervision is necessary if they are to be administered effectively. Alternatively dihydrobenzperidol (Droleptan) and phenoperidine (Operidine) may be used intravenously to provide tranquillity and general analgesia respectively, the majority of cases requiring a retobulbar and facial nerve block using 1% lignocaine. A degree of respiratory depression is sometimes present with this technique. The placidity of the patients during operation, the absence of cough, vomiting and fidgeting, and the post-operative tranquillity, make this 'neuro-leptic' technique an important contribution to intra-ocular surgery. Gamma-OH may be of value for ophthalmic operations under local anaesthesia. 2 g of Gamma-OH may be given orally to a fit adult man an hour before operation. Diazepam (0.2 mg/kg) intravenously is also a useful sedative.

Local techniques. If topical anaesthesia is to be used, 4% cocaine is the most suitable agent as it combines anaesthetic and analgesic properties with vaso-constriction. It has the disadvantage that it dilates the pupil and will only cause analgesia of the cornea and conjuctiva. The ciliary ganglion and nerves must be blocked for more extensive operations on the eye by injecting 2 ml 2% lignocaine with 6–10 units of hyaluronidase through a needle 3.5 cm in length (26 swg). The patient is asked to look up and a small injection is made into the outer third of the lower lid. The needle is pushed through the skin, traversing the gap palpable between the eye and the orbital margin, the injection being made slowly and continuously and the needle advanced tangentially to the globe. As soon as the needle is behind the eye, it is aimed at the apex of the orbit and the major portion of the injection completed. To prevent movements of the lids the facial nerve must also be blocked. A wheal is produced just anterior to the external ear by injecting a little lignocaine with a 3.5 cm needle; injections are made backwards, to block the branches of the facial nerve supplying the orbicularis, and forward, to numb the lid edges.

General anaesthesia

Some authorities make a plea for general anaesthesia, claiming that it brings benefits both to the surgeon and the patient. It allows the surgeon to perform in a relaxed atmosphere and it is undoubtedly kinder to the patient. The disadvantage of general anaesthesia, however, can be great, particularly if the anaesthetic is administered by an anaesthetist who is not skilled in ophthalmic anaesthesia. But, provided care is taken with premedication, induction and maintenance of anaesthesia, problems during and after surgery can be as few as with local anaesthesia.

Effect of pre-anaesthetic drugs on the eye. For many years there has been argument as to whether atropine is dangerous in ophthalmic surgery; in fact, it is probably only dangerous for the patient with narrow angle glaucoma. Morphine, pethidine, and the barbiturates lower the intra-ocular pressure. Observation of pupil size, as affected by intravenously administered atropine and neostigmine during reversal of curarization, suggests that the pupillary changes notes are not deleterious in intra-ocular surgery.

Effect of general anaesthetic agents on the eye. As already stated, general anaesthesia for intra-ocular surgery still presents a topic of controversy. Most ophthalmic surgeons use general anaesthesia for extra-ocular surgery and for intra-ocular surgery in children. The use of general anaesthesia for cataract extractions on adults is increasing. It has been pointed out that the full co-operation needed from a patient under local anaesthetic cannot be achieved in a state of sedation, however complete the pre-operative instructions. In addition, the frequency of senility or deafness as barriers to complete co-operation in patients commonly subject to cataract operations, makes the effective employment of local techniques difficult in these subjects.

There are several factors influencing intra-ocular pressure, which tends to be influenced by the same factors as affect the intra-cranial pressure. Any straining during intubation or during maintenance of anaesthesia, as well as hypoxia, hypercarbia, or transient hypertension, will tend to cause the intra-ocular pressure to rise. Lowering of the blood pressure below 90 mmHg, lowering the arterial carbon dioxide tension, and reduction of central venous pressure will all contribute to a reduction of intra-ocular pressure. Halothane, chloroform, hydroxydione and trichloroethylene, all cause a significant decrease too. Suxamethonium causes the intra-ocular pressure to rise, probably largely due to a vascular effect arising from dilatation of choroidal vessels, but also due to a transient squeezing effect caused by contraction of the extra-ocular muscles.

The evidence suggests that the pressure in the glaucomatous eye does not rise with suxamethonium in the way that the pressure in the normal eye does. There may be a difference between open and closed angle glaucoma. Smooth endotracheal intubation is a pre-requisite for a satisfactory general anaesthetic in intra-ocular surgery; however, because of the marked transient rise in intra-ocular pressure associated with the use of suxamethonium this drug is perhaps better avoided. The use of acetazolamide (Diamox) – 500 mg in 5–10 ml water intravenously – to avoid the elevation of pressure associated with suxamethonium has been suggested. Suxamethonium also produces dilatation of conjunctival vessels and enophthalmos and it should never be used with an open eye (e.g. eye injury), because of the very real danger of loss of vitreous.

There is yet another hazard associated with the use of suxamethonium in eye surgery – apnoea in patients following its use after ecothiopate eye drops have been used. An organophosphorus compound, ecothiopate iodide, is used as an ocular hypotensive agent, being of value in chronic, simple and aphakic glaucoma, and in the treatment of some forms of strabismus. It is also used to decrease the accommodation effort in accommodative estrophia. In the form of eyedrops, it has been shown to depress plasma pseudocholinesterase to dangerously low levels within a few days of commencing therapy. Curare and gallamine relax the extra-ocular musculature, bringing the intra-ocular pressure down. Some authorities have suggested the use of muscle relaxants, retrobulbar injection and the 'lytic cocktail' to produce a state of semi-consciousness and akinesia. Curare has been used to prevent eye movements in conscious patients, using a dose of the order of 7 mg, but this cannot be recommended, as even in this dose it may be distressing to the patient and give rise to underventilation.

Sorbitol, dextran, urea, gycerol, and mannitol have been used with success in glaucoma. The place of halothane and methoxyflurane in ophthalmic surgery has been studied, and no difference has been found between the two as regards respiratory depression, post-operative restlessness, vomiting and the need for analgesia. With methoxyflurane there is slightly better cardiovascular stability than with halothane; there is also a reduced tendency to bleed and a smooth emergence from anaesthesia in children. Methoxyflurane and trichloroethylene have disadvantages, however, that induction and emergence are slow, there is less pronounced ocular hypotonia than with halothane and prolonged vomiting occurs in rare cases.

Diathermy for detached retina. Clearly where this technique is employed, non-explosive mixtures must be used.

Aschner's oculo-cardiac reflex. Slowing of the heartrate and cardiac arrest can occur during the manipulation of the eyeball. The reflex has been noted in about 60% of patients undergoing strabismus surgery, occurring when there is traction upon the extra-ocular muscles, particularly in the presence of hypercarbia and hypoxia. Attempts have been made to reduce the incidence of this phenomenon. Retrobulbar injection of 0.5% lignocaine has been tried and it is claimed that this block prevent the reflex in all instances. Intravenous atropine (0.005 mg/kg) a few minutes before the procedure is commenced gives some protection against the sinus bradycardia; however, over half the cases with a normal atropine premedication have the reflex present and thus premedication with atropine affords no reliable protection. Gallamine may be used routinely as a muscle relaxant, and, together with the avoidance of hypoxia and hypercapnia, it greatly reduces the chances of encountering this reflex.

General anaesthetic techniques. We are of the opinion that if it has been decided that general anaesthesia is indicated, then the patient should be premedicated with a phenothiazine derivative. The opiates, pethidine and other similar agents which predispose to vomiting should be avoided at all costs. Anaesthesia should be induced with thiopentone and gallamine, the vocal cords sprayed with 4% lignocaine and a well lubricated oro-tracheal tube passed, at all times avoiding coughing and straining. Anaesthesia should be maintained with nitrous oxide, oxygen and/or halothane, giving supplemental doses of gallamine as and when required and ventilation should be controlled with moderate over-ventilation and adequate oxygenation. Hypotensive techniques may be necessary, particularly in the operation of dacryocysto-rhinostomy.

Effects of general anaesthesia on the post-operative period: it is of the greatest importance that recovery is rapid and complete, without restlessness, nausea and vomiting, coughing or straining. This is of particular importance in relation to detachment of the retina. Drugs known to cause nausea and vomiting should at all times be avoided, i.e. morphine, ether, etc. Where there is a history of nausea and vomiting in association with general anaesthesia, local techniques should be seriously considered. Some eye operations carry quite a high incidence of nausea and vomiting (and the consequent fear of loss of the vitreous) even under local anaesthesia, therefore prophylactic medication should be employed. Where the patient has a cough before operation, every effort should be made to treat the underlying condition beforehand: patients with upper respiratory tract infections must on no account be subjected to general anaesthesia. Endotracheal intubation should at all times be carried out with great care in order to avoid post-operative tracheitis. The incidence of vomiting varies between 30–40% after cataract surgery, so patients who are candidates for this operation and who have associated degrees of glaucoma are best handled under local anaesthesia, following premedication with a sedative and anti-emetic. It has been shown that thiethylperazine (Torecan) has a high degree of effectiveness as an anti-emetic in ophthalmic surgery, provided that narcotics are not given. It is moreover, free from sedative, hypotensive and potentiating effects.

Anaesthesia for ear, nose and throat surgery

Operations upon the ears, nose and throat, demand that the surgeon has full access to the surgical field, so that the anaesthetist and his equipment are inevitably situated at some distance from the upper part of the body. In order to prevent rebreathing and increased resistance to breathing, unidirectional valves may be employed. These have the disadvantage of noise and distraction to the surgeon, and may stick during controlled ventilation. Closed circuit circle equipment attached beneath the operating table enables the anaesthetist to manage the anaesthetic satisfactorily. In addition, where operations on the nose and throat are concerned, the airway has to be shared with the surgeon, and there is the risk of the inhalation of blood. The operations on the nose and throat are characterized by a significant tendency to haemorrhage; vomiting also is a common sequela in the post-operative period following ear operations. An early return of the protective cough reflex is important particularly following operation on the upper respiratory tract.

Operations upon the ear. In view of the intricacy of some of the operations the surgeon must have a clear field, with minimal disturbance of vision by the presence of blood.

Mastoidectomy. This operation, which may be necessary when an acute infection is present, calls for a quiescent patient, a free airway, and no straining. The patient may be toxic and pyrexial, and may have respiratory tract infection. In the case of a child, particular care must be taken to avoid overheating and the possibility of convulsions; atropine premedication and diethyl ether are probably best avoided in such patients. All patients undergoing this operation should have a secure airway produced by an oral endotracheal tube. Topical anaesthesia of the larynx will reduce straining which would otherwise be likely to occur in association with the slight movement of the head in such operations.

Myringotomy. It should be remembered that these patients are usually children and, again, may be toxic and pyrexial from infection. This is a procedure which in the past was performed under ethyl chloride sprayed on to the mask; however, ethyl chloride should be avoided and anaesthesia produced with nitrous oxide/oxygen/halothane, with or without an intravenous induction.

Anaesthesia for middle ear surgery. Such operations are often extremely intricate and call for absolute immobility on the part of the patient. Great attention should be paid to bleeding at the operative site; there should be an unobstructed airway, no straining and adequate oxygenation and carbon dioxide elimination. Moderate hypotension may be achieved with the use of halothane, or more profound hypotension by using ganglion blocking agents: methoxyflurane anaesthesia has been employed. In order to produce local vaso-constriction, some surgeons use pledgets of cotton wool soaked in adrenaline; great care must be taken to minimize the systemic effects of adrenaline in such cases, and agents such as halothane and trichloroethylene must not be permitted. When nitrous oxide has been employed, it is a wise precaution to turn it off some minutes before the middle ear is closed, in order to prevent it accumulating under the flap.

Anaesthesia for ultra-sonic irradiation of the labyrinth. Irradiation of the labyrinth with ultrasound is now established as an effective treatment for patients suffering from Meniere's disease which has not responded to conservative treatment. It is vital for the successful performance of the operation to observe nystagmus and ocular deviation during the ultrasonic irradiation. Furthermore, the integrity of the facial nerve must be ensured by continual observation of the facial muscles. Vertigo and nausea during the procedure can be most distressing for the patient and may seriously imperil the operation. As it is essential to perform the irradiation with the patient conscious, he should be interviewed preoperatively and the nature of the procedure explained. The patient may be premedicated with atropine 0.6 mg and in order to reduce the vertigo and nausea, prochlorperazine (Stemetil) 12.5 mg is given. Anaesthesia can be induced with a sleep dose of methohexitone, followed by 50 mg suxamethonium. Topical anaesthesia is applied to the larynx and upper trachea, and a cuffed endotracheal tube passed into the larynx. Anaesthesia is maintained with nitrous oxide/oxygen and intermittent methohexitone. The mastoid area is infiltrated with 1:80 000 adrenaline in lignocaine. When the bone over the lateral semi-circular canal is removed and the surgeon ready to irradiate, the endotracheal tube is removed and the patient allowed to wake up before irradiation commences.

Tonsillectomy

Apart from enabling the surgeon to have full access to the operative site, it is essential that the tracheo-bronchial tree is not contaminated with blood or pus. There should be full and immediate recovery of the cough reflex following the termination of general anaesthesia.

Premedication. As most of the patients are likely to be children some form of sedation is desirable but not essential. Trimeprazine (Vallergan) (2 mg/kg up to 80 mg) is considered by some to be the drug of choice. As pentobarbitone and certain of the phenothiazine derivates are ant-analgesics and may give rise to post-operative restlessness they are best avoided. If suxamethonium is to be employed, or ether to be used, it is desirable to administer atropine. Opiates and similar agents should never be used for premedication as they obtund the cough reflex.

General anaesthesia. For many years, it has been customary to maintain general anaesthesia by peroral insufflation of the inhalational agents, using the side tube on the Boyle-Davis gag. Maintenance of general anaesthesia using diethyl ether or halothane may become difficult in the adult patient as sufficient concentration of anaesthetic mixture in the mouth may be difficult – or impossible – to achieve. This disadvantage can be circumvented by insufflating the anaesthetic mixture into the trachea by means of a gum elastic catheter passed between the vocal cords. More recently, endotracheal intubation has been used and this is increasing in popularity. The Doughty modification of the Boyle-Davis gag allows the presence of an endotracheal tube in the mouth without interfering with the operative site: cuffed tubes may be used. Endotracheal intubation has the certain advantage that the patients may be maintained at a much lighter level of anaesthesia, with resultant swifter recovery from anaesthesia when required; in addition the maintenance of a given level of anaesthesia is more certain and predictable than with the peroral technique.

Induction may be produced either with an intravenous or inhalational technique. Intubation in children should be carried out using suxamethonium and a Magill armoured tube passed under direct vision. Nasal intubation should be avoided, particularly in patients with enlarged adenoids; especial care should be taken with young children who, as a consequence, have an obstructed nasal airway. Closure of the mouth by the anaesthetist as he supports the chin may produce serious respiratory obstruction, when an inhalational technique is being used.

In adults a streamlined cuffed nasal endotracheal tube may be employed. The patient should then be placed on the operating table with a sandbag under the shoulders, and the head extended in such a way that the operative site is at a lower level than the laryngeal aperture.

Using such a posture, together with efficient suction, the surgeon can prevent the inhalation of blood by constant visualization of the pool of blood forming under the influence of gravity. Packing is unnecessary. If used, the Doughty tongue plate together with gag is inserted when relaxation of the jaw muscles is adequate. General anaesthesia at a light plane can be maintained by halothane, but some anaesthetists maintain anaesthesia by using neuro-muscular blocking agents and artificial ventilation. Alternatively intermittent suxamethonium, with artificial ventilation may be used. Blood loss should be as low as possible, bleeding vessels being controlled as divided by dissection. There should be no hurry or time limit on the operation, no patient being removed from the operating table whilst bleeding is going on.

If tonsillectomy is performed by means of the guillotine, the following technique may be employed. The patient, usually a child, is induced by the conventional methods and anaesthesia deepened to such a degree that the operation can be performed as he lightens. Immediately the surgery is complete (this taking usually not more than two minutes), the child is turned into the left lateral or semi-prone position and allowed to recover in the presence of the anaesthetist with suction ready to hand.

Before removal from the table, the cough reflex must be present. The insertion of an airway and over-enthusiastic suction should be avoided, the patient being turned to one side in the semi-prone position. In this position, the child should be placed in a cot, actually in the theatre, with a pillow under the thorax, thus allowing the head to be in a slightly head down posture. The patient should be carefully observed by a nurse, whilst the next operation proceeds. As soon as the anaesthetist is satisfied with the patient's condition, the child should be returned to the recovery ward especially set aside for this purpose, and not returned to the ward where other patients are awaiting tonsillectomy.

Tonsillectomy for peritonsillar abscess. 'Emergency' tonsillectomy for acute infections of the tonsil is sometimes employed in the presence of abscess formation. This can be an extremely hazardous procedure from the anaesthetic standpoint, as rupture of the abscess during induction of anaesthesia and intubation could seriously imperil the patient's air passages and infect the lung. From the surgical standpoint, enucleation of the tonsil is apparently facilitated by the infection, and haemorrhage is surprisingly small. Great care must be taken in selection of these cases, as trismus is frequently present and further extension of the infection may involve the soft tissues of the neck. Suction apparatus must be at hand during induction, which should be carried out following pre-oxygenation using the thiopentone/suxamethonium sequence, with careful intubation and packing, taking care not to rupture the abscess.

Post-operative sedation: although opiates and their derivatives depress ventilation and the cough reflex, morphine is a very satisfactory post-operative sedative – an i.m. dose of 0.2 mg/kg is advised. In older children and adults, pethidine 1.5 mg/kg may be used.

Post-tonsillectomy haemorrhage: in a report on 72 deaths associated with post-operative haemorrhage during the period 1957–61, 52 cases could be attributed to anaesthesia for the surgical control of haemorrhage. Many of these patients are shocked and anaemic and may have swallowed large quantities of blood which, for some reason, tends to make them even more collapsed. The patient should be taken immediately to the anaesthetic room, a blood transfusion set up prior to induction of anaesthesia and, in an adult, the stomach emptied if at all possible, prior to induction. He should be placed in the lateral position on the operating table with the head lowered. The anaesthetist should clear the airway by gentle suction to the nose and pharynx, passing a rubber catheter through the nose if need be, but only removing loose clots, as vigorous suction may re-start haemorrhage. Oxygen should be administered: no ethyl chloride should be used, and muscle relaxants are generally not necessary. Indeed, these patients require very little in the way of general anaesthesia, which is usually satisfactorily induced with nitrous oxide/oxygen and halothane. Endotracheal intubation can be carried out according to the individual preference of the anaesthetist, and is probably safest particularly if the stomach is to be emptied under anaesthesia. As soon as the patient is settled a sandbag is placed under the shoulders and the Boyle-Davis gag inserted. After careful suction and ligation of the bleeding points by the surgeon, intermittent aspiration should be applied to the tracheo-bronchial tree, at the same time as the chest is auscultated. If necessary bronchoscopy can be carried out. Post-operatively the patient should be carefully observed, oxygen administered and morphine 0.2 mg/kg administered intramuscularly. The chest should be examined next day.

Blood loss and tonsillectomy: Particular care should be taken to ensure that patients are not unduly anaemic pre-operatively, as appreciable blood loss has been reported by some workers in relation to routine tonsillectomy. This loss may exceed 10% of the blood volume in children.

Laryngoscopy. This procedure may be necessary for diagnostic purposes. In the first place the surgeon may wish to establish the nature of the movement of the vocal cords and, secondly, he may wish to remove tissue for histological purposes. For visualization of movement the patients are best under relatively 'deep' halothane anaesthesia. Where a biopsy is to be carried out, cessation of movement is sometimes a help, in which case a paralysing dose of muscle relaxant, together with the technique of perlaryngeal insufflation and/or oxygen diffusion apnoea, is the method of choice. A rapid return of the cough reflex is desirable. For microsurgery of the larynx a Pollard tube or small catheter may be required. Ventilation occurs either through the tube or round the catheter.

Pharyngolaryngectomy. Extensive and mutilating operations are sometimes necessary for the eradication or palliation of carcinoma of the pharynx, larynx and upper oesophagus. The conditions necessitating such operations may be associated with respiratory obstruction, infection of the tracheo-bronchial tree, anaemia, and cachexia. The nature of the operations vary in their extent but usually they are associated with block dissection of the glands of the neck. A thorough pre-operative evaluation is essential with a kind, tactful, and sympathetic explanation to the patient as to what is likely to be done. Where there is pre-existing anaemia and lung infection, these should be treated. Pre-operative respiratory obstruction may require preliminary tracheostomy under local anaesthesia, particularly if there is evidence of respiratory decompensation. A knowledge of the growth and the bounds of its involvement are essential factors in reaching a decision as to whether or not to perform pre-operative tracheostomy. Apart from the risks of laryngeal obstruction, there is a very real danger of forcing neoplastic tissue down into the tracheo-bronchial tree at intubation. Laryngoscopy, oesophagoscopy and biopsy are essential preludes to surgery. Provided that there is no respiratory obstruction, anaesthesia can be induced with thiopentone and maintained with nitrous oxide/oxygen, relaxants and controlled ventilation. The patient is usually placed in a 10°–15° head-up tilt and the arterial and venous blood pressure and the ECG should be monitored. A block dissection of the neck is carried out, care being taken to avoid reflex bradycardia when dissection is carried out near the carotid sinus. Certain authorities employ deliberate hypotension. After pharyngectomy is performed, the trachea is dislocated from the endotracheal tube and connected to a sterile cuffed tracheostomy or Montando tube; sterile connectors are then connected to the anaesthetic tubing under the towels. This procedure needs to be swiftly carried out to enable controlled ventilation to be continued. Occasionally it is necessary to replace a section of resected oesophagus with a colonic transplant, passed upwards through the mediastinum: this will require good abdominal relaxation to enable the colon to be mobilized. The pleural cavity is not usually opened, but care should be taken to avoid complications such as tension pneumothorax, by continual vigilance. Throughout the operation attention should be paid to blood replacement and at the termination of operation efficient and intensive nursing is required, remembering that humidification of the tracheostomy is essential and that tight bandages should be avoided.

Nasal operations. Operations such as those for the correction of deformed nasal septum, the Cauldwell-Lac operation, the removal of adenoids and dachryocystorhinostomy are associated with the loss of appreciable amount of blood. Full protection of the airway must be ensured. The operation of adenoidectomy is usually associated with tonsillectomy, and the anaesthetic technique is similar. Other operations on the nose require the passage of a cuffed endotracheal tube passed orally, and as an additional safeguard, the packing of the naso-pharynx with a gauze roll soaked in saline or glycerine (but *not* liquid paraffin BP). Some surgeons not only infiltrate the operative site with adrenaline solution, but occasionally call for a deliberate reduction in blood pressure.

Technique for intranasal operations under local anaesthesia: the advantage of local anaesthetic technique is that a bloodless field is more readily obtainable. Nasal anaesthesia can be achieved by the direct application of the drug to the nasal mucous membrane by spraying, painting and packing, or by blocking nerves as they enter the nasal cavity. These methods are only successful if no deformities exist. Moffett (1947) makes up a solution containing 2 ml 8% cocaine HC1, sodium bicarbonate, and 1 ml of 1 in 1000 adrenaline, claiming that sodium bicarbonate renders the cocaine chemically stable and enhances the anaesthetic action. The patient is placed in three clearly defined position for 10 minutes at a time:

(1) With the patient lying on the left side with a pillow under the left shoulder and the head 45° with the vertical, one third of the solution is drawn into a syringe: then a drop is allowed to fall on to the anterior part of the nasal septum. The remainder of the syringe is divided equally between the two sides of the nose by introducing a needle along the floor of the nasal cavity and squirting half the contents into each. This manoeuvre blocks nerves from the spheno-palatine foramin.

(2) A second third of the solution is equally divided between the two sides, the nose pinched and the patient rolled over on to the face with the head well flexed. This picks off the nasal branch of the naso-ciliary nerve and the mucous membrane of the anterior ethmoidal and frontal sinuses.

(3) The same position is adopted as for (1) but with the patient lying on the opposite side and the last $\frac{1}{3}$ of the solution employed as before. Finally, 1–2 ml 1% procaine are injected along the base of the septum. Some surgeons then prefer to follow this technique with a general anaesthetic.

Anaesthesia for plastic surgery

The anaesthetist may be called upon to provide anaesthesia for plastic operations on patients of all ages. The younger patients, in particular, may be suffering from congenital abnormalities which affect not only the operative site, but other parts of the body, such as the heart and central nervous system. The anaesthetist should take care, therefore, to make a complete examination of his patient; this is particularly important in a plastic surgery unit, where the surgical team are likely to be preoccupied by the condition presenting for surgery. In such a unit he has to play the important role of 'physician to the surgical team'. The patients have often to undergo repetitive procedures and a number may, in addition, be suffering from underlying psychiatric disorders that require drug therapy.

The anaesthetist must ensure that full surgical access is available, that there is minimal bleeding and that rapid and undisturbed recovery takes place. In many instances, the anaesthetist and surgeon will be sharing the same region of the body, namely the nose and the mouth, and it is clearly important for the well-being of the patient that frank and relaxed rapport exists between the two and that an air of co-operation pervades the theatre. The anaesthetist must ensure that there is no danger of aspiration of blood in operations on the nose and mouth. In operations on the head and neck it is particularly important that the patient does not cough or strain with the inevitable movement that takes place: an effective topical anaesthetic should, therefore, be applied to the larynx and trachea. In operations on the face, particularly in the region of the nose and mouth, it is important that the endotracheal tube does not distort the tissues. A well staffed and efficient recovery ward, in the closest possible proximity to the operating theatre, is absolutely essential for the successful outcome of major plastic surgery.

Operations for congenital defects

The commonest defects presenting for surgery are cleft palate and lip, birth marks which may well affect the mouth, hypospadias, and defects of the hands and ears.

Cleft lip and cleft palate. This operation is best performed at about 3 months of age, particularly if there is a large premaxillary defect which is likely to disturb feeding and be upsetting to the parents. The operation should be directed towards the closure of the lip and the anterior portion of the palate. If the defect on the lip is bilateral then one side should be closed at a time, at an interval of about six weeks. If the pre-maxilliary defect is large, then the first aim should be to produce a 'Cupid's bow' and the cleft dealt with at nine to eighteen months with the object of producing normal speech. In cases where there is insufficient tissue to enable the surgeon to repair the defect, pharyngoplasty may be necessary, in which case it is best to wait until the patient is two years old.

Pharyngoplasty presents a very real challenge to the anaesthetist's skill. In the first place the adenoids must be removed, as the surgeon utilizes the site for the establishment of a graft: adenoidectomy should be performed at one year, followed by pharyngoplasty at two years. In all cases the pre-operative haemoglobin should be at least 10 g per 100 ml. Throat swab culture should be negative; haemolytic streptococci will inevitably lead to a breakdown of the palatal sutures. Cases with double clefts are usually undernourished and attention should be paid to improving the nutritional status in the weeks prior to operation. In addition, all these patients are particularly prone to respiratory tract infection.

All cases should be intubated; the very young can be intubated whilst conscious and the rest either with the aid of neuromuscular blocking agents or whilst breathing spontaneously under halothane or ether anaesthesia. Where the anatomy does not allow effective artificial ventilation of the lungs the use of relaxants for intubation is particularly hazardous. The anaesthetist must therefore assure himself that artificial ventilation will be possible, before employing a muscle relaxant. The endotracheal tube must be sterile and it is wise to have a number of different sizes available prior to induction of anaesthesia. Opinions differ as to whether the patient should be permitted to breathe spontaneously or to be subjected to controlled ventilation. This is a matter of individual preference, but provided that adequate oxygenation and carbon dioxide elimination take place the technique is immaterial. The Ayre's T-piece is suitable for both methods, and if allowing spontaneous respiration, either the divinyl-ether/diethyl-ether mixture (VAM) or halothane are excellent adjuvants to nitrous oxide/oxygen mixture. Care should be taken to avoid excessive heat loss and, in very young infants, the operation should be of short duration. Prior to intubation, a careful aspiration of the upper air passages should be carried out, and the child should be awake and crying at the end of the operative procedure. Feeding should take place as soon as possible after operation.

Pharyngoplasty is usually undertaken at two years of age or over. Large palatal defects cannot be closed by using local tissue, and pedicle flaps have to be swung in, using the inner aspect of the upper arm as a donor site. Grossly hypertrophied turbinates make nasal intubation dangerous, if not impossible. The tube pedicle is attached to the upper lip, or the corner of the mouth, and three weeks later severed from the arm and stitched to the posterior paryngeal wall. If the patient has teeth, the pedicle is either threaded through an acrylic cylinder or a cap splint with bite block is applied. Extubation is carried out after thorough pharyngeal suction with the patient at a very light plane of anaesthesia, and a nasopharyngeal tube is inserted to maintain the airway until full recovery. The final operative stage, surprisingly, is not as complicated as may appear at first sight. Anaesthesia should be induced with either an intravenous agent (in the older patients) or an inhalational (in the younger age group), in which case a pharyngeal airway is slipped down beside the pedicle, using if need be some topical anaesthesia. Once the patient is asleep, the surgeon severs the pedicle from its attachment to the lips and the anaesthetist can proceed to intubate at leisure.

Traumatic injuries

These may consist of compound injuries involving the face, maxillae and mandible, resulting from gunshot wounds, traffic and industrial accidents. They may be associated with other injuries to the body such as crushing of the chest wall, head injury, and major abdominal trauma: the patients may be severely shocked and even unconscious. In injuries involving the face, the first duty is to achieve a clear airway. Fractures of the middle third of the face involve the maxilla, and this may be forced backwards embarrassing the airway, so the patient should be managed in the semi-prone position for transport, with a stitch through the tongue if necessary. If he is unconscious, intubation may present no real problem apart from clearing the airway of debris or displaced fragments of bone.

Where the subject is conscious, the problem is a great tax on the skill and ingenuity of the anaesthetist. Clearly, intubation cannot safely be carried out under relaxants, as access to the larynx cannot be guaranteed and inflation by face mask will very likely be impossible. If the injury is associated with injury to the chest, tracheostomy may be advisable before other surgery. Intravenous induction may be hazardous, but the anaesthetist experienced in this field realises that trespass into the well-recognized dangers of anaesthesia associated with this type of work may have to be undertaken, because there is very often no other course open. However, before embarking on anaesthesia, adequate and reliable suction, selection of tubes and laryngoscopes, bougies, and above all, an assistant are essential.

Induction should take place with the patient in the Trendelenburg position. Particular care should be taken to avoid vomiting and, therefore, the stomach should be emptied by the passage of a stomach tube prior to the termination of anaesthesia. Complete toilet of the wound must be carried out, broken bone being fixed with wire, and the defect closed as a primary procedure by approximation of mucous membrane to skin. (A stitch may be passed through the dorsum of the tongue and a naso-pharyngeal tube left in the situ.)

Post-operatively, the patient should be carefully nursed in the semi-prone position with the uppermost leg flexed. Wire cutters and suction equipment should be at the bed head with proper instructions as to their use and the foot of the bed should be elevated. Breathing exercises should be instituted as soon as possible. (The defect is replaced later by skin, bone and tissue graft.) If fixation is carried out by interdental wires and splints, a thorough toilet of the naso-pharynx should be carried out and all packs removed. The patient must be within a few minutes of consciousness at the termination of the procedure.

Traumatic injuries to the limbs will require both primary and secondary treatment. Fixation may create difficulties in the immediate post-operative period, and again when the subject requires a subsequent anaesthetic for secondary treatment. A closed fracture can lead to a considerable loss of circulating blood volume, for instance a closed fracture of tibia up to about 500 ml and a fractured pelvis up to 2000 ml or more.

Burns

In the first place the percentage of surface area of the body which has been involved by burns must be assessed: to this end Wallace (1951) introduced the 'Rule of Nine'. The head and face are treated as 9%; the front and the back of the body each 18%; the arms 9% each; the legs 18% each and the perineum 1%. The rate and loss of plasma and therefore the severity of shock are roughly proportional to the area burned: adults with less than 15% involvement do not tend to become severely shocked; children are less able to compensate, and their critical area amounts to about 10%. Knowledge of the area involved enables the anaesthetist to predict the rate and total quantity of protein-rich fluid loss. Adults with 15% or more, and children with 10% or more, require intravenous therapy immediately and this should be continued for at least 36 hours in the form of colloid.

The minimum volume of plasma to be replaced can be calculated as follows:

$$\text{Volume in ml} = \frac{\%\ \text{surface area of burn}}{2} \times \text{body weight in kg}$$

This volume is repeated at successive periods of 4, 4, 4, 6, 6 and 12 hours from the time of burning and the administrator is guided by the presence or absence of restlessness, the colour and temperature of the skin, blood pressure and pulse rate, urine volume and character, nausea and vomiting, presence or absence of gastric retention, and the haematocrit. An average of 0.5% or more of the red cell mass is lost for each 1% of surface area affected by a deep burn, and the replacement of 1% of the total blood volume with bank blood for each 1% of body surface area involved is recommended. The importance of adequate oral fluid intake in patients with lesser degrees of burns cannot be over-emphasized. The airway may be involved and make induction difficult. As stated, many of the patients presenting for general anaesthesia will be severely shocked and therefore great care should be taken with general anaesthetic agents, particularly intravenous agents such as thiopentone. Halothane/oxygen or cyclopropane/oxygen induction is preferable to the use of intravenous agents, but small amounts of pethidine may be given towards the end of the operation.

Many plastic surgeons do not use operative treatment under anaesthesia on burns subjects for several days after the incident, consequently the patients will have been treated for shock and fluid depletion well before surgery; in all but minor cases an intravenous infusion should be set up from the commencement of anaesthesia. In many cases the face and lips will be burnt, and in some the respiratory tract may be involved, so we feel that intubation is best avoided unless there are strong indications for it. There have been many reports of cardiac arrest associated with the use of suxamethonium in the presence of burns, particularly in children, and it would appear unwise to give this drug in such cases. The cause of these episodes is obscure; they may be due to sympathetic overactivity, depleted cholinesterase, leak of potassium out of cells, vaso-vagal inhibition associated with intubation, hypovolaemia or metabolic acidosis.

Cases of severe burns often require multiple anaesthetics for debridement and grafting. Intravenous procaine, Dolitrone and Sernyl, have all been employed for dressing burns and during the last few years a drug similar to Sernyl – ketamine – has been introduced. This agent produces similar conditions to Sernyl and may be administered either intravenously or intramuscularly. It might thus be of use in producing anaesthesia for cases of burns, particularly as it is claimed that the patient is able to maintain his airway without mechanical aids. It is particularly important after ketamine administration not to allow the patients to be disturbed in any way during the first few post-operative hours, as this increases the incidence of distressing dreams. Recently methoxyflurane/air, and nitrous oxide/oxygen (Entonox) inhalations have been found to be of great value for the dressing of burns. Restlessness is often due to a low cerebral perfusion and calls for increased intravenous fluid. Because of the severe degree of peripheral vascular 'clamp-down', drugs injected intravenously may not be absorbed at all, so any analgesics that might be given, should be injected intramuscularly with due caution. Patients who have been exposed to a smoke-filled atmosphere must be observed in hospital for 24 hours, because of the danger of respiratory complications. These may call for immediate tracheostomy, aspiration and oxygen therapy.

Work is at present being done to evaluate the use of the alpha blocking agent, phenoxybenzamine, to reverse the severe vasoconstriction, as it is believed that this increases perfusion in the bowel, liver and kidney, reduces pulmonary congestion and improves skin survival. The dose used is 1 mg/kg body weight, given in 250 ml intravenous infusion fluid, over 1–2 hours. When the desired effect, judged by clinical observation of satisfactory skin perfusion, is obtained, the administration is stopped.

Cancer of the head and neck

Cancer of the face may create difficulties when general anaesthesia is required, because, apart from the difficulty of creating an airway, the anaesthetist may be unable to use a face-piece. Oedema of the tumour may produce respiratory obstruction and, if cytotoxic agents are being perfused, they are often administered in conjunction with dyes, and difficulties may be experienced in judging the patient's true colour. Epodyl, which is sometimes used in the perfusion, may produce hypotension. It should be remembered that certain patients who have received radiotherapy may have a tendency to bleed easily in response to very slight trauma; nasotracheal intubation, in particular, may precipitate almost uncontrollable haemorrhage. Skin cancer, rodent ulcer of the face and epithelioma of the lips, may involve the plastic surgeon in varying degrees of surgical complexity: neoplastic processes involving the floor of the mouth, mandible and maxilla may require extensive and mutilating operations, with subsequent plastic repairs; infra-orbital tumours or involvement of the mandible may require surgery to cross the midline; loss of the mandible or a section of it may produce excessive mobility of the tongue, with resulting obstruction. The mandibular defect may be temporarily corrected by a steel bar. Block dissection of the neck may be necessary. In some of these cases tracheostomy is desirable.

Cosmetic operations

Face-lifts, removal of 'eye bags', mammoplasty and rhinoplasty are often demanded, when some of the patients may well be suffering from underlying related psychiatric disorders. The procedures themselves can be regarded as luxury operations, but unfortunately may be associated with excessive bleeding, so that hypotensive techniques are often required.

Hypotensive anaesthesia: this can be of exceptional value in a small number of cases by diminishing bleeding, shortening the time of operation and lessening the need for transfusion. It is, in our view, of great value for jaw resection and block dissection of the neck. Local infiltration with vasoconstrictors is to be preferred, wherever possible, to hypotensive procedures. Much can be done to reduce bleeding by correct positioning of the patient and attention to such detail as minimal resistance to breathing, and adequate carbon dioxide elimination.

Patients presenting with difficulties of intubation

This may arise where there is restricted opening of the mouth. Trismus may be present as a result of spasm of the masseter, pterygoid, or temporalis muscles. Restricted movement of the jaw may result from fractures of the mandible or malar bone, or as a result of injuries to the growing condyle and consequent lack of development of the mandible:

a recessed chin is thus caused. Temporomandibular joint dysfunction commonly presents in the female patient, usually associated with such dental trouble as bite abnormality. Here, as a last resort in treatment, operations on the temporomandibular joint may be performed. Fracture of the zygomatic arch often results in the coronoid process of the mandible impingeing on it, thus restricting movement. Microstoma occasionally arises congenitally, but it more commonly results from irradition or from burns, when the nostrils may also be involved. The mouth may need to be widened by incising the angles of the mouth before intubation is possible.

Flame injuries from children's inflammable nightdresses. These often require skin grafts to the region of the neck below the mandible. As primary grafts sometimes contract and cause approximation of the chin to the sternum, repeated skin grafts are necessary to overcome this deformity, and on each occasion, after induction of anaesthesia, the surgeon can greatly assist the anaesthetist by deliberately cutting the adhesions and thus freeing the neck, enabling intubation to proceed prior to the commencement of surgery.

The Abbé flap procedure, where the lower lip is attached to the upper by a minute flap in order to correct a defect, often poses a problem for the anaesthetist. In fact, once the patient is asleep the unwanted end of the flap can be separated by the surgeon, covered in gauze, and the patient intubated normally.

Jaw deformities. These again present a challenge to the anaesthetist. The Treacher-Collins syndrome is associated with a receding chin, which makes it extremely difficult for a tube to be passed. Abnormal and undeveloped ears, abnormalities of the eyes and maxillae and cleft palate are sometimes present.

Pierre-Robin syndrome: cleft palate is often present, the tongue is excessively mobile, the mandible underdeveloped and breathing difficulties are sometimes encountered during the first few weeks of life, particularly when the infant lies supine. The respiratory difficulties are overcome by fixation of the tongue to the mandible.

Klippel-Feil syndrome: these patients have short, web necks, cervical spine abnormalities and cleft palates.

Intubation in the syndrome referred to above demands not only skill, but luck! Before embarking on the anaesthetic the anaesthetist should arm himself with as many varieties of laryngoscopes as possible, a variety of tubes of a number of sizes, gum elastic catheters, and filiform bougies. Even if the vocal cords cannot be seen, provided the epiglottis can be displaced from the posterior pharyngeal wall it may be possible to pass a small bougie into the larynx and thread an endotracheal tube down over it. For adults, using a local anaesthetic, a Tuohy needle may be passed through the crico-thyroid membrane and through it a sterile catheter threaded, pushing this upwards into the naso-pharynx and hooking it out through the external nares. An endotracheal tube can now be passed around it. It is advisable when difficulties with intubation are anticipated to avoid the use of neuromuscular blocking agents and maintain spontaneous respiration with halothane.

Post-operative care: in many of the patients who have had operations on the jaw, the mandible will have been immobilized by wiring and cap splints, so a pair of wire cutters must always be available by the bedside of these patients in case the wires need to be cut in an emergency. A well organised, well staffed recovery unit is essential. The patients should be nursed on their sides and if need be the airway maintained with a naso-pharyngeal tube. Undue restlessness must be avoided, particularly if flaps are maintained by immobilized limbs, as the involuntary muscular movement commonly associated with halothane can seriously jeopardize the successful outcome of the operation. The post-operative administration of pethidine can sometimes overcome this risk, but on the whole this hazard is best avoided by using a technique such as nitrous oxide/oxygen and a relaxant and controlled ventilation and by immobilizing the Abbé flap with a barrel bandage.

Leprosy. In the days before sulphone therapy, leprosy was unfortunately a common condition in certain countries. Apart from affecting the nervous system and the superficial tissues of the body it can affect the epiglottis, aryepiglottic folds, arytenoid cartilages and the vocal cords, with the result that the larynx becomes shrunken and fibrosed. Tracheostomy was therefore sometimes called for. The condition is also sometimes associated with pulmonary tuberculosis. The anaesthetist may be confronted with these cases for reconstructive surgery. Owing to the low infectivity of this disease transmission is unlikely, but the anaesthetist should take care to ensure that all equipment is sterilized following use, and is well advised to wear rubber gloves. These patients sometimes receive steroid therapy, and the anaesthetist should take particular care to enquire about this. In view of the fact that the skin of the face, external nares and lips may be affected, difficulties may be created in maintaining an airway, particularly if endotracheal intubation is employed.

Epidermolysis bullosa. This rare hereditary condition is characterized by the formation of bullae and vesicles in the skin in response to pressure, trauma and friction, the lesions also occurring in the mouth, pharynx and occasionally the larynx. As it is essential that trauma to the skin and mucous membranes be avoided; no strapping should be used. These patients have often received steroid therapy, so steroid supplement should be given to cover the period of operation. Owing to the association of this condition with porphyria, barbiturates should be omitted in the premedication and induction of anaesthesia, and endotracheal intubation should be avoided if possible. A smooth inhalational induction should be employed, the mask being separated from the face by muslin gauze soaked in 0.5% hydrocortisone. For dental work the patient should be placed in a head-down position so that packs may be eliminated.

Orthopaedic surgery

No age group is exempt from orthopaedic surgery. In view of the posture adopted for some of these operations, impairment of ventilation and blood flow may occur. Massive blood loss may be associated with some of the formidable operations and the surgeon may request hypotensive techniques to help in his work. Tourniquets may be applied to the limbs to exsanguinate the operative field. Problems for the anaesthetist may also arise in the correction of scoliosis, with a laminectomy, which requires special posture and control of bleeding, and with a fractured neck of femur which occurs particularly in the aged. Psoas transplantation is sometimes employed in the correction of disabilities associated with spina bifida, and the operation may carry with it considerable blood loss in the small debilitated child.

The problem of anaesthesia for manipulative procedures has not been adequately solved. Many of these patients are outpatients and require anaesthesia and relaxation of short duration with rapid recovery. It has been the practice in some centres to administer a bolus of thiopentone to these patients followed by swift manipulation. Fundamentally this practice is wrong; it does not take into account the individual susceptibility of the patient to the agent and, as a result, significant falls in blood pressure and respiratory depression undoubtedly occur. On the other hand, careful induction followed by suxamethonium may well be associated with regurgitation of stomach contents, more particularly so if inflation of the lungs is carried out. The logical outcome would be to follow induction by endotracheal intubation, with respiratory control. Suxamethonium carries, in addition, the disadvantage that a high incidence of muscle pains is associated with its use. There is no ready solution to this problem. The use of propanidid, methohexitone or althesin instead of thiopentone may reduce the degree of cardiovascular depression associated with the technique of bolus injection. We recommend the use of 0.6 mg atropine intravenously, followed by the barest sleep dose of thiopentone. Anaesthesia is then maintained by nitrous oxide/oxygen and halothane, which produces entirely adequate relaxation very soon. As the surgical procedure is short recovery is rapid and usually trouble-free.

During the fixation of a prosthesis to the hip joint cement is commonly packed into the reamed out marrow cavity of the femur. This procedure has on occasion produced severe cardiovascular collapse. As it is possible that this is due to the solvent used it is recommended that evaporation should be allowed before insertion.

The anaesthetist is very often involved in the management of patients with multiple and severe fractures resulting from road and industrial accidents. Each case will present its own problem, especially as regards head, neck, and chest injuries, but all have one feature in common, namely hypovolaemic shock.

Urological surgery

A large proportion of urological procedures is carried out on the older age groups. Many of these patients have co-existing cardio-vascular and respiratory disease; in addition, certain types of renal disease are associated with hypotension. Some of the patients will require regular review, and cystoscopic examination for this purpose is frequently carried out as an outpatient. Some suffer a chronic blood loss from bladder lesions, as a result of which they become anaemic. Regard should be paid also to the fact that certain agents used in anaesthesia are excreted via the kidney, as impairment of renal function may potentiate the effect of these agents, e.g. gallamine.

Prostatectomy may be carried out by a direct supra-pubic approach or via the transurethral route. In both instances bleeding may be troublesome, though the average case does not require deliberate hypotension or blood transfusion. Some authorities do, however, employ deliberate hypotension or spinal anaesthesia in order to reduce the necessity for blood transfusion and to avoid the use of a catheter in the post-operative period. Transurethral resection of the prostate requires constant irrigation to enable the surgeon to visualise the operative site; the use of water for this purpose must be avoided as intravascular haemolysis may occur.

Cystoscopy may be employed for diagnostic purposes and also to enable fulguration to be carried out. In view of the fact that many of these patients are outpatients, either topical or caudal anaesthesia may be employed.

Operation upon the kidney. Kidney disease is often associated with electrolyte imbalance, hypertension and associated heart disease, so caution should be exercised with general anaesthesia. Controlled ventilation should be employed, the patients usually being operated upon in the lateral position.

Kidney transplantation. Patients requiring kidney transplantation may be suffering from severe weight loss, asthenia, anaemia, hypertension, metabolic acidosis, uraemia, hyperkalaemia and hyponatraemia. Because of the short excision-transplant time for the donor kidney, the operation is usually urgent: the patients are potentially extremely ill but this electrolyte imbalance is not usually a problem as regular dialysis corrects it. However many are anaemic. They will possibly be receiving an immunosuppressive drug such as azathioprine. If the patients are already receiving steroids they should be given additional cover, but premedication should be minimal. It is suggested that induction should be carried out using thiopentone or cyclopropane, pancuronium for relaxation, and maintenance with oxygen/halothane or nitrous oxide/oxygen. No gallamine or decamethonium should be given as these are excreted in the urine. Nephrectomy is usually carried out through a subcostal incision and is frequently associated with splenectomy: anastomosis of the donor kidney to the iliac artery and vein requires an incision in the iliac fossa. Heparin must be administered before transplantation and reversal is required at the end. Hydrocortisone 200 mg and mannitol 20 g intravenously may be given when the transplant is in situ. In view of the high levels of potassium often encountered in these patients, rapid transfusion of stored blood should be avoided; blood pressure and ECG should be monitored continuously. During the immediate post-operative period, the patient must be in an intensive care unit, with respiratory support if necessary.

11 *Anaesthesia and the Endocrine System*

The pituitary adrenal axis

Hypopituitarism and adrenal cortical hypofunction. Hypopituitarism tends to be more common in women, as its most frequent cause is post-partum necrosis. It may also arise as a result of irradiation of the pituitary gland, in relation to neoplasia of the gland itself, or to cancer elsewhere in the body. Adrenalectomy may be carried out for the removal of tumours of the adrenal cortex or medulla, or for the treatment of inoperable cancer, particularly of the breast. Hypofunction of the adrenal cortex may be associated with Addison's disease, or result from prolonged administration of cortico-steroids. Apart from disturbances in water and electrolyte balance, patients with pituitary and adrenal hypofunction have a diminished reaction to stress. Steroid replacement therapy is essential in adrenal deficiency conditions and in hypopituitarism; additional cortisone cover will be necessary in these cases, before, during, and after anaesthesia and surgery. Particular care must be taken with intravenous agents such as thiopentone.

Bilateral adrenalectomy and oophorectomy is sometimes undertaken for the management of carcinoma of the breast. These patients are often severely ill, cachetic and anaemic, with widespread metastases. Great care should be taken in moving these women, who are not only in great pain, but may develop pathological fractures. Pleural effusion and secondary involvement of the lungs are frequently present. Ventilation of the lungs may be impaired by effusion, which should be cleared by tapping and drainage prior to the induction of anaesthesia. Steroid cover should be instituted prior to the operation (see below). Ventilation should be controlled throughout the duration of the operation and blood loss replaced.

Tumours of the adrenal cortex

Tumours of the adrenal cortex may result in deficient or excessive function. However, adenomata and carcinoma do not necessarily produce an alteration in function.

Primary aldosteronism (Conn's syndrome). This condition, which is more common in women than men, produces a clinical picture caused by the metabolic effects of aldosterone. It is characterized by hypertension, a deficiency of potassium causing episodes of generalized or localized muscular weakness, polyuria and retention of sodium.

Removal of the source of the excessive aldosterone secretion causes dramatic disappearance of the symptoms. This entails the removal of an adrenal tumour, or bilateral subtotal adrenalectomy for those with apparently normal or hyperplastic glands. Additional cortisone cover is not normally necessary for these patients unless bilateral adrenalectomy is to be performed. Careful attention should be paid to the correction of electrolyte balance prior to anaesthesia.

Cushing's syndrome. This condition may rarely result from a tumour of the pituitary, but more commonly in association with a tumour or hyperplasia of the adrenal cortex. In the absence of a tumour of the pituitary, adrenalectomy is the present treatment of choice.

The syndrome is more common in women than men. The symptoms vary from tiredness, alteration of appearance, obesity and menstrual disturbances, to symptoms resulting from hypertension. The associated osteoporosis may result in pathological fractures and care should be taken in positioning the patient.

Replacement therapy with steroids is necessary prior to, during and after operation. It is customary to start cortisone acetate therapy intramuscularly 2 days before an operation in a dose of 200 mg/day. On the day of the operation, 300 mg is administered in divided doses and this dose is maintained until the third post-operative day. Oral therapy is then commenced, gradually reducing the dose to approximately 12.5 mg 8-hourly or 12-hourly at fourteen days. The operative procedure is dictated by whether a tumour has been located pre-operatively. Acute adrenal crisis may arise post-operatively and is characterized by collapse, hypotension and tachycardia. It is treated by the immediate injection of at least 100 mg hydrocortisone intravenously, and if necessary, noradrenaline (4 mg in 500 ml isotonic saline infusion) or metaraminol (15–100 mg in 500 ml isotonic saline).

The thyroid

Thyrotoxicosis

There are two principle types of thyrotoxicosis, both of which are characterized by over-secretion of thyroid hormone. Primary thyrotoxicosis is usually in young adults (mainly females) in whom there has been no previous goitre. Nervousness, exophthalmos, increased metabolism and tachycardia are the main clinical features.

Secondary thyrotoxicosis is usually found in older patients and the onset is often insidious. A goitre may have been present for many years, nervous manifestations are less pronounced and exophthalmos is generally absent or slight. Patients who are severely affected may have atrial fibrillation, and right sided heart failure. Tachycardia, nervousness, excessive restlessness, tremor, and loss of weight are all signs of excessive secretion of the thyroid gland, which gives rise to an increase in metabolic rate. This gland is asymmetrical and frequently nodular.

Very occasionally, myasthenia gravis may accompany thyrotoxicosis and is seen only in those with diffuse goitres. These patients respond to neostigmine. Treatment of thyrotoxicosis usually causes some improvement in the myasthenia, but rarely cures it.

Pre-operative treatment should be directed towards the establishment of an euthyroid state. Careful sedation, together with sympathetic understanding, will help to allay the patient's anxiety whilst anti-thyroid drugs are achieving their effect. Carbimazole 30–60 mg per day or propyl thiouracil 50–400 mg/day are the anti-thyroid drugs commonly in use to produce the euthyroid state. Patients receiving such treatment may, in addition, receive iodine for fourteen days prior to operation, in order to produce a firm gland. Potassium iodide tablets 60 mg/day or Lugol's Iodine 1 ml daily may be prescribed. The operation is carried out as soon as it is judged that the optimal response has been achieved. There is a current trend to treat cardiovascular involvement with β-adrenergic blocking agents along with the anti-thyroid drugs.

Pre-anaesthetic medication. Provided an euthyroid state has been achieved sedation need not be excessive. If on the other hand nervousness is still a feature, full use should be made of sedative agents. Tribromoethyl alcohol (Avertin) at one time enjoyed much popularity for this purpose, but there is now little place for its use, apart from the occasional case of severe thyrotoxicosis. It is usually given in the form of a freshly prepared solution at 40°C by the rectal route, with a dose based on 80–100 mg per kg body weight, 15–20 minutes prior to the induction of anaesthesia. Atropine should be avoided where there is tachycardia.

Anaesthetic technique for thyroidectomy. Induction with intravenous thiopentone, followed by full relaxation with suxamethonium, allows for good conditions for endotracheal intubation. (Some anaesthetists may wish to visualize the vocal cords during spontaneous respiration prior to intubation, however). In order to prevent straining on the endotracheal tube, a thorough application of topical anaesthetic solution to the larynx and upper trachea is advisable – the endotracheal tube being well lubricated with local anaesthetic ointment. Maintenance of anaesthesia may be achieved by controlled ventilation using nitrous oxide/oxygen mixture, with neuromuscular blocking agents to produce relaxation, or spontaneous ventilation using trichloroethylene, diethyl ether, or halothane. The employment of these agents is influenced by the use of infiltration of the operative site with adrenaline, or of diathermy. If exophthalmos is present great care must be taken to protect the eyes from damage – if necessary the eyelids may be stitched together for the duration of the operation. At the termination of general anaesthesia, the surgeon may wish to visualize the vocal cords in order to assess whether any damage has been done to the recurrent laryngeal nerves.

Patients verging on thyroid crises occasionally require immediate surgery; such patients will require thorough sedation. It has been suggested that the inhibition of the end organ (tissue) response to circulating catecholamines provides a rational basis for the management of the acute hyperthyroid patient. Effective adrenergic blockade can be accomplished by using both β- and α- 'blockers' and treatment with reserpine (0.5–1.0 mg daily) or guanethidine (50–150 mg daily) can also be used. If these agents are used, great care should be exercised with general anaesthesia. Suppression of the amount of circulating thyroid hormone cannot be quickly achieved, but intravenous iodine can be employed first (sodium iodide 5.0%, 1.0 g slowly), with the immediate commencement of anti-thyroid drugs. Hydrocortisone therapy is thought to be necessary to compensate for the excessive metabolism of cortisone associated with the hyperthyroid state. Sedation should be freely employed. Hyperpyrexia is treated by ice-packs and chlorpromazine 25–100 mg i.m. while the fluid and electrolyte balance is corrected by the oral or intravenous administration of solutions containing plenty of glucose.

Myxoedema. Hypothyroidism seriously delays the metabolism of drugs and renders the patient unduly sensitive to them. The operative risk is further increased because of secondary changes in the pituitary/adrenal glands, which impair the normal response to stress. Great care should be taken if any attempt is made to correct the hypothyroid state in the pre-operative period by the administration of thyroid hormone, particularly in patients over the age of 50 years and in those in whom there is a history of angina pectoris or evidence of atherosclerosis.

Enlargement of the thyroid, retrosternal goitre, carcinoma of the thyroid. These conditions can give rise to severe respiratory obstruction. It may be necessary to intubate such patients under local anaesthesia, prior to the induction of general anaesthesia.

All patients with thyroid disease when seen pre-operatively should be assessed in the supine position, to ensure that there is no obstruction to ventilation, as well as having radiographic investigation, to exclude retrosternal prolongation. Post-operatively, the anaesthetist should be aware of the possibility of collapse of the trachea following extubation.

Diabetes mellitus

There are two main types of diabetes. Firstly, the type which occurs characteristically in middle-aged obese patients. This type is generally controlled by dieting, but occasionally may need control with oral anti-diabetic agents or small doses of insulin. Some of these diabetics not on insulin or oral agents may undergo an operation without specific treatment for diabetes, but if time allows, dieting, particularly if the patient is obese, will prove of undoubted value. The second type usually has an acute onset, and is associated with an absolute deficiency of insulin, which necessitates the restriction of carbohydrate intake and the administration of insulin. The latter may arise at any age, but is commonest and most severe in the young. Diabetes may also occur in association with thyrotoxicosis and pituitary and adrenal hypofunction. Many patients with diabetes, particularly in the older age groups, suffer from impairment of peripheral flow, and this may be associated with hypertension, gangrene and infection. Coronary artery disease or pathology of the kidney may further complicate the picture for the anaesthetist.

General management. There are four main groups of diabetic patients likely to present for surgery:

(1) Patients on oral anti-diabetic agents. These are usually on a diet and are receiving phenformin, metformin, tolazamide, chlorpropamide (Diabenase) or tolbutamide (Rastinon). It is well to remember that the half-lives of the two latter agents are 30 hours and three hours respectively. These patients should not receive the drug on the day of operation and the blood sugar should be monitored both during and after operation: intravenous glucose is given if the blood sugar is low.

(2) The well-controlled diabetic. For elective surgery it is usually unnecessary to change from long-acting to soluble insulin preceding operation, unless a long period of parenteral feeding post-operatively is envisaged. Fletcher *et al.* (1965) studying 56 operations on 47 diabetic patients, of whom 30 were controlled by insulin, and 17 by oral anti-diabetic agents, showed that complicated regimes were unnecessary for minor or moderate surgery. From midnight on the day prior to operation until after the operation the patients were starved and received no specific treatment or intravenous glucose. Premedication was with Omnopon and scopolamine and

anaesthesia was induced with intravenous thiopentone and maintained with nitrous oxide/halothane. Post-operative insulin is given on the basis of blood sugar and urine (see below).

Mild diabetics on insulin may either be managed along the lines outlined above or, alternatively, as follows, particularly if the operation is in the afternoon. Sufficient glucose is given intravenously to cover the normal morning insulin, on the basis of 1 unit of soluble insulin to 2.5 g carbohydrate. The urine should be tested pre- and post-operatively, and then four hourly, using catheterization if necessary. The following is a rough guide to insulin requirements:

if sugar is absent or	+ (0.25%)	: give no insulin
if sugar is	++ (0.5%)	: give 10 units insulin (soluble)
if sugar is	+++ (1.0%)	: give 15 units insulin (soluble)
if sugar is	++++ (2.0%)	: give 20 units insulin (soluble)

It is essential to take carbohydrate by mouth or intravenously immediately following an operation: as soon as possible post-operatively, carry on with the normal treatment for the diabetes. It must be stressed that the above is only a rough guide for a fairly well controlled diabetic on average insulin dosage. Where the operation is of a major nature, it is wise to stabilize the patient on soluble insulin for several days prior to anaesthesia and surgery. Patients with uncontrolled diabetes, often associated with sepsis, are likewise best treated by soluble insulin.

(3) Some patients may not be ketotic but have a very high blood sugar. This condition is associated with severe dehydration and accompanying hypernatraemia. Blood sugar is usually corrected by relatively small doses of insulin and dehydration by fluid replacement.

(4) For the severely ketotic, where possible, the operation should be postponed and an attempt made to correct the ketosis and electrolyte disturbance with insulin, glucose, electrolytes and water.

Soluble insulin may be administered intravenously together with saline – lactate solution (sodium 130 mEq/l; chloride 104 mEq/l; lactate 30 mEq/l). Provided that there is heavy glycosuria, there is little need to administer glucose. Care must also be taken to observe the plasma potassium level, as potassium will return to the cells under this treatment: when this occurs a solution containing 20 mEq/l of sodium; 30 mEq/l potassium; 5 mEq/l magnesium; 45 mEq/l chloride; 10 mEq/l phosphate; and glucose may replace the former solution. Bicarbonate solution is advocated by some for the correction of metabolic acidosis. To err on the side of safety, a trace of glucose in the urine is a helpful guide. The operation should be delayed as long as possible in order to give the dehydration and electrolyte imbalance the maximum chance of correction. To prevent the onset of hypoglycaemia, blood glucose levels are of value when operating upon an uncontrolled diabetic, and when the operation is of a major nature in the hitherto controlled diabetic. Post-operatively, there may be vomiting or pyrexia: this too may upset the picture, so that the help of a physician in any major procedure is invaluable.

General anaesthetic agents: diethyl ether has been shown to increase the blood glucose twofold in half-an-hour and by the same amount in the second hour. Similar changes are seen with methyl-*n*-propyl ether and with cyclopropane, but the changes with halothane are, by comparison, negligible. Chloroform, ether, and cyclopropane should be avoided in the diabetic. α-blockers, tolazoline (Priscol), phentolamine (Rogitine), β-blockers and ganglion blocking agents interfere with the normal blood sugar response to stress and adrenaline and tend to make the patient sensitive to insulin.

Islet-cell tumour of the pancreas: Fraser (1963) reported alarming episodes of hypotension and cyanosis during and after an operation on one of these tumours. Such tumours of the pancreas involving the beta-cells and giving rise to hyperinsulinism, may be benign or malignant, the former being more common. Whipple's Triad describes a history of repeated attacks of hypoglycaemia with concommittant blood sugar levels under 50 mg/100 ml, and relief of these attacks by Glucose administration. Hargadon and Ormston (1963) suggest that an intravenous infusion should be set up before the patient leaves the ward. A basal blood glucose level is determined and this is repeated before and after induction of anaesthesia, and at intervals throughout the operation. The signs under anaesthesia of excessive insulin activity are sweating, tachycardia, hypertension, or hypotension, dilated pupils and cyanosis. They advise an adequate premedication to allay anxiety, no thiopentone and no halothane. General anaesthesia is provided by nitrous oxide/oxygen and relaxation by D-tubocurarine.

Porphyria

Schultz (1874) first described this disease of metabolism involving pyrolle pigments which take part in respiratory metabolism. In 1906 (three years after the introduction of barbiturates), Dobrschansky described a typical case of acute intermittent porphyria, apparently caused by the prolonged administration of diethylbarbituric acid. The acute intermittent form of porphyria is most commonly aggravated by barbiturates. Symptoms and signs include abdominal pain, constipation, vomiting, tachycardia, arterial hypertension, mental symptoms and, less frequently, motor or sensory disturbances. Death is due to respiratory paralysis. Attacks may be precipitated by the following drugs, which should, therefore, not be used: salicylates, sulphonamides, oestrogens, griseofulvin, chloroquin and methyldopa.

Many cases have been reported to develop acute episodes in close association with thiopentone anaesthesia. They may have peripheral neuropathy or even quadriplegia with bulbar paralysis, and death may supervene. IPPV may be required in these patients. Although it has been stated that with the South African variety, porphyria variegata, thiopentone anaesthesia may not cause untoward effects, most workers strongly affirm that all barbiturates are absolutely contraindicated in any case of porphyria. An inhalational induction should be used, although the eugenol derivatives (e.g. propanidid) or althesin may be considered. Patients suffering from symptomatic porphyria (acquired or cutanea tarda porphyria) who have a defect in their precursor metabolism are, however, not likely to develop fulminant attacks on exposure to barbiturates.

Rheumatoid arthritis

Because of the high incidence of this debilitating disorder, patients often present for incidental surgery. They may, in addition, present themselves for the orthopaedic correction of some abnormality connected with the disease.

Ankylosis and arthritis of the small joints of the larynx, the cervical spine and temporomandibular joints may create problems for the anaesthetist in the maintenance of a patient's airway. Intubation may prove extremely difficult. Ankylosis of the costovertebral joints may also create problems in regard to the adequacy of ventilation, particularly in the post-operative period, and the presence of amyloidosis may seriously imperil the efficient detoxication and elimination of agents from the body. Restriction of the movement of the joints may create damage during posturing of the patient. Many of these patients will have received or will be receiving steroid therapy which may well impair adrenal cortical activity.

Management. A careful examination should reveal restriction of the movement of the joints and, if there is any suspicion regarding the larynx, the case should be referred to an ENT surgeon for further examination. These patients are often anaemic and careful preparation may be necessary to ensure an adequate haemoglobin content of the blood. Patients with history of steroid therapy should be managed along the lines outlined on page 5. Kidney and liver function should be investigated. In the post-operative period these subjects should be carefully observed for any evidence of respiratory insufficiency.

Phaeochromocytoma

Phaeochromocytomata are tumours of the sympathetic nervous system which secrete quantities of the catecholamines, adrenaline, noradrenaline and dopamine. The tumours may arise in the adrenal medulla or in extra-adrenal chromaffin tissue elsewhere, e.g. along the sympathetic chain in the chest or abdomen, or in the organs of Kohn and Zuckerkandle which lie along the abdominal aorta. Such widespread distribution may lead to difficulty in localization. About 10% of the tumours are bilateral or multiple and about 10% malignant; other tumours of the nervous system, such as neurofibromata and neuroblastomas, occasionally secrete catecholamines. This latter neoplasm is likely to be present in any young child with a mass in the retropleural or retroperitoneal regions or in the epidural space.

The abnormality presented by the patients can be accounted for by the known physiological effects of adrenaline and noradrenaline. High blood pressure with associated cardiovascular disease is not uncommon, though normotension and paroxysmal hypertension may occur. Slowing or acceleration of the pulse rate is associated with this condition and anxiety and hyper- metabolic states, gylcosuria and excessive sweating similar to thyrotoxicosis are often present.

Diagnosis. Many tests have been devised to assist in the diagnosis. The so-called 'provocative tests' are now considered dangerous and unnecessary.

Histamine 0.01–0.05 ml in saline has been given intravenously and methacholine chloride 20–25 mg subcutaneously has also been used. Tetraethyl ammonium chloride 300–500 mg, dibenamine 7 mg/kg in 300 ml 5% glucose/saline, phenoxybenzamine (Dibenyline) 0.5–2.0 mg/kg in 300 ml glucose/saline, benzodioxane (Piperoxan) 0.25 mg/kg intravenously, and tolazoline (Priscol) 25–100 mg intravenously, intramuscularly, or orally, have all been tried. The following test seems to be preferred – a fall in blood pressure, following the intravenous administration of 5 mg phentolamine (Rogitine) intravenously, is confirmatory evidence of phaeochromocytoma. These tests are now being superceded by tests of blood and urinary catecholamines and, if considered necessary, perirenal insufflation with air and radiographic evidence of tumour may be elicited.

Spontaneous attacks of hypertension may be provoked by coughing, straining and bending down. Hyperventilation, hypercapnia, and hypoxia can trigger off an attack, as can histamine release from various drugs (e.g. D-tubocurarine). Alteration in posture and positioning on the operating table and surgical manipulation can also be responsible. In addition to the danger of spontaneous attacks of hypertension, the sufferer may develop profound and intractable hypotension, following the removal of a tumour. It has been observed that these patients have a greatly reduced circulating blood volume, due to the vasoconstrictor action of the catecholamines, and the sudden release of vasoconstrictor tone leads to the fall in blood pressure. Although noradrenaline is mainly a stimulator of alpha-receptors, it has, together with adrenaline, inotropic and chronotropic effects upon the heart which may lead to dysrhythmias and heart failure.

Anaesthetic management

There have been many reports in the literature regarding the anaesthetic management of these cases.

Pre-operative sedation. It is of the greatest importance that these patients do not get excited, as this can lead to stimulation of the tumour. Sedation should be given during the days before operation and the night before and immediately pre-operatively. Meprobamate (Equanil) 800 mg, chlordiazepoxide (Librium) 50–100 mg, and diazepam (Valium) 10 mg are all suitable sedatives. Narcotic analgesics which may provoke histamine release are best avoided in the premedication and chlorpromazine, though having an adrenergic blocking effect, has been thought to contribute to post-excision hypotension, and is probably best avoided. Perphenazine (Fentazin) 5 mg and promethazine (Phenergan) 50 mg can be given as premedication, intramuscularly.

Adrenergic blocking agents. The place of these agents in the pre-operative preparation of patients suffering from phaeochromocytoma has been much debated. It has been suggested that pre-operative therapy with adrenergic blocking agents leads to difficulties in restoring blood pressure to normal after the removal of the tumour. However, continuous alpha-adrenergic blockade in the pre-operative period would appear to be in the best interests of the patient, despite this objection, as it leads to a general improvement in the overall general condition. By removing vasoconstriction the adrenergic blockade is capable of improving the blood volume deficit over a few days even without blood transfusion. Phenoxybenzamine is the most suitable of the alpha-blockers for pre-operative therapy. Doses should be determined by the individual response to an initial test dose of 50 mg intravenously, and the drug is administered for at least four days pre-operatively, by mouth, in doses up to 240 mg/day bearing in mind that the effects lasts for about 24 hours. The last dose should therefore be terminated 24 hours before the induction of anaesthesia. Alternatively 500 mg phenoxybenzamine may be given in 300 ml dextrose as a slow intravenous infusion. The blocking of α-receptors in the presence of high levels of catecholamines tends to over-activate the β-receptors, with the result that the inotropic and chronotropic effects on the heart become pronounced. Therefore the combination of α-receptor blockade with β-receptor blockade has been advocated. Propranolol 5 mg intramuscularly, or 20 mg orally, should be given along with the phenoxybenzamine, the dose being adjusted according to the heart rate. Other β-blockers may be used (see page 120).

Anaesthetic technique. A few hours prior to induction, a slow intravenous infusion of phentolamine may be set up and further doses of β-adrenergic blockers given intravenously in divided doses according to the heart rate. Not all anaesthetists follow this course particularly if the blood volume has been expanded. At all times straining, hypoxia and hypercarbia should be avoided. Gallamine should be avoided because of its tendency to cause tachycardia, and curare because it causes histamine release in certain subjects. Diallylnortoxiferine (Alcuronium) can be used without this worry and possibly pancuronium despite its tendency to cause hypertension. Suxamethonium has disadvantages in that it is a stimulant of sympathetic ganglia and, because of increased pressure from muscle fasciculations following its administration, it may lead to an increased output of catecholamines. After pre-oxygenation the induction of anaesthesia follows, using thiopentone given cautiously at a slow rate. Pancuronium 4–6 mg is then administered and the larynx and trachea are sprayed with 4% lignocaine, a well lubricated endotracheal tube is passed and the patient ventilated with nitrous oxide/oxygen mixture. Controlled ventilation is maintained, using if necessary further doses of pancuronium to maintain relaxation. Some authorities have employed halothane or methoxyflurane for maintenance of anaesthesia, but we feel that this technique is fundamentally unsound, in view of the effects of halothane in particular on the myocardium, and prefer small doses of phenoperidine or fentanyl given intravenously as a supplement.

Monitoring: careful attention should be paid to the venous pressure which should be monitored as a routine. Blood pressure, pulse rate and the ECG should also be closely followed and blood loss must be measured throughout the procedure.

Blood volume: if the patient has received routine α-adrenergic blockers in the pre-operative period together with blood transfusion, the tendency to develop hypotension following the removal of the tumour will be greatly diminished. The deliberate attempt to increase the circulating blood volume is undoubtedly beneficial to the patient. Careful replacement of blood loss during the course of the operation will be facilitated by attention to the venous pressure. However, even with attention to these details, disturbing hypotension occasionally occurs. To counter this, an infusion containing noradrenaline (Levophed) may have to be administered intravenously. Very rarely it may be found necessary to replace further quantities of blood and to administer nor-adrenaline for 24 hours or so.

5-Hydroxytryptamine (Serotonin)

5-HT (Serotonin) occurs widely in the body and is present in particular in the chromaffin cells of the gastro-intestinal tract, the spleen, platelets and brain. Increased levels of 5-HT in the plasma are found in association with carcinoid tumours affecting the small intestine, ovaries, testes, and bronchus, argentaffinoma of the lung, non-tropical sprue, intestinal lipodystrophy and occasionally in association with thrombosis and mental deficiency. Amongst many factors morphine and reserpine are known to cause its release. The reported prolongation of barbiturate narcosis in mice by the administration of 5-HT has been confirmed by Wulfsohn and Politzer (1962), who found that this potentiation of effect occurred also to chloral hydrate, diethyl ether, and chloroform. Monoamine oxidase inhibitors, by preventing the breakdown of 5-HT by amine oxidase were also found to prolong the effect of all these agents.

Carcinoid syndrome: the syndrome is characterized by release of 5-HT giving rise to a widespread disturbance of smooth muscle, manifesting itself as watery diarrhoea, asthma, and skin blanching with alternating hyper- and hypo- tension. Attacks may be precipitated by alcohol, morphine and monoamine oxidase inhibitors. The pulmonary and tricuspid valves may become coated with a white fibrous layer affecting the endothelium, giving rise to stenosis of these valves, and resultant right-sided heart failure, with cyanosis, raised jugular venous pressure and oedema.

Histamine in anaesthesia

Several substances used in anaesthetic practice have been blamed for causing histamine release, which is of particular importance in those patients who are hypersensitive to its action. D-tubocurarine, trimetaphan, and pethidine, have been particularly implicated. In patients such as asthmatics, these substances should be avoided, and suxamethonium, gallamine, pancuronium, or alcuronium used when relaxants are required (see page 53). Recently it has been reported that propanidid can cause sudden collapse associated in some instances with an urticarial type rash : this is possibly a histamine release phenomenon.

12 *Neurosurgical Anaesthesia*

In the past, neurosurgical anaesthesia was deemed to be shrouded in mystery and was often approached with a mixture of dread and apprehension. But how did it differ from other forms of anaesthesia? Perhaps the main difference lay – and still lies – in the effect of imperfections of anaesthetic technique on the surgical result. In abdominal surgery an error in anaesthetic technique hinders the surgeon at the time, but once corrected, good operating conditions are restored. The same is not true of neurosurgical operations. A short period of hypoxia, hypercarbia and straining, leads to swelling of the brain which will persist for an appreciable time: the operation will certainly be made more difficult and in some cases impossible.

The high penalties exacted for imperfections in anaesthetic technique, combined with the lack of basic knowledge of the pathology of cerebral oedema, frequently deterred neurosurgical anaesthetists from readily employing new methods and new agents. It also discouraged them from modifying techniques which had, in their hands over the years, given fairly good results: trivialities were sacredly observed, although the reasoning behind them had long since been forgotten. In recent years, however, much of the detailed folklore has been set aside and replaced by general principles based on scientific fact. Now even the uninitiated, with a good background knowledge of physiology, can approach a neurosurgical case with confidence.

A smooth induction, followed by a tranquil maintenance without hypoxia or hypercarbia, are the chief ingredients of a successful neurosurgical anaesthetic. None of the techniques discussed later in this chapter will provide good operating conditions if this cardinal rule is disregarded. No apologies are made for repetition; a good technique is a smooth technique, the anaesthetist who ignores this principle does so at his patient's hazard.

Radiological investigations in neurosurgical practice

Some of the radiological investigations performed on neurological patients are only mildly uncomfortable and, with sympathetic handling, can be performed without general anaesthesia. However, in young children, and in adults who cannot co-operate by remaining immobile whilst the films are being exposed, anaesthesia may be necessary even for the simplest procedures. Two investigations, cerebral angiography and air encephalography, are uncomfortable and the service of an anaesthetist is frequently required.

Cerebral angiography

General considerations: this investigation is carried out on a wide range of neurological patients, some of whom are conscious, in good general condition and present few problems, while others are semi-conscious, have papilloedema and may be dehydrated. In the latter group premedicant drugs which depress the respiratory centre must be avoided and no attempt should be made to correct dehydration before surgery. Where the patient has been semi-conscious for some time, sputum may have accumulated in the chest and the opportunity of performing a thorough tracheo-bronchial toilet during anaesthesia should not be missed. Cerebral angiography is often an urgent investigation, upon the result of which future treatment hinges. It is thus rarely advisable, even in extremely ill patients, to defer anaesthesia in the hope of the patient's condition improving.

Anaesthetic requirements

(1) *Immobile patient.*

Coughing may displace the needle from the artery, thus traumatizing the wall of the vessels. Straining leads to venous congestion and increases the liability of haematoma formation, while movement of the head when the films are being exposed distorts the pictures.

(2) *Maintenance of normal blood pressure.*

Hypotension, although it may assist in the detailed radiological demonstration of a highly vascular tumour, makes puncture of the artery by the radiologist more difficult, whilst uncontrolled hypertension in patients with subarachnoid haemorrhage may rupture the aneurysm. A normal blood pressure is generally desirable, especially as hypotension in the presence of raised intracranial pressure predisposes to medullary failure.

(3) *Avoidance of further neurological damage.*

As hypoxaemia, rise in PCO_2 levels, obstruction to respiration or coughing and straining can all precipitate cerebral oedema and increase the neurological damage, they must be avoided. The potent inhalational agents, particularly halothane, raise the intracranial pressure and should only be used with discretion.

Anaesthetic techniques

Local anaesthetic. In some centres local anaesthetic with sedation is employed for carotid angiography. In suitable cases, premedication with an appropriate dosage of a narcotic analgesic is satisfactory or neuroleptanalgesic drugs may bc administered intravenously immediately prior to the investigation. Before attempting the arterial puncture, the radiologist injects a local anaesthetic agent intradermally at the site of the proposed puncture and also to the side of and behind the artery: excessive injection of local anaesthetic solution into the neck may obscure the vessel. The chief disadvantage of carrying out the investigation on a conscious co-operative subject is the occurrence of a burning sensation on the side of the face and retrobulbar pain following the injection of the contrast medium, so that the patient may move and the quality of the films suffer. However, the technique is frequently satisfactory when the investigation is limited to one vessel and a quick puncture is obtained. Local anaesthesia is often considered inadvisable in patients suspected of having had a recent haemorrhage from an intracranial aneurysm, as the stress of the investigation may cause a further bleed by raising the arterial blood pressure. Vertebral angiography by retrograde femoral catheterization using the Seldinger technique can also readily be performed under local anaesthesia in co-operative patients following appropriate sedation.

General anaesthesia. This is preferred in many centres for carotid angiography, and is generally considered essential for anterior cervical puncture of the vertebral artery, because of the proximity of the sensitive cervical plexus to the artery and the technical difficulties of this puncture.

Premedication. Avoid respiratory depressants in the presence of raised intracranial pressure. Atropine only is satisfactory.

Induction. A rapidly acting intravenous induction agent and short acting muscle relaxant is satisfactory for intubation with a non-kinkable tube. (If non-kinkable tubes are not available, a nasal tube is preferable to an oral tube.)

Maintenance. In the past spontaneous respiration was often employed, in the belief that observation of the respiratory pattern was of value in recognizing changes in the patient's intracranial condition during anaesthesia. Nitrous oxide and oxygen were supplemented with halothane, trichloroethylene or a narcotic analgesic. Recently the hazard of using halothane and other inhalational agents in intracranial disease has become recognized and the use of muscle relaxants with controlled ventilation for angiography has been strongly advocated, especially in patients with cerebral tumours.

An added advantage of hyperventilation is that the tumour circulation is better defined : this is because the blood flow to the tumour is unaffected by the lowering of the arterial carbon dioxide tension, whilst the circulation to the rest of the brain is reduced. On the other hand, in patients who have had a subarachnoid haemorrhage and in whom spasm of the intracranial vessels is present, the circulation to the brain is already slow. A further reduction in blood flow as might occur with hyperventilation, might not be an advantage. For this reason some neurosurgical anaesthetists prefer spontaneous ventilation if the patient has had a recent sub-arachnoid haemorrhage.

As X-ray apparatus is rarely spark proof, explosive agents should never be used for the maintenance of anaesthesia in radiological departments.

Possible complications

(1) *Circulatory changes*

With modern contrast media, change in blood pressure following their injection is uncommon, but when it occurs it is generally in patients with pre-existing cerebral vascular spasm, often associated with subarachnoid haemorrhage. The pressure may either rise or fall and, in either case, it is an indication of cerebral ischaemia. In most cases no specific treatment is necessary but, if a low blood pressure persists, vasopressors may be indicated.

(2) *Haematoma*

Haemorrhage from the punctured vessels is normally controlled with ease by digital pressure, but small haematomata are not infrequent and they seldom give cause for worry. A large haematoma, on the other hand, will displace the trachea and respiratory difficulties may result, requiring re-intubation and perhaps surgical evacuation of the haematoma.

(3) *Medullary failure*

In patients with markedly raised intracranial pressure, respiratory arrest may occur after intubation, or later following injection of contrast medium or saline. The anaesthetist must exclude the more common causes of apnoea before notifying the neurosurgeon that the respiratory centre has failed. Controlled respiration should be instituted and the intravenous infusion of an osmotic dehydrating agent commenced to reduce the pressure : it is probable that immediate craniotomy will be necessary.

(4) *Increase in neurological deficit*

(a) In patients with cerebrovascular disease, or following subarachnoid haemorrhage, angiography may precipitate further neurological damage. This is thought to result from an increase in spasm of small intracranial vessels adjacent to the pathological area. Injections of lignocaine and papaverine around the major vessels in the neck have been advocated by some, in the hope of reducing this hazard, but the value of this is in doubt.

(b) When carotid stenosis is present, discretion is obviously necessary in compressing the opposite carotid. In these patients spontaneous respiration is clearly indicated for the maintenance of anaesthesia, so that at the end of the investigation, following withdrawal of the needle from the artery, the respiration as well as blood pressure and pulse rate can be carefully observed. Once the radiologist is satisfied that bleeding from the puncture site has ceased, the patient should be extubated under adequate anaesthesia to avoid coughing.

(c) The anaesthetist may be requested to compress the carotid on one side while contrast media is being injected into the other, in order to demonstrate the degree of cross circulation to the opposite hemisphere – a manoeuvre which, if gross hypertension occurred, could rupture an aneurysm in patients suffering with subarachnoid haemorrhage. The effect on the blood pressure depends on the site and duration of compression: hypertension is greatest following prolonged compression of the common carotid and least after brief compression in the region of the carotid body. The latter site is to be preferred, but the pulse rate and blood pressure should be carefully monitored.

(5) *Intrathecal injection of contrast medium*

This is a rare but serious complication of vertebral angiography, generally not recognized until the films are developed when it is observed that the contrast medium has entered the cisterna magna instead of the vessels. There are no symptoms or signs at the time of injection but later severe tonic spasms and hypertension may develop quite suddenly and can prove fatal. The recommended treatment consists of irrigation of the subarachnoid space to remove the contrast medium as soon as the condition is recognized and control of any spasms with curare and controlled ventilation.

Pneumoencephalography

The initial stage of this investigation is carried out with the patient in the sitting position. Lumbar puncture is performed and some cerebro-spinal fluid withdrawn and replaced with air; the gas passes up the subarachnoid space and, if the head is suitably positioned, enters the ventricular system through the foramina in the floor of the fourth ventricle. Air encephalography, by changing the pressures within the skull, may lead to ischaemia of the vital centres and medullary failure in patients with increased intracranial pressure. In such cases, pneumoencephalography must be avoided and the ventricles outlined by ventriculography (via a burr hole) employing either air or a contrast medium.

The presence of gas inside the cranium, especially if it lies over the surface of the brain, is unpleasant and often distressing to the patient. Severe headache with nausea and vomiting is common and the assistance of an anaesthetist is frequently requested to provide relief: this can be provided by general anaesthesia or by sedation and analgesia.

General anaesthesia. Premedication will depend on the anaesthetist's preferences, but drugs which would predispose to hypotension in the sitting position should be avoided. Anaesthesia is normally induced with a rapid acting intravenous induction agent and a short acting muscle relaxant: the larynx is sprayed with topical anaesthetic and, as the head will be placed in extreme flexion during the procedure, the trachea should be intubated with a non-kinkable tube. Anaesthesia is maintained with nitrous oxide/oxygen supplemented by a non-explosive inhalation agent.

Although halothane is more liable than trichloroethylene to cause postural hypotension, it is still the author's preference for patients in the sitting position. It is important to raise an anaesthetized patient gradually to the sitting position, and if this is done, vasopressor agents are seldom necessary.

Sedation and analgesia. Various combinations of sedative and analgesic agents have been tried, usually by the intramuscular route. Papaveretum and scopolamine, chlorpromazine and pethidine, barbiturates, etc., are beneficial but, unless they are administered in a dosage which produces a semi-stupor and an unco-operative state, pain relief is inadequate and vomiting remains a problem. Neuroleptanalgesia has been a major advance in this field. The author, when employing this technique, prefers to estimate the required dosage more on the patient's general condition and age than on a weight basis. Droperidol 2–3.5 mg and either phenoperidine 1–2 mg or fentanyl 0.05–0.1 mg are given intravenously initially: after 5 minutes, the patient is positioned and, if sedation or analgesia proves inadequate, further smaller increments of the analgesic agent may be given, the respiratory rate being observed and not allowed to fall below 12/min. (Levallorphan and nalorphine are both effective in antagonizing the respiratory depression and, unfortunately, they also antagonize the analgesic effect.) Where sweating, nausea or vomiting occur, further droperidol (less than 1 mg) is indicated, provided the blood pressure is stable. If further sedation is undesirable or the blood pressure unstable, cyclizine lactate 5 mg may be tried instead of droperidol. Employing the technique described, hypotension is seldom a problem and responds readily to vasopressor agents. However, occasionally the combination of droperidol and analgesic has led to dramatic falls in blood pressure which have not responded to vasopressor agents until the patient has been placed supine. Delayed respiratory depression has been reported and careful observation of these patients post-operatively is necessary. The intramuscular use of droperidol is not satisfactory in adults as the dosage required (20 mg) will result in Parkinson-like tremors and other excitory phenomena in a proportion of patients, 24–48 hours later. It is doubtful if neuroleptanalgesia is a suitable technique for the radiologist to employ single-handed.

Complications of pneumoencephalography

1. Postural hypotension: this is seldom a major problem, unless the patient is in a poor general condition with a low blood volume.
2. Respiratory disturbances: there are two circumstances where respiratory disturbances may occur:
   (a) Respiratory irregularity or arrest may occur in the presence of a grossly raised intracranial pressure when cerebrospinal fluid is taken off, or after air has entered the cranium and upset the internal dynamics. Controlled respiration should be initiated and a dehydrating agent administered intravenously: immediate craniotomy may be indicated if the lesion has been localized. This complication can be avoided by never performing a lumbar air encephalogram in the presence of raised intracranial pressure.
   (b) When excess air is injected intrathecally and little fluid withdrawn, the intracranial pressure may rise markedly and embarrass the respiratory centre even in patients without cerebral pathology. The treatment in this case is to ask the radiologist to take off further cerebrospinal fluid. This complication occurs more frequently in the anaesthetized subject, possibly because the nitrous oxide from the blood enters the air bubble more rapidly than nitrogen passes in the opposite direction, thus increasing the tension in the bubble. The secondary rise in pressure from nitrous oxide can be prevented by the radiologist injecting nitrous oxide or oxygen intrathecally instead of air, (the compressed gases in anaesthetic cylinders are sterile), or by the anaesthetist using air as a vehicle for the anaesthetic agents instead of nitrous oxide.

Pre-operative preparation for intracranial surgery and post-operative care of the patient

The neurosurgical anaesthetist frequently commences the care of his patient some days before major surgery is undertaken and his care is continued into the post-operative period, often for several days. The craniotomy itself is but an episode – albeit an important one – in the overall treatment of the patient. During the pre-operative and post-operative days the anaesthetist collaborates with his surgical colleagues in the general care of the patient, paying particular attention to the degree of hydration, the presence or absence of increased intracranial pressure and the condition of the patient's lungs.

The state of hydration. Consider the patient's history. Has there been vomiting? Has fluid and food intake been restricted over the past days or weeks? Has he received a dehydrating agent? An adequate history and an accurate fluid intake and output chart, in conjunction with the specific gravity of the urine, haemoglobin, electrolyte balance and blood urea estimation should give a reasonably accurate picture of the state of hydration. *If increased intracranial pressure and papilloedema are present, no attempt should be made to correct even gross dehydration before operation.* Dehydration in these circumstances is a safety mechanism and rehydration would precipitate failure of the vital medullary centres. Of course, where the intracranial pressure is normal, there is no objection to at least partial rehydration before operation.

The intracranial pressure. Headache, neck stiffness or papilloedema suggest increased intracranial pressure. If any of these are present, depression of the vital centres by drugs, e.g. opiates, or indirectly by intravenous infusion, should be avoided pre-operatively. In some respects the respiratory centre acts as an on-off switch. It can be under severe stress, yet tidal volume, vital capacity and rate may be normal and the patient may be conscious and only slightly irrational; but, if small quantities of respiratory depressant drugs are given, apnoea and unconsciousness may ensue. In suitable cases, the intracranial pressure can be lowered and the neurological deficit reduced by (a) the restriction of the fluid intake to the body, (b) the administration of tubular or osmotic dehydrating agents, (c) the administration in massive dosage of adrenal glucocorticoid steroid, e.g. prednisolone 160 mg daily, (d) hyperventilation, or (e) ventricular tap.

The care of the lungs. The anaesthetist with his knowledge of respiratory physiology and his specialized skills is well prepared to advise on the care of the patient's pulmonary system. The condition of the lungs and their response to physiotherapy and antibiotics, the level of consciousness, the physical status of the patient and the presence of emphysema or obesity will guide the anaesthetist as to the possible need for tracheostomy, either pre-operatively or later in the post-operative period. Tracheostomy should, if necessary, be performed early rather than late and certainly before respiratory distress has actually occurred. Particularly in the immediate post-operative period hyperventilation may be of value, either to ensure a normal arterial carbon dioxide and oxygen tension or to relieve the patient of the labour of breathing spontaneously.

Immediate pre-operative care. Before surgery is contemplated, the majority of patients will have been in hospital several days, during which time various investigations, including some with anaesthesia, will have been carried out. Thus before making his final pre-operative visit, the anaesthetist will have had the opportunity to gain the patient's confidence, assess his mental outlook and obtain some prior knowledge of his possible reactions to major surgery. Pre-operative sedation will frequently be unnecessary and may be detrimental, atropine 0.6 mg i.m. being generally given to dry up secretions and to produce partial blockade of the vagus. The drug therapy the patient is receiving should be reviewed at this stage.

Anaesthesia for craniotomy

From the anaesthetist's view point, the problems associated with craniotomy can be considered under three headings:

- the positioning of the patient
- the maintenance of a low intracranial pressure
- the replacement of blood loss

Operations on the posterior fossa present special problems and will be considered separately.

Positioning of the patient

Surgical access. The first consideration in positioning any patient for surgery is to ensure that the surgeon has the best possible access to the operative site. In the case of a frontal craniotomy the patient is placed supine with the brow up. For a temporal lobectomy the body can remain supine, but the head should be rotated 30° towards the opposite side and a small pillow placed under the shoulder adjacent to the occiput, to relax the sternomastoid muscle. For a parieto-occipital lesion the body should recline in the lateral position, with the head in the horizontal plane.

Free venous drainage. The second consideration is to provide free venous drainage from the head, the absence of which will raise the intracranial pressure (cf. the Queckenstedt manoeuvre) and will also increase operative haemorrhage. Free venous drainage can be obtained by elevating the head relative to the heart and avoiding compression of the veins in the neck. Obstruction to the neck veins can occur from tight clothing, from over flexion of the neck, or from compression by the sternomastoid when the head is rotated laterally without turning the body. (When the head is to be placed in the horizontal plane, the patient should be positioned on his side.)

Respiratory obstruction. It is frequently necessary to flex the head and as kinking and obstruction of the endotracheal tube can thus occur, a non-kinkable tube, either a nylon spiral armoured tube or the specially designed Oxford tube, should be employed. Flexion and backward displacement of the head shortens the distance from the teeth to the carina and care should be taken that the endotracheal tube does not enter the right bronchus. Once surgery has commenced, re-intubation would be extremely difficult and special precautions should be taken to ensure that the tube remains in the trachea. The author, in addition to using waterproof strapping, prepares the attachment areas of the face and tube with comp. mastic paint (BPC) to provide a firm grip and avoid damaging the sensitive skin of a child or elderly person. It is also valuable in patients with greasy unshaven skin.

Iatrogenic injury. The patient should be positioned so that he does not harm himself during a prolonged operation.

Straining of joint ligaments: joints, e.g. elbow and wrist, should be retained in a neutral position, preventing any strain on the ligaments. In this respect, the lumbar area should not be overlooked; the arch should either be supported, or the lower limbs raised to obliterate the hollow. Lack of support to the lumbar area with the table flat and the patient supine is considered to be a frequent cause of backache following prolonged operations.

Damage to superficial nerves: compression of superficial nerves on bony or table protruberances should be avoided, e.g. by protecting the lateral popliteal nerve in the lateral position.

Venous thrombosis: post-operative venous thrombosis in the lower limb is reduced by elevating the limbs without over extending the knee joints and supporting the heels, thus avoiding compression of the calf muscles and stagnation of the blood.

Pressure necrosis: in prolonged operations, areas on which the support of the body is concentrated may become ischaemic and should be massaged regularly, during surgery, to restore the circulation. Examples: the lower ear in the lateral position, the forehead in the prone cerebellar and the knees in the knee-elbow position for lumbar laminectomy. The author is aware of cases where necrosis in these areas has occurred following 6–8 hour operations. Rubbing the areas with oils prior to positioning, and with spirit post-operatively, appears to be beneficial.

The maintenance of a low intracranial pressure

There are two ways to tackle this problem; first, by avoiding factors which increase the intracranial pressure and second, by taking active measures to reduce the pressure.

Factors tending to raise intracranial pressure. Anaesthesia increases the intracranial pressure, but the effect of the anaesthetic agents themselves – in the absence of respiratory depression – is not of prime importance. The important factors are the blood tension of carbon dioxide and the cerebral venous pressure, a rise of either of which markedly increases the intracranial pressure. Hypoxia has a similar effect. Obstructed respiration, coughing on the endotracheal tube or straining will result in a fall in arterial oxygen tension and a rise in arterial carbon dioxide tension and venous pressure; the increase in brain volume which ensues will persist for some time, perhaps changing the entire course of the operation. Resistance to expiration also raises the intracranial pressure by increasing the mean intrapulmonary pressure and obstructing the venous return to the heart. Such unnecessary resistance during spontaneous respiration can be avoided by the use of a low spring tension in the expiratory valve, or, better still by employing an Ayre's T-piece.

Respiratory depression of pharmacological or pathological origin also produces a rise in arterial carbon dioxide tension in addition to a fall in arterial oxygen tension. Drugs which depress respiration must be used with caution, both pre-operatively and during maintenance of anaesthesia, if it is intended for the patient to breathe spontaneously during the operation.

All the inhalational agents which are employed to supplement nitrous oxide/oxygen anaesthesia raise the intracranial pressure, but their effect is not of prime importance, provided the pre-anaesthetic intracranial pressure is low and the arterial carbon dioxide tension during the anaesthetic is kept within the normal range. If the arterial carbon dioxide tension is allowed to rise, or if there is a pre-existing raised intracranial pressure of pathological origin, then the addition of inhalational agents, particularly halothane, will produce a sharp rise in intracranial pressure. This rise can be prevented, or reversed, by the infusion of the osmotic dehydrating agents mannitol or urea. However, some anaesthetists prefer to supplement nitrous oxide with an agent which has been shown to have little or no effect on the intracranial pressure, e.g. thiopentone, droperidol, phenoperidene or fentanyl. In practice a marked rise in intracranial pressure can be avoided by:

smooth anaesthesia
a clear airway with minimal resistance to expiration
free venous drainage from the skull
the avoidance of hypoxia and hypercarbia
the judicious use of inhalation anaesthetic agents

Active methods of reducing brain volume. Several methods are available to reduce brain volume in the operating theatre:

controlled ventilation
cerebral dehydrating agents
hypotensive techniques
hypothermia

Controlled ventilation is beneficial in three ways: it lowers a raised arterial carbon dioxide tension; increases the capacity of the venous reservoir; and permits the use of minimal quantities of anaesthetic agents.

Lowering a raised arterial carbon dioxide tension to a normal physiological level will have a marked effect on the intracranial pressure, but a further reduction to below this level will be of limited value and the additional cerebral vasoconstriction produced may even be a disadvantage. Considered from its effect on the arterial carbon dioxide tension, controlled ventilation is only of practical value in reducing brain volume where the blood tension of carbon dioxide is initially high. However, if controlled ventilation is obtained with muscle relaxants the abdominal musculature is paralysed, thus reducing the intra-abdominal pressure and increasing the capacity of the inferior vena cava; the ease of venous return from the cranium is thus improved and the brain volume reduced. The reduction in venous pressure depends, not on the control of respiration which in theory raises it, (by increasing the mean intra-thoracic pressure), but on the relaxation of skeletal muscle. In clinical practice, therefore, it is important, in order to obtain maximal benefit from controlled respiration, to retain muscular relaxation throughout the operation by ensuring continuous neuro-muscular blockade. During the anaesthetic, a fall in tidal volume, or unexplained change in pulse rate or blood pressure, suggests the possible need for the further administration of a muscle relaxant. Where the central venous pressure is being monitored this is a most sensitive guide. Complete muscular relaxation with artificial ventilation providing a near normal arterial carbon dioxide tension is probably the ideal state. The use of a negative phase in the cycle is helpful, but not essential.

Cerebral dehydrating agents. The intravenous infusion of hypertonic solutions increases the osmotic pressure of the plasma relative to the tissue, water is drawn out of the tissues into the blood stream and the size of an organ such as the brain, is reduced; concurrently, the intracranial pressure falls before there is a significant diuresis. Indeed it can occur without a diuresis.

As the brain is surrounded by a rigid box, any reduction in brain tissue must be compensated for by a rise in volume within the cranium of cerebrospinal fluid and blood. Although the total volume of the intracranial contents is not measurably reduced after hypertonic solutions, some reduction must actually take place as the intracranial pressure falls. Several hypertonic solutions have been employed to produce cerebral dehydration.

Hypertonic saline and dextrose. Both are effective in reducing brain volume but as both rapidly leave the circulation to enter the tissues, their concentration in the tissues soon equals that in the plasma, the differential osmotic effect is lost and the organs return to their original size. Following this, as the saline is excreted and the dextrose metabolized, their concentration in the tissues becomes greater than that in the blood, fluid is then drawn into the tissues, and the brain becomes larger than before. This is known as the rebound phenomenon. Significant rebound with these two solutions occurs within 3–4 hours: they are thus unsuitable for clinical use.

30% Urea in fructose. As urea enters the extracellular compartment only slowly, rebound, if it occurs (the evidence is contradictory) is delayed for about 12 hours. Clinically it has proved satisfactory and efficient. The entry of urea into the brain substance is facilitated by respiratory acidosis and inhibited by respiratory alkalosis. For reducing brain volume, urea solutions are administered intravenously in a dosage of 1.5 g/kg over a period of not less than 20 minutes. More rapid transfusion may lead to haemolysis of the red cells and haemoglobinuria.

Precautions should be taken to avoid the solutions leaking around the vein or necrosis and ulceration are produced. In the average adult the infusion of hypertonic solutions result in an increase in blood volume of about 1 litre, and, if given before surgery, bleeding from the incision is increased. It has been suggested that such infusion should be withheld until the first burr hole is made; in practice, it is advisable not to depend on any rule of thumb but rather to vary the technique according to the tempo of the surgery, administering the solution early for a quick surgeon and later for his slower colleague.

Contraindications to hypertonic urea:

(1) Renal insufficiency or damage.
(2) General body dehydration.

General body dehydration can be considered a relative contraindication. It is true that, following urea, a diuresis is produced, more fluid will be excreted than was administered and further general dehydration will result; this can be prevented by an appropriate transfusion of fluid and circulatory collapse avoided. It is the author's practice, in the presence of dehydration, to give a dehydrating agent at the beginning of the craniotomy, reducing the brain volume, and extra fluid (blood or plasma) subsequently during the course of the operation, to prevent a serious fall in blood volume post-operatively.

Mannitol 20% or 25%. Mannitol appears to have all the advantages of urea without some of the disadvantages; certainly, it is less irritant to the tissues and extravasation may have less serious sequelae. Mannitol increases the blood flow to the kidney and this property has led to its use in vascular surgery to protect the kidney from the effect of ischaemia and in the treatment of oliguria and anuria. Thus a case can be made out to permit the employment of this agent to reduce brain volume in patients with renal damage. Further, as mannitol does not enter the cells, the rebound phenomenon is less than with urea and it is thus particularly useful in cases where a surgical decompression is not being performed. Red blood cell agglutination may occur and, for this reason, blood and mannitol should not be mixed in the infusion set.

(Storage: 20–25% solutions of mannitol are supersaturated and will crystallize out at low storage temperature; the crystals will, however, re-dissolve on warming.)

Triple or quadruple plasma and hypertonic sucrose. Both can be employed. The former is difficult to dissolve and there is a risk of serum jaundice, but is useful when it is desired to reduce the brain volume and at the same time increase the blood volume for a prolonged period. Sucrose has been suspected of producing tubular damage of the kidney.

Hypotensive techniques. These techniques probably reduce brain volume by lowering the venous pressure and not primarily by their effect on the arterial system, as the mean arterial pressure must normally be reduced to below 65 mmHg before the blood flow through the brain is reduced. Additional advantages of a hypotensive technique are a bloodless field for the surgery and a reduction of blood loss. Where it is employed, the systolic arterial pressure should be raised to at least 100 mmHg before the dura is closed, to ensure that no potential bleeding points are concealed.

Hypothermia will reduce the intracranial pressure, but it is seldom employed primarily for this purpose.

The replacement of blood loss at craniotomy. Blood loss can be considerable during cranial operations, but provided the hazard is appreciated and stored blood is available for replacement, it should not cause the anaesthetist undue worry. (Even a slight haemorrhage continuing over a period of hours can mount up and trap the unwary.) On the other hand, the loss can be acute and difficult to control quickly, particularly at three periods during the operation. The first is after the cutting of a burr hole, because if damage to a superficial vessel occurs it may not be possible to control the haemorrhage until the bone flap has been raised; secondly on raising the bone flap, if a vascular tumour is attached to the dura at its centre, and the tumour vessels become torn; and thirdly during the removal of a tumour attached to a venous sinus, or where the tumour extends deeply and involves major vessels.

When major blood replacement is necessary, the appropriate quantities of calcium and bicarbonate should be given.

General principles of anaesthesia for craniotomy

Having considered the problems involved, we are now in a position to suggest some general principles around which the anaesthetic technique can be built.

Premedication. If papilloedema is present, drugs which depress the respiratory centre should be avoided: atropine 0.6 mg is frequently employed. Do not correct general body dehydration pre-operatively.

Induction. Induce anaesthesia intravenously as this is safe and pleasant for the patient. Facilitate intubation with a non-kinkable tube by the use of short acting muscle relaxants. Spray larynx and upper trachea prior to intubation with a local anaesthetic agent to assist in obtaining a smooth transition to spontaneous respiration. Strap the endotracheal tube carefully in position and ensure a clear airway at all times.

Maintenance. Continue light anaesthesia by the inhalation agents nitrous oxide/oxygen, appropriately supplemented if necessary. Avoid explosive agents, as the surgeon will wish to use diathermy.

Brain volume may be reduced by: controlled ventilation using muscle relaxants. The use of the dehydrating agents mannitol 20%, or urea 30% in fructose (1.5 g/kg).

Complications during craniotomy

Respiratory arrest. In patients with grossly raised intracranial pressure, the induction of anaesthesia may lead to respiratory arrest of central origin. (It should be noted that some patients with a very high intracranial pressure are not unconscious and ventilation is not depressed pre-operatively.) Once the anaesthetist is satisfied that the respiratory arrest really is of central origin, and not related to a complication of the anaesthetic, the surgeon should be notified, controlled ventilation commenced and a dehydrating agent given. Surgery should not be delayed.

Fortunately, during the actual operation, respiratory arrest rarely complicates intracranial manoeuvres above the tentorium cerebelli, but when it occurs it is a grave omen and is seldom amenable to treatment.

Hypotension. Unexpected hypotension during an operation is generally the result of a low blood volume from general body dehydration or from blood loss. In either case, transfusion is indicated and vasopressor agents are best avoided. The possibility of steroid deficiency should not be overlooked in patients with secondary cerebral tumours, as secondary deposits in the adrenal glands also are not uncommon. Less frequent causes of hypotension are damage to the hypothalamus, or air embolism from an open venous sinus.

Acute oedema of the brain. With modern anaesthetic techniques, this complication should rarely be seen. It occurs when the dura is incised and the oedematous brain under pressure herniates through the opening, the veins of the exposed brain become compressed on the bony or dural margin and further oedema develops. The surface of the brain ruptures and the surgeon is faced with the vicious circle of more oedema – more venous congestion – more oedema.

Treatment of the condition once it has occurred is most difficult and the prognosis is poor. The patient should rapidly be given an osmotic dehydrating agent and placed on controlled respiration, but the most successful line of treatment is prevention, ensuring that the intracranial pressure is low before the dura is opened.

Particular operations

Hypophysectomy. Patients undergoing this operation should be given steroids (cortisone acetate 100 mg b.d.) for 48 hours pre-operatively, which should be continued in the post-operative period, gradually reducing to a maintenance dose after ten days. In addition, hydrocortisone hemisuccinate 100 mg i.m. is often administered during the operation.

Hypophysectomy is sometimes performed in the management of carcinomatosis for breast neoplasms. Such patients are frequently anaemic, cachexic and may have pleural effusion and secondary deposits in bone; careful pre-operative preparation is essential. Special care should be taken in positioning these patients, in view of the risk of causing pathological fractures.

Generally a frontal craniotomy will be performed; the patient is placed supine with the neck flexed, but less so than for a frontal lobectomy; in this position the frontal lobe will tend to fall away from the orbital plates, improving the surgical exposure. With modern techniques, access to the pituitary fossa should be readily obtained without undue retraction of the brain. In the past such retraction was often necessary and damage to the hypothalamus (retractor ischaemia) was a potential hazard. Hypothalamic trauma can be recognized while operating, by the occurrence of unexpected hypotension, but the effect is often delayed until the post-operative period. Diabetes insipidus is another complication of this operation; an accurately kept fluid intake/output chart in the immediate post-operative period assists early diagnosis and demonstrates the effectiveness of pitressin.

Meningioma. A meningioma is pathologically a simple tumour and successful removal should give the patient many years of useful life. It is, however, highly vascular and the frequent attachment to dural sinuses makes blood loss at operation a major problem. Adequate cross-matched blood (6–8 units) should be available before the operation is commenced, a second intravenous infusion may prove helpful and the advisability of employing a hypotensive technique should be considered. Severe blood loss may occur at four points during the operation; (1) when a major vein draining the tumour is damaged whilst making a preliminary burr hole; (2) where the surface of the meningioma is torn on raising the bone flap; (3) when the deepest part of the tumour is being dissected out; (4) and finally when the tumour is being dissected off a venous sinus. The anaesthetist should attempt to transfuse ahead of blood loss until the tumour has been removed and the bleeding controlled. Appropriate quantities of calcium and bicarbonate should be given if large and rapid transfusions of blood have proved necessary.

Temporal lobectomy for the removal of an epileptic focus. The surgeon will require to record the EEG by placing electrodes directly on the cerebral cortex, both before and after the removal of brain tissue. General anaesthesia would interfere with the EEG tracing, so local anaesthesia with sedation is generally employed until the epileptic focus has been satisfactorily removed. Sedation can be provided by phenothiazine derivatives and an analgesic drug, the neuroleptanalgesic drugs being suitable, as the object of the exercise is to produce tranquillity and yet retain the co-operation of the patient. It is important that the anaesthetist should have good rapport with the patient and obtain his confidence pre-operatively. A few extra minutes when positioning the patient to ensure his comfort will be well rewarded during the subsequent hours of the operation. The patient is placed on his side supported by pillows and sand bags; pressure on the point of the shoulder is avoided by flexing the lower arm at right angles to the body and supporting the limb with an arm board; the patient supports his upper trunk on his thoracic cage. The lower limbs should be elevated and separated by a pillow. Elevation of the legs in relation to the trunk reduces the incidence of cramp in the lower limbs which may occur after 2–3 hours of surgery; cramp can be very severe and extremely resistant to treatment so, though massage is frequently beneficial, additional analgesia and sedation may be required. Prevention of cramp is more simple than the cure! Once the successful removal of the focus has been confirmed by EEG it is no longer necessary for the patient to remain conscious. The induction of anaesthesia is not as difficult as the position on the table would suggest and, after pre-oxygenation, unconsciousness is induced with a sleep dose of thiopentone sodium (100 mg will usually suffice). Topical anaesthesia is applied to the upper nostril and pharynx, and the injection of 1 ml 4% ligocaine intratracheally anaesthetizes the larynx; further thiopentone is given if required, and a 'blind' nasal intubation performed. If intubation of the trachea proves difficult, the tube is withdrawn to the pharynx and nitrous oxide, oxygen and halothane administered: the tube is later advanced into the larynx, guided by the respiration.

Surgery of Intracranial Aneurysms. In addition to the usual problems of craniotomy, the anaesthetist must avoid episodes of hypertension which may result in rupture of the aneurysm before the dura is opened. Hypertension is most hazardous after the intracranial pressure has been lowered by hypothermia or a dehydrating agent, possibly because in these circumstances the outside support of the aneurysmal sac is minimal. Halothane may be administered judiciously during the course of the anaesthetic to maintain normotension. Circulatory arrest may be required by the surgeon to facilitate the dissection around the neck of the aneurysm, whilst avoiding rupture of the aneurysm itself. It may be obtained locally by the application of temporary clips to the cerebral vessels feeding the aneurysm, or centrally, by either occluding the major vessels to the head within the chest, or by internally pacing the heart to produce cessation of the circulation with a rapid normal rhythm or with deliberately induced ventricular fibrillation. Where there is the possibility of temporary circulatory arrest being employed, hypothermia is essential. Moderate* hypothermia (29°–31°C) is generally obtained by surface cooling and the administration of drugs to prevent shivering and vaso-constriction. Where profound hypothermia is required an extra-corporeal circulation must be employed. Surface cooling can be obtained by immersing the patient in a bath containing ice cold water, by surrounding him with ice bags, or by circulating cooled air over him. With all of these techniques, vaso-constriction is difficult to avoid and surface cooling in a water bath at 25°C has much to recommend it. Employing this technique, it has been claimed that vaso-constriction and metabolic acidosis do not occur; in addition, the temperature differential between the organs and also the 'after drop' is reduced, without substantially increasing the cooling period.

Circulatory complications with dehydrating agents are more prone to occur under hypothermia than under normothermic conditions, but, as the agents are more potent at lower temperatures, they are effective at approximately half their normal dosage.

Hypotensive techniques during craniotomy. With the advent of the operating microscope in neurosurgical practice renewed interest has been taken in hypotensive techniques. Intra-arterial pressure monitoring is now more frequently available and thus the accurate measurement of the arterial blood pressure is both feasible and convenient. Sodium nitroprusside is currently popular for reducing the blood pressure; it is administered either by drip in a 0.05–0.1% solution or by syringe employing a slow injection pump. The chief advantages of this drug include an evanescent action – a great comfort when sudden severe haemorrhage can occur – and controllability; tachycardia occasionally occurs, in which case β-adrenergic blockade may be employed.

Indications for hypotensive. The general rule still applies – hypotension should only be used to make an operation possible or safer for the patient and not simply to make an operation technically easier. A hypotensive technique may be considered in patients free from evidence of cardio-vascular or cerebro-arterio-sclerotic disease and in whom major surgery is being undertaken. Such a bloodless field is then essential for the safe removal of a vascular lesion or for a delicate dissection using the operating microscope. The blood pressure should only be lowered for as short a period as is required and only as much as is required by the procedure: As a guide a mean arterial pressure of 65 mmHg will be tolerated by most patients for a period of hours, but it can be lowered to 30 mmHg for periods of up to 20 minutes with reasonable safety. A hypotensive technique should not be undertaken in the presence of raised intra-cranial pressure, otherwise perfusion of the brain could become inadequate.

Posterior fossa exploration

An exploration of the posterior fossa presents some special problems to the anaesthetist. These arise from: the position of the patient during surgery and the effect of interference on the medullary centres.

Position of the patient: the relative popularity of the two positions commonly employed, the 'prone cerebellar' and the sitting or 'chair' position, has waxed and waned over the years, but at the present time the pendulum has swung in favour of the prone position. The sitting position gives better surgical access than the prone, but has two definite disadvantages, postural hypotension and air embolism.

Postural hypotension. When a subject under general anaesthesia is raised rapidly to the sitting position, a marked fall in blood pressure may ensue, particularly where the patient is elderly, dehydrated, or has an unstable vasomotor system. However, if the patient is raised gradually, the circulation usually has time to adjust to the new environmental conditions and hypotension is not a serious problem unless drugs which depress the autonomic system, e.g. chlorpromazine or anti-hypertensive drugs, have been administered pre-operatively. For the maintenance of anaesthesia, trichloroethylene, which is considered to have less effect on the blood pressure than halothane, is preferred by many anaesthetists, but the author has administered halothane for several years with the patients in this position and has seldom been seriously concerned by hypotension. Halothane has the advantage of permitting limited movement of the head during positioning, without producing breath-holding from laryngeal stimulation.

During positioning, if the blood pressure does fall appreciably, the patient should be returned to the horizontal plane; after normotension has returned, he can be raised again, more slowly and with frequent pauses to allow the circulation to stabilize. A 'G' suit or pressure bandage to the lower limbs may be employed to prevent pooling of blood in the extremities. The use of vasopressors may help initially and seldom need be repeated once the patient is postured, but, as they complicate the assessment of the patient's general condition and can delay the recognition of a small air embolism, the author feels they are best avoided.

Air embolism is a serious hazard of the sitting position, occurring whenever the venous pressure is low and the walls of a cut vein are held apart by the surrounding tissue. During an operation, these conditions may be present in the suboccipital venous plexus, the epiploic vein and in a venous sinus.

Prevention of air embolism:

diathermy of open veins

waxing of the bone edges

avoiding accidental damage to vessels

compressing the veins in the neck regularly during the operative approach or producing a resistance to expiration to raise the venous pressure and demonstrate any open veins

recently, investigations have been made with a pressure suit which unlike the better known 'G' suit also enclosed the abdomen and chest: this could be of real value

avoiding too light a plane of anaesthesia and irregular deep respiration, which sharply lowers the central venous pressure

controlled respiration: in the British Isles, controlled ventilation in the sitting position is generally feared as a potent cause of air embolism, but at least one North American centre does not agree and the practice has now spread to this country as well

Diagnosis of air embolism: with a massive air embolism, the patient makes a gasping respiration even under controlled respiration (the gasp being the result, not the cause, of the air embolism); the blood pressure falls to zero and the typical 'mill wheel murmur' is heard on auscultating the heart.

Small air embolisms produce a much less dramatic picture, but, as they may herald a larger embolism, their early diagnosis is important. An air embolism should be suspected if respiration becomes irregular, or the blood pressure falls by 10 mmHg, or the heart rate rises by 10 beats per minute in circumstances where air embolism is possible and there is no other obvious cause for the change: the diagnosis can be confirmed or refuted by compressing the veins in the neck. It has been claimed that continuous monitoring of the heart with an oesophageal stethoscope provides an early and certain diagnosis of embolism. More recently it has been demonstrated that even minutes quantities of circulating gas (less than 1 ml) can be detected by ultra-sound employing the Doppler principle. This is a major advance and one which could well be instrumental in swinging the pendulum back in favour of spontaneous respiration and the sitting position.

Treatment: the classical method of treatment is to lower the head, raise the feet and turn the patient onto his left side. (Animals in the lateral position tolerate air better than when supine, possibly because in this position the outflow from the right ventricle is no longer the highest point and the air lock is removed.) The chief disadvantage of this line of therapy is the unavoidable delay in getting the patient into the lateral position, during which time there is no effective circulation. The author has employed external cardiac massage, which can be commenced in the sitting position with good effect. The essence of success is early diagnosis and prompt treatment.

Once a small air embolism has been detected the neck should be squeezed to prevent further air entering the great veins and also to demonstrate to the surgeon the site of entry of the air. In the majority of cases this is all that is required, the surgeon seals the open vein by diathermy or wax and no further treatment is needed. If, however, a large embolism does occur the arterial blood pressure falls precipitously and it is in these circumstances that external cardiac massage is indicated. If the patient's condition does not rapidly improve with massage the table should be levelled and preparations made for thoracotomy to remove air directly from the heart. The author does not favour the blind needling of the heart through the intact chest wall, nor does he feel it necessary or justifiable to routinely place a catheter in the superior vena cava before operation, as has been advocated, so that if embolism did occur the air could be aspirated immediately.

Air embolism is a serious complication and is the reason why many anaesthetists and surgeons now prefer the prone position. However, with meticulous surgery and a vigilant anaesthetist, the hazard can be reduced to acceptable proportions.

Prone cerebellar position: in this prone position, neither air embolism nor circulatory instability is likely to occur, but surgical access is not as good as in the sitting position; in addition, ventilation may be embarrassed, especially in the obese subject. Under ordinary circumstances, controlled ventilation would be considered mandatory for prolonged operations in the prone position, but the neurosurgeon may wish to be advised of any changes in the respiratory pattern when he is operating on or near the floor of the fourth ventricle. Thus, spontaneous ventilation must be permitted, except where the lesion is laterally placed in the cerebellar hemisphere. However, in some centres respiratory monitoring is not considered essential and all posterior fossa explorations receive muscle relaxants and controlled ventilation. (See below for the place of monitoring.)

The patient is supported on his shoulders, upper chest and pelvis; the abdomen should be unsupported to allow free excursion during both inspiration and expiration; the neck is extended and the head flexed at the atlanto-occipital joint (but not so flexed as to obstruct the jugular veins). Finally, the upper part of the body is elevated to place the operational site higher than the heart to facilitate venous drainage. During prolonged operations the points providing most support to the body may become ischaemic, but greasing such points before positioning and regular massage during the operation is helpful in preventing permanent damage.

The effect of interference on the medullary centres. Interference resulting in ischaemia of the vital medullary centres may arise from: general increased pressure below the tentorium; compression or obstruction to the supplying or draining vessels; and direct interference with brain tissue on the floor of the fourth ventricle. Either respiratory or cardiovascular changes may be produced by the ischaemia.

Respiratory changes: with mild ischaemia, the respiratory pattern becomes irregular. When the posterior inferior cerebellar artery or its territory has been interfered with a Cheyne-Stokes pattern of respiration without actual apnoea is observed; when the anterior inferior cerebellar artery is involved an irregular spiky pattern is produced; in severe ischaemia complete apnoea occurs. One of the most sensitive means of observing and recording these changes is by the use of the Hewer Respirometer. This simple apparatus will demonstrate many irregularities which would pass unnoticed if monitoring consisted simply of observing the reservoir bag. The author employs the respirometer routinely in adults during posterior fossa explorations and has found it invaluable.

Changes in respiratory patterns may be observed immediately following the induction of anaesthesia in patients with increased intracranial pressure or in similar circumstances when the head is postured in flexion. In both cases, if apnoea results anaesthetic causes should be excluded, controlled ventilation initiated, a dehydrating agent given and the craniotomy expedited. If the posterior fossa is already open when the irregularities occur, the surgeon should be notified immediately, as these changes may be the result of retraction of the brain to expose the tumour, or of retraction of the tumour itself interfering with the blood supply to the vital centres. While the surgeon is in the best position to appreciate the cause of the damage and may be able to prevent it occurring, the anaesthetist, being aware of the character of the respiratory changes in conjunction with changes which he may observe in the cardio-vascular system, should be willing to advise on their seriousness.

Changes in the cardiovascular system: a rise in the systolic blood pressure is frequently an early sign of interference with the blood supply to the vital centres, but it can also occur from other causes, such as stimulation of the cranial nerves or of sensitive areas of dura under light anaesthesia. Thus a rise in blood pressure on its own is not of great significance.

Bradycardia and ventricular irregularities are more important. They are often of short duration, just three or four beats, and are readily overlooked unless the ECG is being carefully monitored; a change to nodal rhythm may also occur. These ECG changes are of serious portent and suggest the possible advisability of interrupting the surgery. On the other hand, the anaesthetist should not be lulled into a false sense of security by the absence of ECG changes, as respiratory arrests can occur without any cardiac derangements. However, in such cases, with efficient controlled respiration, it is unlikely for the arrest to be permanent.

The place of monitoring during posterior fossa surgery. It has been claimed that the electrocardiogram will detect changes due to manipulation in the region of the medullary centres just as early as careful scrutiny of the respiratory excursion will suggest insult to these centres. Many anaesthetists have accepted this view and now routinely employ controlled respiration for posterior fossa explorations, monitoring only the heart and circulatory system. However, the evidence in support of this theory is inconclusive : it has been shown by other centres that respiratory changes, as demonstrated by a direct-writing spirometer, frequently occur without any changes in the electrocardiograph and only rarely have electrocardiographic changes been observed before the onset of respiratory irregularities. Indeed, respiratory arrest can occur, can persist for many minutes and require manual ventilation without any evidence of electrocardiographic changes. It must, however, be admitted that many of the respiratory changes are minor and would pass unnoticed without special equipment and that it could be argued they may be without practical significance. Perhaps serious permanent damage to the brain stem does not occur without electrocardiographic changes being produced, but at the present state of our knowledge it would seem unwise to make this assumption. The author believes an excellent case can be advanced for the use of spontaneous ventilation and both respiratory and cardiac monitoring during posterior fossa exploration in the sitting position.

The pertinent points in anaesthesia for posterior fossa exploration may be summarized :

(1) Employ spontaneous ventilation in both prone and sitting positions.
(2) Be wary of embolism and hypotension in the sitting position.
(3) Ensure (a) unobstructed ventilation with a non-kinkable tube,
(b) reliable fixation of the endotracheal tube, and
(c) an efficient intravenous infusion.
(4) Reduce intracranial pressure with a dehydrating agent.
(5) Monitor ventilation and ECG and inform the surgeon of changes.

The intracranial pressure should not be lowered by dehydrating agents in 'by-pass' operations, e.g. Torkildsen's operation or the insertion of a ventriculo-atrial shunt, as the surgeon requires a moderate CSF pressure in order to position the tube in the ventricle. Rapid release of cerebrospinal fluid at these operations may embarrass the vital centres, but the effect is only temporary and no specific treatment is generally necessary.

Spinal operations

The chief problem in spinal operations is to prevent excessive venous oozing obscuring the operative field. Most of the troublesome haemorrhage is from the veins around the vertebral canal, as they have few valves and faithfully reflect pressure in the vena cava. To obtain a dry field, the anaesthetist must maintain a low pressure in these large vessels and this can best be done by posturing the patient and providing complete abdominal relaxation.

Posture during surgery. For operations in the lumbar area, the lateral or prone position may be employed. The former allows blood to drain out of the wound, away from the operative site; also, by breaking the table as for a renal operation and flexing the upper limb with knee to chest, a lumbar disc can be removed without performing a laminectomy. For other lesions in the lumbar area and all lesions in the thoracic and cervical region the prone position gives better surgical access.

In the prone position, the patient should be supported on his upper chest and superior iliac spines, the abdomen being allowed to hang free. Obstruction to abdominal excursions will raise the intra-abdominal pressure within the vena cava; the venous bleeding from the wound will be increased. The table should be tilted to position the operation site at the highest point, thus further improving the venous drainage. Various modifications of this position can be employed satisfactorily provided that free excursion of the abdomen is permitted. The 'Mohammedan praying position', with the knees tucked under the patient, is the most effective in removing the lumbar lordosis but, in the obese subject at least, respiratory movements are embarrassed.

Abdominal relaxation. Relaxation of the abdominal muscles which reduces the intra-abdominal and intra-caval pressure, can readily be obtained with muscle relaxants and controlled respiration, or with spinal and epidural anaesthesia.

Other methods of reducing bleeding: reduction of venous oozing is most important and, provided it is at a minimum, additional methods are generally unnecessary, though they are considered useful in some centres. Local infiltration with vasoconstrictive agents is very effective and gives a cadaver-like appearance to the wound. Halothane should be avoided when vasoconstrictor agents have been employed. Arterial hypotension by ganglion blocking agents, spinal and epidural anaesthesia are also effective. With all techniques a rise in arterial carbon dioxide tension must be avoided.

Cervical Explorations

The sitting position may be employed, since this reduces the venous pressures to a minimum and allows blood to escape freely from the wound. There is, however, a potential hazard of air embolism and the prone position is generally preferred. Unilateral damage to the autonomic tracts in the cervical (or bilateral in the thoracic area) may result in hypotension. The hypotension is temporary and associated with generalized vaso-dilatation, needing correction only when it is gross, or in a patient with cardiac disease or cerebral arteriosclerosis. Post-operatively, respiratory insufficiency may be present from damage to the upper cervical cord. Thus careful observation of the patient in the recovery ward is essential, with facilities for assisted ventilation at hand. Chest complications in these cases are frequent.

Cordotomy for intractable pain

All the problems of a cervical exploration are present and, in addition, the surgeon may wish the patient to be awake during the actual cordotomy in order that he may evaluate the degree of pain relief produced and the motor damage caused with each cut into the cord. The patient is anaesthetized for the first part of the operation and local anaesthetic agents are injected during the exposure, as if the patient were awake. Before the cordotomy general anaesthesia is discontinued, but the difficulty remains of getting the patient sufficiently awake and co-operative for the testing; several techniques have been suggested and apparently work well in their protagonist's skilled hands, but the tyro often finds them less effective. Pre-operative sedation is generally avoided or kept to a minimum and the patient is not told that testing will be carried out in the conscious state, until he has reached the anaesthetic room. Unnecessary concern is thus avoided. Anaesthesia can be induced with an intravenous agent and an orotracheal or a naso-pharyngeal tube of the correct length inserted after a topical anaesthetic has been applied to the nostril and throat. Anaesthesia can be maintained with nitrous oxide and oxygen supplemented by either halothane, a methohexitone 'drip' or analgesic drugs; controlled ventilation with muscle relaxants has also been employed. Before testing, anaesthesia is discontinued, spontaneous ventilation restored, if necessary, and the endotracheal tube withdrawn into the pharynx, (a naso-pharangeal tube being left *in situ*). It may be necessary to wait several minutes for the patient to recover consciousness sufficiently for testing: after testing, anaesthesia is re-induced. It is claimed that some of the patients are amnesic for the entire procedure while the remainder are not disturbed by the ordeal. In many centres it is felt that the testing under such conditions is not of sufficient accuracy to warrant the possible distress to the patient and the entire operation is performed under general anaesthesia.

Anaesthesia in patients with neurological disease

From the medico-legal point of view spinal, epidural and regional anaesthetic techniques are often best avoided in patients with neurological disease, particularly in conditions in which relapses are frequent and unpredictable – e.g. disseminated sclerosis. In these circumstances the anaesthetic procedure might easily be blamed for any incidental change in the patient's neurological state. Chest infections are prone to occur in patients in whom there is loss of muscle tone, paresis or blurred consciousness. However, a rapid recovery from general anaesthesia at the end of the surgery, adequate post-operative analgesia without over sedation and efficient physiotherapy should prevent serious complications.

Neurological disease *per se* seldom provides any particular problem for the anaesthetist in the operating theatres. Barbiturates should not be employed in acute intermittent porphyria and only with extreme caution in myotonia congenita, a condition in which any form of anaesthesia is hazardous. Again, in Huntington's chorea the respiratory centre may occasionally be abnormally sensitive to barbiturates.

An interesting complication is seen in patients with complete transection of spinal cord above T6. At cystoscopy, when the bladder is distended with fluid, a marked rise in systolic blood pressure occurs, presumably from a 'mass reflex' of the spinal cord below the lesion. The hypertension may give cause for concern to the uninitiated. See also amyotrophic lateral sclerosis (page 64), mysthenia gravis (page 65), poliomyelitis (page 64), familial periodic paralysis (page 64) and multiple sclerosis (page 64).

Anaesthesia for electro-convulsive therapy (E.C.T.)

The purpose of anaesthesia in this instance is to protect the patient from the side effects of the therapy which include fractures of the spine and long bones, prolapsed intervertebral disc, avulsion of the teeth, hypoxia and para-sympathetic over-activity.

Premedication. Atropine is best given intravenously before induction to partially block the powerful vagotonic action of the convulsion.

Anaesthesia. A rapidly acting intravenous induction agent followed by a short acting muscle relaxant and intermittent positive pressure respiration, without endotracheal intubation, is all that is required. The patients are ventilated with air or oxygen, a special rubber prop is positioned between the upper and lower gum to protect the teeth and the electrical therapy administered. Following the tonic phase of the convulsion, artificial ventilation is continued until spontaneous ventilation recommences, at which time the patient should be turned onto the lateral position, until consciousness is regained. If a large dose of relaxant is given, little evidence of a convulsion may be seen. This disadvantage can be overcome by inflating a sphygmomanometer cuff on one limb to above the arterial blood pressure, thus preventing the relaxant from entering that part of the body; an unmodified convulsion in one limb is now observed. Many of the patients receiving this form of treatment are elderly and have cardio-vascular disease. The muscle relaxant avoids the hazard of hypoxia during the convulsion, but it should be borne in mind that the nicotinic side effects of suxamethonium will increase the degree of hypertension associated with electrotherapy. It has also been suggested that the type of induction agent employed affects the incidence of cardiac irregularity; in one series of patients with cardiovascular disease the incidence of dysrhythmias was greater following thiopentone than following methohexitone. However, it would seem possible that the difference may be related to the depth of anaesthesia, rather than to the drugs themselves.

Paediatric neuro-anaesthesia

Radiological investigations. General anaesthesia is advisable for all but the simplest of radiological investigations; local analgesic techniques frequently prove unsatisfactory and should seldom be employed. The problems encountered and their prevention and treatment are similar to those discussed in the adult.

Intracranial surgery. Paediatric intracranial surgery is exacting; in particular, blood loss and replacement must be carefully balanced. The dehydrating agents can be administered on a weight to weight basis, (mannitol 1.5 g/kg), but rapid infusion should be avoided and the required quantity should be given over a period of not less than 20 minutes, otherwise haemolysis may result. Generally the body temperature, particularly in infants, should be maintained by artificial means, but in appropriate cases hypothermia can be therapeutically employed. The large surface area relative to weight and the frequent paucity of adipose tissue permits a rapid fall of temperature on cooling; in addition, the 'after drop' is small.

The two most common neurosurgical operations in children are for the insertion of a Spitz-Holter valve and for the treatment of meningomyelocoele. For the former, conventional anaesthesia with spontaneous ventilation is satisfactory, but the anaesthetist may be requested to interpret the ECG tracing while the catheter is positioned in the atria. In the latter operation, the chief problems are the age of the patient (under 12 hours), the measurement and replacement of blood, and the maintenance of body temperature. Intermittent positive pressure ventilation is advisable.

Stereotactic procedures

The patients may be under general anaesthesia or sedated during the preliminary stages of the operation, but it is necessary when the actual lesion is being produced, for them to be awake and co-operative, capable of obeying commands and of carrying out simple actions. In addition, the tremor and rigidity in persons with Parkinson's disease should not be ablated by the drugs employed. Many of the elderly patients are frail and have cardio-vascular disease, so anaesthesia or sedation in the sitting position is liable to be associated with postural hypotension. The anaesthesia or sedation required is governed by the surgical technique employed, which varies markedly between different centres. The operation is performed in either two stages or one.

Two stage operations. The first stage is performed under conventional general anaesthesia, with spontaneous ventilation. It consists of lumbar encephalography to locate the exact position of the globus pallidus, followed by a burr hole to permit access to this area of the brain by a probe. A heavy frame to steady and control the probe is then positioned on the patient's head and, with the aid of radiology, the probe is correctly positioned in the brain. The position of the probe in relation to the frame and of the frame in relation to the skull is recorded, so that on a subsequent day they can be accurately replaced. After this has been accomplished, the apparatus is removed from the patient's head, anaesthesia is discontinued and the patient returned to the ward. Some days later the patient is brought back to the theatre and the equipment repositioned; neither anaesthesia nor sedation is necessary, as the lesion in the brain can now be made in a fully conscious, co-operative patient. The problems from the anaesthetic point of view during the first stage are the age, and frequent debility of patients, and the sitting position. It is not necessary to have an awake, co-operative patient at the end of this stage of the procedure.

One stage operations. In most centres, the operation is performed in one stage and now the problem is more difficult, for the patient must be kept comfortable during the first part of the procedure and yet be awake and co-operative, with the tremor and rigidity present, when the stereotactic lesion is being made. If small quantities of the air are injected through a burr hole (ventriculogram) instead of via the lumbar route, headache and nausea is less frequent. The procedure is now only mildly uncomfortable and, as the patient is really enthusiastic to have the best result from the operation, it can be satisfactorily performed in many cases without any form of anaesthesia or sedation. However, where pneumoencephalogram is employed as a preliminary, some method of pain relief is essential. Various techniques have been advocated; endotracheal anaesthesia with nitrous oxide and oxygen, with minimal halothane and spontaneous ventilation; nitrous oxide and oxygen, muscle relaxation and controlled ventilation; or methohexitone 'drip' without intubation. Prior to making the lesion, anaesthesia is discontinued and the patient allowed to waken up, but, although consciousness is rapidly regained, the return of the tremor and rigidity is often delayed and an appreciable time may elapse before the patient is sufficiently co-operative for testing.

Neuroleptanalgesia appears to give more satisfactory results. The patient may sleep during the earlier part of the procedure and the absence of tremor during sleep will be appreciated by the surgeon especially during the delicate operation of placing the probe. When the time comes to make the lesion the patient is readily aroused, becomes fully co-operative and – very conveniently – the tremor and rigidity return. At the present time droperidol and phenoperidine or fentanyl are the agents most frequently employed to obtain the neuroleptanalgesic state. Continuous infusion of 'althesin' is currently under investigation and is giving highly satisfactory results.

Pre-operative preparation. Drugs which effect the stability of the circulatory system should be avoided, e.g. antihypertensive agents and phenothiazine derivatives. Opiates and similar drugs are also best avoided, as they depress respiration and predispose to postural hypotension. Whether the anti-Parkinson drugs should be stopped pre-operatively is controversial. If they are discontinued, the patient's condition will deteriorate before surgery; on the other hand, their continued action may make assessment of the result of surgery difficult. The chief side effects with these drugs are their para-sympathetic action. In addition it has been suggested that one of them, benzhexol, may potentiate the action of thiopentone.

Head injury

In the British Isles it has been estimated that each year 25 000 persons receive head injuries sufficiently severe to require admission to hospital. Relatively few are admitted direct to Neurosurgical Units, which are generally concentrated at major cities and provide a service to a large region. Indeed, it is neither practical nor necessary for the majority of these cases to be treated in such specialized units: only a small minority will require surgery. What is really required is efficient conservative treatment, (which should be available locally) and facilities for simple surgery. In both spheres the anaesthetist, with his special training and expertise has a specific role to play, thus it is important that every anaesthetist should be familiar with the problems involved in the treatment of acute head injury.

Conservative care of head injury

Prevention of further neurological damage. The first consideration in the conservative treatment of head injury is to ensure that no further neurological damage is produced. In practice, this means that the respiratory system must continue to function efficiently.

Respiratory problems in head injury. Over the past 25 years clinicians have stressed the detrimental effect of airway difficulties in patients with head injury. Hypoxia and hypercarbia accentuate the changes already produced in the permeability of the brain capillaries by the trauma. Laboured respirations raise the venous pressure. Both factors produce further cerebral oedema, a further increase in the intracranial pressure and more irreversible neurone damage. Efficient ventilation must be ensured and the respiratory tract protected, not merely during any operation, but continuously commencing as soon as the patient comes under medical or nursing care. In the majority of cases, satisfactory control of the airway can be obtained by posture and the insertion of an oral airway, but in some cases endotracheal intubation or tracheostomy may be necessary.

Posture: the best position in which to nurse unconscious patients, both during transportation to hospital and in the wards, is the lateral decubitus. This position prevents the tongue falling backwards and obstructing the pharynx. It also ensures that any blood, vomit, mucus or cerebrospinal fluid in the pharynx, drains out through the mouth, instead of entering the trachea and soiling the bronchial tree. Inhalation of vomit is a potential hazard in these cases, as a meal or alcohol may have been consumed just prior to the accident and gastric emptying is frequently delayed.

Tracheal intubation becomes necessary in cases where simple means, such as an oral or nasal pharyngeal airway, have been ineffective in ensuring clear respiration, or where it is necessary to protect the trachea from soiling. An oral or nasal tracheal tube will be satisfactory, and a tracheostomy can be avoided where it is considered that unconsciousness will be of short duration. In these circumstances, the patient will soon regain the power to control his own airway without assistance, and the endotracheal tube can be dispensed with before laryngeal damage is produced. Nasal intubation is convenient; it permits the tube to be stabilized in position with certainty, is less likely to kink than an oral tube and allows pharyngeal toilet to be performed with ease, but it has certain disadvantages. In the adult, the lumen of the internal nares is appreciably smaller than that of the trachea and, in the majority of patients, passage of a tube that is adequate in size from the respiratory and tracheal point of view would induce haemorrhage from the nasal mucosa, which might find its way into the trachea. Furthermore, it is a fallacy that naso-tracheal tubes cannot kink. In the adult, then, oral intubation with a Portex or unkinkable flexo-nylon armoured tube is to be preferred. Biting of the tube can be prevented by the use of a London Hospital or a Thornton prop, the latter being more difficult to insert, but kinder to the teeth. In children, the lumen of the nares and trachea are of comparable diameter and nasal intubation is satisfactory. The tube designed by Jackson Rees is very suitable in this situation.

Tracheostomy. In addition to its use simply to obtain a clear airway or to protect the trachea, tracheostomy may be indicated under the following circumstances in patients unconscious from head injury:

- in patients with pre-existing chest disease
- in association with severe chest injury – e.g. fractured sternum
- with other associated injuries which interfere with physiotherapy – e.g. fractured femur, pelvis, spine and mandible

in cases where physiotherapy has failed to keep the chest clear of secretions
where endotracheal intubation is damaging the larynx
in the presence of a raised arterial carbon dioxide tension
in patients requiring prolonged IPPV

Tracheostomy has been advocated in all cases which do not show imminent signs of recovering consciousness, but tracheostomy is not without its hazards. Of special importance is the possibility of it acting as a source of general ward infection, if the patient cannot be nursed in isolation.

It is the firm belief of the author that the operation of tracheostomy should always be carried out with an endotracheal tube *in situ* and general anaesthesia employed if necessary. There is a major distinction between a rushed haemorrhagic operation on a moving patient with congested veins and the calm, unhurried, dry surgery on the intubated subject.

Oxygenation. Efficient oxygenation of the blood is of the greatest importance in preventing further neurological damage in patients unconscious from head injury. It is frequently not appreciated that if the arterial oxygen tension is measured in such patients while breathing air, they will be found to have hypoxaemia, although they are hyperventilating. Added oxygen can be given by mask – or by nasal catheter, but it is also vital to ensure that the respiratory passages are free of obstructions, including sputum.

Controlled ventilation. This is probably employed much less frequently than is warranted. It is indicated in cases of severe chest injury in association with unconsciousness, pulmonary oedema of central origin and blood gas analysis showing a rise in arterial carbon dioxide levels. In addition, it has been claimed to be of value in reducing neurological damage in patients with severe head injuries, even without the above indications. Its mode of action in these circumstances is uncertain; possibly it acts in several ways by ensuring efficient oxygenation of the blood, by removing the effort of respiration and thus reducing the venous pressure, and by allowing easier control of chest infections.

Controlled ventilation therapy should not be employed until the surgeon is no longer concerned with observing the patient's level of consciousness and is satisfied that surgery has nothing further to offer. Phenoperidine 1–2 mg, tubocurarine 10–15 mg, or pancuronium 2–6 mg either intravenously or intramuscularly every 1–2 hours is required to prevent the patient straining against the ventilator. Straining will raise the intracranial pressure and must be avoided.

Resuscitation. A low blood pressure is seldom the result of brain injury, so its presence in patients with closed head injuries should suggest the probability of other injuries. In searching for these the pelvis should not be overlooked. Blood transfusion should not be withheld because of the fear of promoting further intracranial haemorrhage; this hazard is small compared with the damage which will be caused by hypoxia. Over transfusion, however, should be avoided, as should the infusion of simple electrolyte solutions, which will rapidly leave the blood stream and enter the extravascular compartment, especially the traumatized areas of the brain, leading to further oedema and neurological damage. In circumstances where blood is not immediately available, plasma may be employed. The protein in this solution will retain the transfused fluid in the blood stream and not increase the fluid content of the tissues. Patients in whom significant blood loss has not occurred do not require fluid during the first 24 hours. None should be given orally as there is frequently a failure of absorption; in fact, a stomach tube should be passed once the airway is safe, to remove the gastric contents.

In the subsequent days, fluid intake should be restricted to approximately 1500 ml daily. Electrolyte imbalance of central origin occasionally occurs in these cases, so blood electrolyte estimations should be carried out daily and appropriate quantities of electrolytes given preferably by mouth. If they are not being absorbed, the intravenous route must be employed.

Chemotherapy cover should be routine to prevent or control chest infection. Such infection may not only interfere with respiratory function but will accentuate damage to the nervous system.

Physiotherapy. Not only is it of the greatest importance that the chest receive constant attention, but joints must be put through their full range of movements to prevent contractures. In order to provide maximal benefit, a 24 hour physiotherapy service, seven days a week, is required, either by trained physiotherapists or by the nursing staff. Unconscious patients should be nursed on the side, as already stated, and turned every hour during the day and at two hourly intervals during the night. Before and after changes in position, tracheal toilet and percussion of the chest, with more emphasis on vibration than clapping, should be carried out.

Specific treatment of acute head injury

Cerebral dehydration. At first sight, the infusion of dehydrating agents would appear advantageous in reducing the permanent neurological deficit following head injury. The osmotic agents, however, whilst reducing the overall pressure, may not reduce the oedema in the traumatized area, possibly because the impairment of capillary permeability allows the particles to enter the tissues rapidly, with no osmotic differential developing between the blood and tissue fluid. In clinical practice, then, neither mannitol nor urea will lessen the amount of neurological damage unless there is a general rise in intracranial pressure. Mannitol, because it produces less 'rebound', is preferred to urea in the presence of raised intracranial pressure.

Hypothermia by reducing the oxygen requirement, should give a measure of protection to the damaged neurones. Experimental work on animals has, however, shown that it is only of value in reducing the mortality if it is commenced early (within 6–8 hours of the trauma) and this is seldom practical clinically. Also, the induction of hypothermia will confuse the clinical picture and may lead to delay in the recognition of complications which are amenable to surgery. At the present time, hypothermia is seldom employed in the conservative treatment of head injury, except in a few centres where it is used in the treatment of patients with damage to the brain stem. Before hypothermia is induced, bilateral exploratory burr holes should be made to exclude subdural, or extradural, haematomata.

Whilst actual hypothermia is seldom employed, cooling of hyperpyrexial patients is still popular and may be of value. However, as the aim is to reduce the metabolic rate, the common practice of exposing patients to cooling without taking active steps to prevent shivering (which can increase the metabolic rate by 300%) would appear illogical! Indeed, the administration of drugs to prevent shivering may obscure the clinical picture. It is probably best to allow the hypothalamus, within reason, to control the temperature of the patient.

Controlled ventilation. This has already been considered in relation to the prevention of further damage; it may also be of value in reducing cerebral oedema, but experimental evidence is lacking. It could be of particular value in patients in whom hypertonicity is interfering with ventilation but, once again, it should only be employed in the acute stage, after complications amenable to surgery have been excluded.

Steroids. The value of the gluco-corticoid steroids in reducing the final neurological deficit in head injury is under investigation in many centres. Animal work suggests it could be most useful and the clinical impressions seem to bear this out. The dosage of steroid employed is large, 40 mg prednisolone initially and 20 mg 4 hourly. Gastric haemorrhage is a potential complication and, in patients with a history of gastric ulceration, steroids should be administered with discretion.

Surgical intervention. Surgery is required in only a minority of patients with severe head injury. It consists most frequently of bilateral, exploratory burr holes to remove or exclude subdural or extradural haematomata. In some of these patients speed is essential, and time should not be wasted transferring them to other hospitals or awaiting the arrival of a more experienced colleague. Burr holes are all that is required as a life saving measure. If at operation more extensive surgery is considered necessary, a drain can be left in the burr hole and the patient transferred to a neurosurgical unit for further treatment.

Positioning the patient. The patient is positioned supine, with the head and shoulders raised above heart level, to facilitate venous drainage from the head. The operative procedure should be of relatively short duration, approximately 30 minutes and, in these circumstances, the simplest of anaesthetic techniques will suffice.

Local anaesthesia. At first sight, local anaesthesia might appear appropriate, but it will not ensure the unobstructed airway which is essential: nor will it prevent vomiting and, with the patient in the supine position and the larynx unprotected, inhalation of vomit would be almost inevitable. In addition, during the procedure, the patient's level of consciousness may change and extreme restlessness may hamper the surgery and expose the operation site to the risk of contamination.

If general anaesthesia becomes essential during the procedure, induction is, to say the least of it, inconvenient; with the patient supine and the head in the sterile area, general anaesthesia can only be induced safely by stopping the operation, removing the sterile drapes and allowing the anaesthetist free access to the head for endotracheal intubation. Anaesthesia or sedation without intubation should never be considered.

Where a trained anaesthetist is available, the author does not consider local anaesthesia an appropriate technique in acute head injury.

General Anaesthesia. There are 3 essential requirements for these patients:

(1) Control of the airway to avoid hypoxia and hypercarbia.
(2) The avoidance of agents that increase intracranial tension.
(3) Rapid recovery at the end of the procedure to permit re-assessment.

Premedication should consist of atropine only. Drugs which depress respiration are best avoided, until the patient reaches the anaesthetic room. The actual method of induction is not important, provided hypoxia and hypercapnia are prevented. Hypotension in the presence of a raised intracranial pressure is dangerous but, provided this point is appreciated, the barbiturates and relaxant drugs are not contraindicated. Endotracheal intubation with a cuffed non-kinkable tube is essential to ensure control of the airway. The application of a local anaesthetic agent to the larynx and upper trachea will reduce the tendency to coughing and will permit a lighter plane of anaesthesia to be employed, and where maintenance consists of nitrous oxide and oxygen only, recovery at the end of the procedure should be rapid. With halothane, anaesthesia and recovery are swift. It increases the intracranial pressure more than trichloroethylene and both are best avoided when the pressure is raised. Provided the operation is of short duration, spontaneous respiration may be employed, provided oxygenation and carbon dioxide elimination are adequate. If the procedure is prolonged or if the operation is extended to the turning of a bone flap, then controlled ventilation is advisable. An intravenous infusion, if it is not already *in situ*, should be set up before the operation is commenced and cross-matched blood should be available for transfusion.

With an acute subdural haematoma, the underlying brain is damaged and oedematous and a dehydrating agent is often employed to reduce the overall intracranial pressure. Until recently, urea 30% in fructose was most commonly employed, but this has now been superseded by mannitol 20 or 25%; the latter does not enter the intracellular compartment, its 'rebound phenomenon' is less prominent, it is less irritant to the tissues and possibly protects rather than does further damage to the inefficient kidney.

With a chronic subdural haematoma, and some cases of acute extradural haematoma, the brain is simply pushed away from the skull and is not visibly oedematous. In these circumstances, a space is left when the clot is removed, and the haematoma may reform post-operatively, unless the brain is made to re-expand. The infusion of physiological saline will assist re-expansion; a dehydrating agent would hinder the process and should be avoided. Where the age of the haematoma is in doubt and the condition of the underlying brain uncertain, the dehydrating agent can be withheld until the dura is exposed and the state of the brain actually observed.

Specialized surgery

In certain cases where facilities are available, the surgeon may wish to turn a bone flap to ensure haemostasis, or to provide a sub-temporal decompression. This is a major undertaking, both from the surgical and anaesthetic point of view, and is seldom considered outside a neurosurgical unit. The anaesthetist must treat these cases as major neurosurgical problems and employ a technique which will provide maximal reduction in brain volume. If the brain volume and intracranial pressure are not reduced, the brain will herniate through the dura when the latter is incised, compressing and tearing the surface vessels and leading to further rapidly developing oedema and a frequently fatal vicious circle of oedema – venous congestion – oedema. As for all craniotomies, an adequate supply of blood should be available before surgery is commenced. Haemorrhage can be severe and rapid transfusion may be necessary.

The author's preferences for these cases include controlled respiration and the dehydrating agent mannitol.

Anaesthesia for non-cranial surgery in patients with acute head injury

The timing of surgery in these patients is important. If acute haemorrhage is occurring, e.g. from a ruptured spleen, no delay is justified in getting it under control. If, however, the head injury is severe and the other injuries do not endanger life, then it is advisable to observe the patient for 4–6 hours to ascertain that the neurological state is stable or improving. During this time the necessary resuscitation should be carried out; after 4–6 hours if the patient has not deteriorated neurologically, it is unlikely that a well managed anaesthetic will cause damage or conceal a dangerous neurological complication. A well managed anaesthetic would ensure that hypoxia, hypercarbia and hypotension are avoided; the anaesthetist would employ a technique from which the patient would rapidly recover at the end of the operative procedure so that the neurological state could be re-assessed. Drugs which increase the intracranial pressure – particularly halothane – should not be employed.

13 *Outpatient Anaesthesia*

Outpatient anaesthesia demands the rapid conversion from an active alert state into quiet unconsciousness, followed by a rapid emergence and return to full consciousness with complete recovery of cortical as well as normal reflex function. The patient may be extremely apprehensive and have a full stomach. In addition there may be some medical or surgical condition which is a relative, or absolute, contraindication to general anaesthesia. The anaesthetist should assess the patient's fitness for general anaesthesia, paying particular attention to drug therapy. Having determined that there is no medical or surgical contraindication, he should satisfy himself that the patient is adequately prepared: empty stomach and bladder, no history of drugs, no false teeth, no jewellery, etc. Permission must be granted for the anaesthetic and operative procedure and there must be a responsible adult to take the patient home afterwards.

General anaesthesia

The anaesthetic should be conducted in such a way as to produce a rapid onset with rapid recovery and minimal side effects – general anaesthetic agents with a low solubility in blood and of high potency will produce such effects. Cyclopropane and halothane are at the moment nearest to meeting these requirements: however, each used alone has its disadvantages, and nitrous oxide/oxygen/halothane if administered skilfully will produce satisfactory results. We advise the administration of this mixture by full (conventional) face mask. The mixture should contain at least 21% oxygen, and after the first breath the patient should receive rapidly increasing concentrations of halothane up to 3.5%. One cannot overstress the importance of the first breath containing a just detectable concentration of halothane, which is increased in concentration at each subsequent breath. Once anaesthesia has been induced and the appropriate level achieved, the halothane can gradually be reduced in concentration, with the anaesthetist 'feeling his way'. The minimal concentration of halothane should always be given that is adequate to maintain anaesthesia and as soon as the termination of operation is in sight, the halothane should be discontinued. The actual timing of this event will depend on the experience of the anaesthetist and the speed of the surgeon, but with correct timing the patient can be awake within a short time of the end of the operation. Clearly, however, the longer the operation and the deeper the plane of anaesthesia, the longer is the recovery time.

Some anaesthetists will prefer to induce anaesthesia with an intravenous induction agent and, in the past, thiopentone and methohexitone have been employed for this purpose. However, Althesin, or the eugenol derivative propanidid (Epontol), may be considered, as these agents are rapidly broken down in the body and full return of mental faculties occurs more quickly than after methohexitone. With the barbiturates, after-effects may be present for up to 12 hours. We are of the opinion, however, that no patient should be permitted to drive a vehicle or indulge in activities which may result in harm to himself or others, on the day of the operation, whatever the operation, or the anaesthetic. No alcohol should be taken by mouth following methohexitone or other barbiturate anaesthesia.

The use of analeptics to terminate anaesthesia does not appear to have anything to recommend it.

Dental outpatient anaesthesia

The problems confronting the anaesthetist called upon to administer a general anaesthetic for an outpatient dental procedure are manifold.

First of all the anaesthetist is confronted with the problem of anaesthesia for the ambulant patient. Such patients are frequently unprepared, often coming in from the street unaccompanied. The patient, the surgeon and the anaesthetist expect a rapid recovery from the anaesthetic with minimal side effects. Anaesthesia must produce pain relief and sleep without movement, but must at the same time be at a light plane. In addition, the surgeon will be operating in the vicinity of the upper air passages and, in some cases, will have to share the responsibility for maintaining the airway with the anaesthetist. The lungs must be protected from the inhalation of foreign materials. Finally, the posture of the patient has considerable bearing on the successful outcome of the anaesthetic.

Fitness for operation

Clearly a detailed history and examination are impracticable in a busy dental anaesthetic outpatient department. However, a few direct leading questions are fully justifiable, provided that the patient is of an age to understand. Questioning should be directed in such a way as to obtain an answer to the following points:

has the patient had a previous anaesthetic? (if so, discreet questioning may reveal any untoward side-effects that might have occurred)

has the patient had any illness in the past? (if so, details)
does the patient get breathless? what causes the breathlessness?
does the patient get swollen ankles?
does the patient get pain in the chest or arm?
has the patient any difficulty in breathing through the nose?
(common cold? sinusitis? nasal polyps? adenoids? etc.)
is the patient cyanosed?
is the patient anaemic?
is he on drug therapy?

Answers to these queries will usually reveal any serious underlying illness which will call for further detailed questioning and examination. Each case must be treated on its merits, as contraindications will vary according to circumstances and with the degree of disability. The accessibility of the veins should also be assessed, if i.v. anaesthesia is contemplated. Common contraindications – relative and absolute – which may be elicited are set out in Table 13.1.

If the patient is in anything but normal health, the administrator should ascertain the severity of the disorder and, if necessary, obtain appropriate medical or surgical treatment prior to anaesthesia. The list given above is merely a guide and is in no way complete. If any doubt exists as to the advisability of a general anaesthetic as an outpatient, a second opinion should be sought or the patient admitted to hospital for further dental treatment.

Preparation and premedication

Having decided that the patient has no impairment of general health likely to contraindicate anaesthesia (Tab. 13.1):

(1) Make sure there is a responsible adult to accompany the patient home.
(2) Obtain signed consent (see page 435).
(3) Make sure that the bladder and stomach are empty.
(4) Remove all jewellery, wrist watch, and tight clothing.
(5) Get the patient to blow his nose.

The normal patient arriving for a dental extraction under general anaesthetic will be apprehensive. The degree of nervousness will vary – some patients have the ability to suppress outward signs of anxiety. On the whole, widespread sedation is unnecessary for adults, but the judicious use of sedation in selected cases is of great value, particularly if this can be arranged the day before anaesthesia, as adequate sleep the night before an operation is desirable. There is no one agent that is satisfactory for all. Barbiturates – sodium pentobarbitone (Nembutal) 200 mg may be given orally. Methylpentynol (Oblivon), phenothiazines, diazepam

Table 13.1 *Possible contraindications for dental outpatient anaesthesia*

General contraindications

Is the stomach empty? When was the last meal taken? Remember, apprehension will delay gastric emptying and prolonged starvation may predispose to fainting

Is the patient accompanied? Is the patient driving a car?

Is written consent available?

Is the patient receiving any drug therapy: hypotensives, insulin, phenothiazines, amine oxidase inhibitors, barbiturates, steroids, anti-coagulants, etc.?

(In the pigmented races, consider the possibility of sickle cell anaemia, and always screen for abnormal haemoglobin.)

Psychological contraindications

Anxiety state: varying degrees of co-operation

Amentia: No co-operation

Metabolic contraindications

Thyrotoxicosis: Heart disease Nervousness Raised B.M.R.

Myxoedema: Heart disease Low B.M.R.

Disorders of the pituitary-adrenal axis

Steroid therapy Diabetes mellitus

Rare conditions: porphyria, etc.

Cardiovascular contraindications

Congenital heart disease: as well as symptoms and signs of decompensation the risk of sub-acute bacterial endocarditis must be considered

Acute rheumatic fever Rheumatic valvular disease

Hypertensive heart disease and hypertension Bacterial endocarditis

Coronary artery insufficiency Anaemia Hypotension

Respiratory contraindications

Nasal obstruction Recent or old nasal injury

Deliberate occlusion of the nose by previous operative procedure

Common cold Nasal polyps Cleft palate

Deflected nasal septum Repaired cleft palate and hare lip

Conditions which may or may not be associated with trismus:

Ankylosis of the temporo-mandibular joint Ankylosing spondylitis

Ludwig's angina Cellulitis of dental origin

Cellulitis and other infections in the neck which may be spread by handling

Pus draining into the mouth from a burst abscess

Acute gingivo-stomatitis (Vincent's angina)

Enlarged tonsils and adenoids Peritonsillar abscess

Glottic oedema Laryngeal obstruction Tracheal obstruction

Disease of the lung tissue Chronic bronchitis Emphysema

Bronchiectasis: risk of coughing sputum and vomiting

Asthma (history of?): is actual spasm present?

T.B. (active or healed?): degree of disability?

Pneumonia Pulmonary oedema Collapse of the lung

Bronchial carcinoma Foreign body, etc. Air or fluid in pleural cavity

Miscellaneous contraindications

Gastro-intestinal obstruction Pyloric stenosis

Diseases of the central nervous system (e.g. methohexitone contraindicated in epileptics)

Involuntary movements, etc. Myasthenia gravis

Cerebro-vascular disease Severe renal disease

Rarities such as epidermolysis bullosa

(Valium) and other sedative agents can be tried. Children are, inevitably, a particular problem.

All equipment should be checked before the patient enters the surgery. When the patient enters the surgery it is important to place him at his ease and inspire confidence. There should be no noise – all instruments should be placed out of sight, and the number of people in attendance kept to the minimum with the dental surgeon remaining in the background.

Posture. It is still common practice to administer general anaesthetics to dental outpatients with the subject sitting upright in the dental chair. This is in spite of the fact that if fainting occurs in the upright posture and passes unrecognized, grave cerebral hypoxia may occur. Furthermore, it has been confirmed that, even with apparently efficient packing, inhalation of foreign material from the upper respiratory tract can occur. However, in recent years some anaesthetists have carried out the whole procedure with the patients in the supine position. Although aspiration of foreign material may be less likely in the supine position, respiratory obstruction is a complication once the mouth is open, as the maintenance of a patent airway is sometimes difficult to achieve. In addition, regurgitation may occur with the horizontal posture, particularly if respiratory obstruction is present. The adoption of the horizontal position is not altogether popular with dental surgeons, as the posture is not an easy one for the removal of teeth to those unacquainted with this position. However, the routine adoption of this posture should minimize the possible sequelae arising from unrecognized fainting, should this occur during the course of dental anaesthesia. We have found the horizontal position most useful, in particular with small children, where it is often difficult to maintain an upright position for any length of time.

Position in the chair. The patient should assume a relaxed upright posture with the head rest placed under the occiput, assuming a 'sniffing the morning air' position of the head. Fingers should be interdigitated with the hands lying on the lap and the feet dangling on either side of the foot rest; male patients may place their hands in their trouser pockets. The chair should not be tilted backwards, as this will encourage the movement of blood and debris towards the pharynx.

Evidence suggests that the blood pressure rises with the onset of anaesthesia. Fainting, however, is likely to occur through apprehension at the time of induction, or when a high concentration of oxygen is breathed after a period of hypoxia. Should it occur, the patient should be placed immediately in the horizontal position with the feet up and atropine 0.6 mg intravenously, should be given if there is associated bradycardia.

The apparatus should be on the left hand side and slightly behind the patient, with the anaesthetist standing between the patient and the machine.

Apparatus

A large variety of equipment and techniques is available.

Intermittent flow/continuous flow nitrous oxide/oxygen. With McKesson 'Anesthesor Special', Walton Mark V, and Cyprane A.E. machines the proportion of nitrous oxide/oxygen can be controlled by means of a graduated dial. Furthermore the pressure at which flow ceases from these machines can be varied from 0 to 20 mmHg, with the Walton V (see Table 13.2), and from 0 to 40 mmHg with the McKesson, as these machines were originally designed to deliver gas mixtures on demand, thus leading to economy of gases. Both items of apparatus incorporate an oxygen by-pass control, which allows for the emergency administration of 100% oxygen. It is common practice today to administer the mixture by employing at least a few l/min of gas flow continuously throughout the procedure, and this is supplemented by the increased flow which occurs on demand when the patient takes a breath.

Table 13.2 *Performance of Walton Mark V machine*

Pressure (mmHg)	*Flow rate* (l/min): *oro-nasal attachment*
5	20
10	50
15	80
20	110

The Walton Mark V and Cyprane A.E. machines incorporate automatic cut-off valves which, should the oxygen supply fail, cut off the supply of nitrous oxide. There is also an air inspiratory valve which permits the admittance of air in the event of the gas mixture cutting off, and an audible warning of gas failure is now a standard provision on these machines. The McKesson apparatus may have a rebreathing attachment; this was originally designed to conserve gases and to 'foster adequate respirations'; but it is our opinion that there is no justification for the use of this attachment. The reservoir bag should never be employed unless high continuous flows of at least 8 l/min are being used; even under these circumstances, there is a time lag between a change at the machine and the mixture reaching the patient. It should be pointed out

M

that there is considerable variability in the performance of dental anaesthetic equipment.

Continuous flow apparatus. Many types are available on the market. The simplest form available comprises a bank of flow meters receiving gas from cylinders at reduced pressure via reducing valves. The appropriate control of the gas mixture is achieved by adjusting flow through the rotameters and collecting the mixture in a reservoir bag prior to its being inhaled. It is of importance to ensure that the flow of gases is sufficient to prevent rebreathing of exhaled air from the reservoir bag. A non-return valve in the system overcomes the disadvantage of rebreathing and also serves as a useful guide to the minute ventilation of the patient. The Quantiflex control system permits the anaesthetist to preset not only the concentrations but also the flow rate of gases.

Vaporizers

Both the intermittent flow and continuous flow equipment allow the attachment of vaporizers for the administration of adjuvants.

Halothane (Fluothane). There are various vaporizers on the market which enable halothane to be vaporized. The simplest have no temperature compensating devices and therefore have a built-in safety factor, in that as the temperature of the liquid falls with vaporization, the concentration of the mixture vapour leaving the chamber falls. This may have disadvantages, as the delivered concentration may fall sharply, thus producing an inadequate mixture.

Goldman halothane vaporizer: at flow rates of gas of 8 l/min with 20 ml in the cup at a temperature of 21°C, for one minute, the results being shown in Table 13.3.

Table 13.3 *Goldman halothane vaporizer*

Drum position	*Concentration*
1	0·03
2	0·74
3	2·21
on	2·08

McKesson halothane vaporizer Mark II: at flow rates of gas of 8 l/min with 20 ml in the cup at a temperature of 20°C (see Table 13.4).

Cyprane halothane vaporizer: temperature compensated. Designed for both continuous flow and draw-over use.

Fluotec: temperature compensated. Designed for continuous flow.

Table 13.4 *McKesson halothane vaporizer Mark II*

Dial reading	*Concentration*
1	0·05
2	1·05
3	1·84
on	2·80

Halothane IV: temperature compensated.

Marrett nitrous oxide/oxygen/halothane apparatus: Marrett has described a technique for the administration of the above mixture, using a portable apparatus called the Medrex. Anaesthesia is induced by halothane and 100% oxygen, with the occasional use of nitrous oxide, instead of the conventional method of nitrous oxide and oxygen with halothane as a mere adjuvant. The machine is set to a flow of 1 l/min of oxygen and 5 l/min of nitrous oxide (17% oxygen approximately); a full face mask is applied and the patient breathes to and fro through the machine, picking up halothane. After 5 breaths the nitrous oxide is turned off, the halothane concentration control turned up and further rebreathing occurs. Marrett claims that the machine is self controlling in that any depression of respiration, due to relative overdosage with halothane, in turn leads to a diminution in the total quantity vaporized and that there is adequate oxygenation. However, the concentration of halothane within the circuit must at times be very great. If the procedure is to take any length of time, he suggests the change to a nose piece and maintenance with nitrous oxide and oxygen, using the Medrex head.

Trichloroethylene (Trilene). In the Rowbotham vaporizer the vapour strength is controlled by the movement of a lever, but the apparatus is not temperature compensated and it also has the disadvantage of considerable resistance to airflow.

The Goldman halothane vaporizer can be used for trichloroethylene. The readings for a flow rate of 8 l/min are shown in Table 13.5.

Table 13.5 *Goldman halothane vaporizer with trichloroethylene*

Dial reading	*Concentration using 20* ml *at 21*°C *after 1* min
1	nil
2	0·44
3	0·68
on	0·70

Trichloroethylene is sometimes employed as an adjuvant, but patients do not recover as quickly as from pure nitrous oxide/oxygen. They do not feel as well, frequently complain of severe nausea and some actually vomit, and cardiac dysrhythmias may occur.

Cyclopropane. This agent is a potent anaesthetic but unfortunately carries the risk of explosion, as it is flammable; it is on record that sparks have been noticed during dental extractions when the forceps have been in contact with teeth. Non-explosive mixtures of cyclopropane and oxygen, using nitrogen and helium as diluents, have been produced. The CON apparatus developed for the short anaesthesia of mass casualties, has been found to provide a simple and effective method for anaesthesia in the dental chair. The apparatus consists of a face mask, tap, soda lime canisters and reservoir bag: by using a discharge device, the contents of two different 'sparklet' bulbs are delivered into the bag and a mixture containing 40% cyclopropane, 30% oxygen and 30% nitrogen is thereby produced. This mixture is applied by a full face mask and breathing allowed to continue for approximately 1–2 minutes; the mask is removed and a period of anaesthesia remains for approximately two minutes. As cyclopropane carries with its use a high incidence of nausea and vomiting, it is little used in dental anaesthetic practice.

Divinyl ether (Vinesthene). This agent produces rapid induction of anaesthesia with rapid recovery; it is not so irritant as diethyl ether, but it tends to produce salivation and is flammable. However, in the presence of adequate oxygenation it is a safe anaesthetic agent, ideally suited for children. As the sole agent it is administered either on an open face mask or with the Goldman inhaler, or its modification, the Oxford inhaler. These inhalers enable the apparatus to be charged from an ampoule with the tidal volume passing through a chamber to and from a reservoir bag with the addition, if necessary of oxygen. The Oxford inhaler allows for control of the concentration to avoid coughing. Vinesthene can also be used as an adjuvant and is administered with continuous/intermittent flow apparatus using the Goldman drip feed, which accommodates a 25 ml inverted bottle, the drip rate being regulated by a fine adjustment control.

Methoxyflurane (Penthrane). Recently this non-explosive anaesthetic agent has been tried as an adjuvant in outpatient dental general anaesthetic practice. It is claimed that adequate anaesthesia can be achieved more economically than with halothane using 10% Penthrane, but it is likely to be associated with a prolonged induction and recovery time.

Ethyl Chloride and Chloroform. Both these agents have, in the past, enjoyed popularity in the sphere of dental anaesthesia, but there is little justification in their general use in modern anaesthetic practice. In particular, the practice of spraying ethyl chloride on to the mouth pack of a mouth breathing recalcitrant patient is to be strongly deprecated. The use of chloroform as a general anaesthetic agent may still be found to be of value in less developed parts of the world, where expensive equipment and drugs are at a premium.

Nitrous oxide/oxygen techniques

Amnalgesia: this was defined as the condition induced by the administration of a minimal amount of a general anaesthetic drug, or combination of drugs, in conjunction with local block or infiltration anaesthesia of the operating field. Klock (1955) states that there is a very precise and well defined plane of general anaesthesia in the first stage existing between the analgesic and the excitement stage (see ultra-light methohexitone). He achieved this anaesthetic state by delivery of 20% oxygen and 80% nitrous oxide to the patient. The success of the technique appears to be the avoidance of the excitement stage, but if excitement occurs, further oxygen is given. This was the first approach to the problem of achieving adequate anaesthesia with nitrous oxide and at the same time maintaining adequate oxygenation. Tom (1956) departed in detail from Klock's technique in his report, but claimed to be producing the same level of narcosis without hypoxia. Recently there has been a reawakening of interest in this technique and it is currently in favour as a form of sedation for conservative dentistry.

Pre-oxygenation: Mostert (1958) has employed a technique of nitrogen washout with 100% oxygen for two minutes prior to the administration of 100% nitrous oxide for one minute, followed by maintenance with 20% oxygen.

Premixed gases: recently it has been found possible to premix oxygen and nitrous oxide and store these in a cylinder under pressure. In temperate climates these mixtures are delivered in the correct proportions from the cylinders, provided that the concentrations of oxygen are not less than 40%. Such mixtures of gases obviate the need for special sophisticated apparatus and merely a flow meter and halothane vaporizer are required: this equipment is easily portable and adaptations are now available for dental use.

Insertion of gag or mouth prop

After the dental surgeon and the anaesthetist have together examined the correct patient and ascertained which teeth require extracting, and in what order, the anaesthetic can proceed. There are two schools of thought regarding the insertion of a mouth prop. One group inserts the prop prior to induction asking the patient to bite, but this procedure is distracting and most difficult for the patient, particularly if at the same time he is being requested to breathe through his nose. We prefer to induce anaesthesia and, once the patient is asleep, insert the mouth prop. In the past, when anaesthesia was induced and maintained by a mixture of nitrous oxide and hypoxia, it was often advisable to insert the prop prior to induction, as relaxation was often not achieved owing to the masseteric spasm arising from the hypoxia. Today this procedure is largely unnecessary.

Mouth props: many mouth props have been devised, each having its particular merits. It is important that these should neither damage the teeth, nor slip. A central swivel prop is preferred by some, as it allows the extraction of the teeth on both sides of the mouth without change of prop, but, if used incorrectly, it can seriously damage proclinated incisors.

Induction of anaesthesia

Induction of anaesthesia can be achieved by either using intravenous agents, or entirely by the inhalational route.

Intravenous anaesthesia. During recent years much interest has been shown in the use of intravenous agents in dental practice. Much of the disrepute that has accrued to this practice has arisen in association with the use of these agents in the hands of the inexperienced or single operator. There is no doubt that, with intelligent and careful use, intravenous anaesthesia has a part to play in the technique available to the dental anaesthetist. Though, with modern adjuvant inhalational general anaesthetic agents, there is rarely a situation where intravenous agents are the method of choice on clinical grounds alone, particularly for the maintenance of general anaesthesia as the sole agent, intravenous induction is frequently demanded by the patient.

Many ultra-short acting agents are available to the anaesthetist and much work has been done in an attempt to evaluate the relative merits of the various agents. In the past, hexobarbitone, thiopentone and thialbarbitone have been employed, but, more recently, methohexitone sodium (Brietal), propanidid (Epontol) and Althesin have been used and have gained favour because complications are less than with hexobaritone and thiopentone. If methohexitone is to be employed, it is suggested that a 1% solution be used and given on the basis of 1.0–1.5 mg/kg (6–8 mg per stone) body weight: using a slightly larger dose artificial ventilation may be necessary should apnoea occur.

Propanidid (Epontol), a derivative of eugenol and therefore a non-barbiturate, is undoubtedly a very short acting intravenous agent. Both recovery and leaving times compare very favourably with other intravenous agents in common use, there is a marked absence of 'hangover' and the drug appears to have analgesic properties. Unfortunately the solution is viscous, it causes hyperventilation and possibly increases the incidence of nausea and vomiting. Propanidid can be given as 5% solution using 6–7 mg/kg: methohexitone and propanidid should never be mixed together. Althesin may be given in a dose of 0.05–0.075 ml/kg body weight slowly intravenously.

Whilst recognizing that it is not uncommon practice in certain circles to give intermittent or continuous doses of intravenous agents without an inhalational supplement, we feel strongly that this is a practice not to be encouraged in the hands of the inexperienced administrator. It is very difficult to maintain an even plane of anaesthesia, particularly with propanidid, and there is a very real danger of saliva or debris falling on the vocal cords and causing laryngeal spasm. If the patient is allowed to remain at a light plane of anaesthesia, coughing, swallowing and even vomiting can occur: involuntary movements are particularly associated with the administration of methohexitone. As the cumulative effect of intermittent doses of intravenous agents can give rise to cardiovascular and respiratory instability and as it is of paramount importance to maintain an efficient and reliable airway at all times (not readily done by a single pair of hands) it is strongly to be deprecated that the same person operate and administer the anaesthetic.

If the intravenous route is to be chosen it should be carefully ascertained that there are no contraindications. The patient should have been weighed, the approximate dose of intravenous agent worked out on a dose per weight basis and a suitable vein selected. Whilst the injection is being given the assistant should hold the head steady. As soon as the injection has been given the anaesthetist should withdraw the needle, applying a firm pressure with a pad to prevent haematoma formation and rapidly return to the patient's head to present an inhalation anaesthetic mixture for immediate breathing. If he is too slow he will find the patient recovering consciousness, as the effects of the intravenous agent wear off.

Intravenous 'premedication' and 'ultra-light' anaesthesia. The 'Jørgensen Technique' has been employed not only for the removal of impacted teeth, the removal of the remaining upper and lower anterior teeth and trimming the alveolar processes for immediate denture insertions, and for patients with hypertension or coronary arterial disease, but also for patients with inordinate apprehension or fear of dentistry and those with a psychotic history. The two latter groups, however, may often prove to be unsuitable for this procedure.

Method: after a careful history, the blood pressure and pulse are noted and intravenous pentobarbitone sodium (Nembutal) is given extremely slowly, until a stage of light sedation is reached (a dose of 150 mg pentobarbitone is rarely exceeded). The needle is left *in situ*, the syringe is detached and is replaced by one containing 25 mg pethidine and 0.3 mg scopolamine diluted to 5 ml; small quantities of this solution are then slowly administered until the patient becomes detached and withdrawn from his surroundings. He should, however, at no time be unconscious or excessively restless as the aim is to achieve a relaxed state, maintaining the full co-operation of the patient throughout the procedure. The dental conservation work is then carried out using local anaesthesia, where necessary. The only disadvantage of this otherwise ideal technique is that the patient may remain drowsy for some hours. More recently the so-called 'ultra-light technique' has been employed; intermittent doses of methohexitone are given intravenously with the twin object of producing an extremely light plane of anaesthesia and maintaining the full co-operation of the patient. It is claimed that it carries a high incidence of amnesia, recovery being more rapid than with the Jørgensen technique and any tendency to restlessness is met by deliberately lightening the anaesthesia. However, there are great difficulties in avoiding unconsciousness and inaccessibility with associated loss of protective reflexes, so that this technique has severe limitations and potential dangers (Mann *et al.*, 1971).

Diazepam (Valium) in doses of up to 20 mg i.v. given in 5 mg quantities at 1 minute intervals can be given until the subject is drowsy, (a dose of 0.25 mg/kg, is usually adequate). In view of the likelihood of thrombophlebitis the injection should be made into a large vein. Conservation work can then be carried out under local anaesthesia, in a sedated patient without loss of consciousness: the incidence of amnesia is high. Patients should not be permitted to drive for the remainder of the day and should be accompanied home.

Lange has recently introduced the technique of minimal concentration of nitrous oxide for sedation in dental conservation work.

Induction and maintenance of anaesthetic with inhalational agents

Now that potent adjuvants are available it is indefensible to administer a concentration of oxygen to the patient lower than that present in atmospheric air (20%). There is good evidence to suggest that concentrations of 25–30% oxygen should be employed. Induction should commence with a mixture of nitrous oxide : oxygen at least 79% : 21%. Adjuvants available are trichloroethylene, divinyl ether, halothane and methoxyflurane: in our opinion the advantages of halothane outweigh the cost and, provided the halothane is carefully administered, economies can be achieved. Using halothane with adequate oxygenation it is important to introduce the adjuvant at the first breath and, provided a sufficiently low concentration is employed, the smell is not objectionable and the anaesthetic mixture is rapidly inhaled by the patient. A concentration which is just detectable by smell (approximately 0.1%) is first used, rising rapidly to 1.5% in the average patient and 3% in the robust. (Care must be taken to avoid overdosage with the nervous patient who overbreathes). The onset of surgical anaesthesia is characterized by regular automatic respirations; eye signs are extremely unreliable and the opening of the eye to test reflexes is to be deprecated. A technique employing a one way circuit, continuous flow of gases, and a temperature compensated vaporizer leads to economy of gases. There are very real dangers associated with any mis-use of a vaporizer which can deliver high concentrations.

One of us (J.A.T.) employs a system using an intermittent flow Walton V or McKesson machine, with the pressure set to 5 mmHg (flow approximately 8 l/min) and the reservoir bag not in circuit. After settling the patient comfortably in position with the harness behind the head and the expiratory valve loose, the anaesthetic mixture is presented at the nose, with instructions to breathe through the nose quite naturally. After the first few breaths the concentration of halothane is rapidly increased, the nose piece firmly applied and the harness fixed. Prolonged induction should be avoided as it leads to nervousness and salivation. As soon as regular automatic respirations have been achieved, with the accompanying relaxation, the mouth prop is readily inserted by the dental surgeon. Careful packing is the next step and, again, this should be carried out by the dentist in co-operation with the anaesthetist. Anaesthesia is maintained with a nitrous oxide/oxygen mixture, using the minimal concentration of halothane compatible with maintaining a quiescent patient.

The dental pack. The importance of the correct positioning of the dental pack cannot be over stressed. No single factor is of such importance during the course of dental anaesthesia as this one: on it depends the failure or success of the procedure. Imperfect application can lead to mouth breathing, coughing, retching, vomiting and the inhalation of foreign material. We believe that the tongue should be used as the barrier between the operative field and the air passages; by careful placing of the pack lateral to and under the tongue, efficient approximation of tongue to palate can be achieved without forcing the soft palate or tongue against the posterior pharyngeal wall. The placing of the pack on the dorsum of the tongue frequently leads to obstructed airway and is very often an inefficient barrier against blood, pus and other debris. Many packs have been devised. Each has its merits but we have found a pack eight inches long and two inches wide, comprised of a gauze covering with absorbent wool interior, with a strong tape attached, the most suitable for adults.

Procedure: slip the forefinger between the lateral margin of the tongue and alveolus, lifting the tongue upwards and towards the midline. The end of the pack is held between the thumb and the forefinger and middle fingers of the other hand and then inserted into the space produced by the forefinger of the first hand, twisting it so that the tongue is further lifted and the pack falls into the space so created. It is eventually lying somewhat beneath the lateral margin of the tongue and the lingual aspect of the alveolar process of the mandible. This procedure maintains the seal between the dorsum of the tongue and the junction of hard and soft palates, creating an effective seal between the operation area and the air passages, but not causing obstruction. In the 'well' so created the absorbent pack mops up the blood and debris.

The mouth prop and pack having been inserted, a brief pause should be taken so that the airway can be regained. The jaw should be held in a forward and upwards direction by the anaesthetist applying his fingers, or the crook of the forefinger, to the angle of the jaw. (As pressure on the carotid artery or body may result, care must be taken not to press into the soft tissues of the neck.) It should be stressed that close co-operation between the anaesthetist and dentist is essential throughout the operation, as both can help one another in the maintenance of an adequate airway. Adequate suction should be available to remove excess secretions, pus and blood, and every precaution taken to ensure that foreign material is not inhaled; the teeth should be counted on removal from the mouth. According to the progress of the extraction the halothane concentration should be progressively reduced. The pulse must be palpated continuously through the course of general anaesthesia.

Signs of premature lightening of anaesthesia are the formation of tears, salivation, phonation, swallowing and movements of voluntary muscle, and are indications for increasing the concentration of halothane. A frequent cause of lightening of anaesthesia is mouth breathing; nasal obstruction due to a common cold, sinusitis, deflected nasal septum, nasal polyps or enlarged adenoids and tonsils are potent predisposing factors. It is important, therefore, to ascertain that this obstruction is not present before anaesthesia is induced, as the technique may have to be modified.

Nasal intubation. For prolonged maintenance of a nasal airway, a naso-pharyngeal tube may be inserted, but care should be taken not to produce bleeding. The use of a naso-pharyngeal tube in dental anaesthesia has an important place amongst the techniques available to the anaesthetist. In the case of a prolonged procedure, or where there is difficulty in maintaining a good nasal airway, this technique is invaluable. Care should be taken, however, to ensure that there is no nasal obstruction prior to anaesthesia, as insertion of the tube may well cause bleeding or the dislodgement of an obstruction, such as a polyp. It is often useful to spray the appropriate nostril with a long acting vasoconstrictor not containing adrenaline (as halothane is being used) such as oxymetazoline, prior to the passage of the tube. Cocaine should be avoided. Great care must be taken to ensure that there is no possibility of the tube slipping out of reach down the pharynx, either by using a flange or a safety pin placed through the tube. To encourage nasal breathing the tension of the expiratory valve may be increased.

Experience will enable the administrator to decide when to terminate general anaesthesia and thus avoid prolonged recovery time. During recovery the pack should be placed over the bleeding points, the head and body moved forward and careful watch kept on the airway. The gag and pack should not be removed whilst the patient is recovering.

Special Cases

Children. Provided children are treated firmly and sympathetically, anaesthesia can be induced and maintained with nitrous oxide:oxygen 70:30 and halothane supplement. The dilution of the inspired gas with air by mouth breathing is avoided by placing the Goldman nose piece over nose and mouth. With children it is of the greatest importance to provide a mixture to breathe that contains an adequate concentration of oxygen and care should be taken that relative overdosage does not occur through overbreathing.

As already mentioned, it is often easier to induce anaesthesia with the patient in the recumbent position, but if the upright position is adopted then a special chair or modified chair is of great assistance. A nurse may place an arm horizontally across the body at the level of the abdomen to prevent slipping. Divinyl ether (Vinesthene) is an excellent induction agent, and may be given by the Goldman Vinesthene inhaler, with the bag initially filled with oxygen. It must be remembered that children often have obstructed nasal passages and maintenance of anaesthesia by the nasal route may be impossible to achieve. Intermittent oral administration with a full face mask may be necessary in such cases.

It is well recognized that over-anxious parents will frequently affect the general demeanour of children due for anaesthesia: indeed segregation from the nervous mother may be necessary. It need hardly be said that children should not be allowed to see other children recovering from anaesthesia, nor to hear them crying. Many forms of premedication for children have been tried, but firm, sympathetic handling can often replace this need. Certainly, children should not be allowed to dominate the proceedings. Elixir promethazine 10–20 mg according to size of the child, one hour before an operation, is of value, or syrup of trimeprazine tartrate (Vallergan) given two hours pre-operatively in dosage of 1–2 mg/kg body weight may be used. Intramuscular methohexitone (5 mg/kg) used as a 2% solution, results in sleep within 6–8 minutes and is of considerable value. However, by using these forms of sedation consciousness is sometimes lost and the child should then be cared for by someone experienced in the maintenance of the airway.

Trismus. Cases suffering from trismus require special care when contemplating general anaesthesia. The anaesthetist should ascertain whether there is glottic oedema or gross cellulitis in the region of the larynx – if these are present the case should be admitted to hospital and under no circumstances should general anaesthesia be administered as an outpatient. When trismus is present alone, a mouth gag with Ackland jaws should be inserted gently between the molars on the side opposite to where the extraction is to take place, held lightly by the anaesthetist and the jaw not opened until the patient is surgically anaesthetic. Care should also be taken with the position of the nose piece whilst the patient is awake, as the face may be painful and oedematous.

Obesity. Obese patients present particular problems from the point of view of general anaesthesia. Added to these problems is the very real difficulty in maintaining an adequate airway in a patient with a 'bull neck'.

Emphysema and bronchitis. These patients are notoriously difficult to induce with inhalational anaesthetics, particularly in the dental chair, as bronchospasm and excessive sputum production are always present to a varying degree and further complicate the smooth course of anaesthesia. Because of the greatly enlarged functional residual capacity and disturbed ventilation perfusion relationships within the lung, induction with a weakly potent, insoluble anaesthetic agent such as nitrous oxide is often prolonged. If nitrous oxide is the sole agent employed, a state of affairs where the patient is hypoxic but awake may be reached. Consideration should be given to an intravenous induction in carefully selected patients.

The 'resistant patient'. There is no doubt that certain patients have a history of resistance to anaesthesia : some of them may be suffering from emphysema, others may be chronic alcoholics or, for some reason, just have a peculiar resistance to general anaesthesia. With such a history, provided there is no contraindication, an intravenous induction should be considered.

Haemophilia and allied disorders such as purpura and von Willebrand's disease. These patients constitute distinct problems from the point of view of the dentist and the anaesthetist. They require admission to hospital, special care and, in particular, careful anaesthetic management.

The multiple dental extraction. Multiple dental extractions are not infrequently required. It should be borne in mind that a complete dental clearance is often accompanied by a loss of blood which, dependent upon the condition of the gingivae, may approach one pint. To inflict this insult on a patient as an outpatient, together with a general anaesthetic, is not in his best interests, particularly as, in many cases, the patients are old and possibly anaemic. It is our opinion that these cases should be treated in stages and, if need be, under local anaesthesia with or without intravenous diazepam.

Endotracheal intubation. It has been argued that intubation with a cuffed tube protects the patient from the possible aspiration of blood and debris. We do not dispute this fact but consider that the situation where excessive blood loss occurs and excessive operative time is spent, can be avoided by careful selection and management of cases, as outlined above. There is no doubt that certain procedures will require time and unhurried conditions: under ideal circumstances these patients should be admitted to hospital for treatment and not dealt with as ambulatory cases. It should be borne in mind that a sore throat following intubation is not an infrequent occurrence and, in certain cases, can be severe and incapacitating. The use of suxamethonium carries very definite disadvantages and it is doubtful if its use on a dental outpatient in the average dental surgery can be justified: prolonged apnoea, associated with its administration, is not the rarity that might be supposed, and muscular pain can be very severe and incapacitating. Certainly endotracheal intubation in the dental surgery should not be contemplated unless adequate equipment, suction and recovery facilities are available.

Anaesthesia in situations outside hospital

In domiciliary obstetrics and in civil or military disasters an anaesthetic may be required at short notice, in any one of a variety of unusual situations.

Anaesthetic technique. With the reservation that extreme caution is necessary when administering a general anaesthetic to the casualty, who may be suffering from obligaemic shock or have a full stomach, induction may be carried out by the use of methohexitone, propanidid or althesin followed by suxamethonium and endotracheal intubation with a cuffed tube, provided suction apparatus is at hand. Intubation is the only way to guarantee a free and uninterrupted airway, and is of particular importance if the patient is to be cared for whilst under general anaesthesia by an assistant acting under the supervision of a superior. Maintenance can be assured by using halothane or trichloroethylene with controlled ventilation if necessary. Gallamine, pancuronium or D-tubocurarine may be used for relaxation and artificial ventilation with air using an Oxford bellows or an Ambu bag (oxygen enrichment being highly desirable but not absolutely essential). Portable equipment has been devised for this work and is described on page 32.

14 *Local Anaesthetic Agents and Techniques*

Local anaesthetic agents

The great disadvantage of local anaesthetic agents is their toxicity. Many deaths and near-deaths have been reported in the literature relating to situations where, clearly, a relative overdosage has been administered to the patient. Some local anaesthetic agents are more toxic than others and some are more rapidly absorbed from one site than another. This rate of absorption can be reduced by combining the anaesthetic with a vasoconstrictor such as adrenaline, thus allowing larger doses to be used. One of the problems is to obtain adequate anaesthesia without exceeding the maximum safe dose: this dose is best obtained by relation to the body weight of the individual, the age, and physical status, and the total quantity determined by these factors and carefully measured prior to the commencement of the procedure should, under no circumstances, be exceeded (see Tables 14.1 and 14.2).

Side effects of local anaesthetic agents

Met-haemoglobinaemia: shortly after the introduction of prilocaine, cases were reported of cyanosis in relation to the use of this agent, most of them having occurred when more than 600 mg of prilocaine have been used. Cyanosis only becomes evident when 5%–6% of the total haemoglobin is present as met-haemoglobin. Met-haemoglobinaemia can occur not only with prilocaine but also with lignocaine and procaine, if sufficient quantities are administered. Lignocaine and prilocaine are derivatives of aniline, and as such their metabolites may well provoke met-haemoglobinaemia. Met-haemoglobin disappears spontaneously within 24 hours but may nevertheless be disturbing to those concerned. In addition, a parturient may well transmit the metabolites to her child, with the result that the baby, when born, may have a persistent cyanosis which causes difficulties in correct diagnosis and care. In the patient suffering from met-haemoglobinaemia who is not anaemic there are no clinical signs of deficiency in oxygen transport. The condition can be treated by the intravenous administration of 1 mg/kg of methylene blue.

Table 14.1 *Local anaesthetic agents*
Recommended maximum quantity for a fit 70 kg male

Agent	*Route‡*	*Concentration* g/100 ml	*With adrenaline* ml	mg	*Without adrenaline* ml	mg
cocaine	topical only	20		—	1	200
	topical only	10		—	2	200
	topical only	5		—	4	200
amethocaine	topical	0·5		— —	8	40
	topical	2·0		—	2	40
	lozenge	—		—	—	60
	infiltration	0·05	400	200	—	—
	epidural or nerve block	0·1	100	100	—	—
	heavy spinal	1:200 in 6% glucose		—	0·5–2·0	—
	light spinal	1:1500		—	6·0–18	—
nupercaine	topical	2·0		—	2	400
	ointment	1·1 and 2·0		—	—	—
	lozenge	—		—	—	1
	nerve block and infiltration	0·1	120	120	—	—
	heavy spinal	1:200 in 6% glucose*		—	0·5–2·0*	—
	light spinal	1:1500 in 0·5% isotonic saline		—	6·0–18	—
procaine	infiltration	0·5	200	1000		up to 1000
	nerve block	1·0	100	1000		up to 1000
		2·0	50	1000		up to 1000
		3·0	30	1000		up to 1000
	intravenous	0·1–1·0		—		up to 1000
	spinal	5·0		—	0·5–2·0	—
	spinal: crystals dissolved in CSF	5·0		—	—	50–300
lignocaine	ointment	5		—	—	—
	topical	4		—	5	200
	jelly	2		—	—	—
	infiltration	0·5	100	500	40	200
		1·0	50	500	20	200
		2·0	25	500	10	200
	epidural or nerve block	1·0–1·5	10–50	100–750	—	—
	spinal†	5% in 3·0% dextrose		—	0·5–2·0	100
prilocaine	topical	4		—	10	400
	infiltration	0·5	120	600	80	400
		1·0	60	600	40	400
	nerve block	2·0	30	600	20	400
		3·0	20	600	—	—

Agent	Route‡	Concentration g/100 ml	With Adrenaline ml	With Adrenaline mg	Without Adrenaline ml	Without Adrenaline mg
	epidural	1·5	15–25	225–375	15–25	225–375
	spinal	5·0 in 5% dextrose		—	—	—
mepivacaine	infiltration	1·0–1·5		—	20–15	200
	nerve block	2		—	10	200
bupivacaine	nerve block	0·25	56	140	56	140
		0·5	28	140	28	140

* No longer manufactured in the U.K. Available through Ciba temporarily.

† Not yet passed by Committee of Safety of Drugs for use in spinal anaesthesia.

‡ Many of the proprietary spinal anaesthetics have now become extremely limited, although the formulae are still in *Martindale*. As a result of manufacturers discontinuing their proprietary materials the basic chemicals often vanish. However, although some of the preparations listed above are no longer readily available in the U.K., many are still available in other countries of the world.

Table 14.2 *Local anaesthetic agents: potency and duration*

Agent	*Relative potency (frog sciatic nerve)*	*Average onset time* (min)	*Duration of epidural analgesia* (min)
lignocaine	1	5·0	97–156
mepivacaine	1	6·5	149
prilocaine	1	6·5–7·3	97–135
amethocaine	4	6·6–14·5	145–334
bupivacaine	4	5·8–10·8	196–423

Bupivacaine is said to be much longer acting than lignocaine: 0.5% bupivacaine with 1 in 200 000 adrenaline (Marcain) has a duration of action approximately 3–4 times that of lignocaine (see Table 14.2). It would appear that a dose of 2 mg/kg in any four hour period should not be exceeded in a fit 70 kg adult, i.e. 25–30 ml of 0.5% solution Marcain or 50–60 ml of 0.25% solution Marcain. 0.5% Marcain is equivalent to 2% lignocaine. Solutions: bupivacaine 0.25% or 0.5% without adrenaline (Marcain plain); bupivacaine 0.5% with adrenaline 1 in 200 000, and 0.25% with adrenaline 1 in 400 000.

Toxicity. See Table 14.3. Many tragic and totally unnecessary deaths have occurred because of complete disregard of the safe dose of these agents. Some, such as cocaine, amethocaine, and nupercaine are notoriously dangerous. Prilocaine, although having the same potency as lignocaine is less toxic and gives a lower blood level. It also is slightly longer in dura-

Table 14.3 *Local anaesthetic agents: characteristics of toxicity*

Agent	*Blood level* (μg/ml) *at which toxic side effects seen*	*Epidural analgesia* *Dose* (mg)	*Maximum blood level* (μg/ml) *resulting*
prilocaine	Not known	400 without adrenaline	2·74
mepivacaine	6·0	50–62·5 with adrenaline (single injection)	0·3
		50 no adrenaline	0·64
lignocaine	10·0	400 no adrenaline	4·0–4·3
		400 with adrenaline	2·30–3·09
bupivacaine	1·6	1·45 mg/kg with adrenaline (single injection)	0·33
		174·5 continuous	0·44

tion of action than lignocaine. The margin of safety with lignocaine is greater than with bupivacaine and mepivacaine. Intravenous mepivacaine and bupivacaine in equipotent doses show no difference between the systemic toxicities and rate of disappearance from the blood. Toxic signs with lignocaine are seen when blood levels exceed 10 μg/ml. The plasma levels are related to total dose, and rate of administration, but not to the concentration of solution when given by the epidural route. Cumulation with bupivacaine and lignocaine is less than with mepivacaine (Carbocaine). Mepivacaine tends to produce higher blood levels than lignocaine. Some sites, too, are particularly vulnerable because of the rapidity of absorption in relation to specific agents – for example, amethocaine is very rapidly absorbed from the urethra and the lung. The toxicity of local anaesthetic agents can be reduced by limiting their absorption through the addition of a vasoconstrictor. Such a practice not only enables more of the agent to be used, but also prolongs its effect. Prolongation of effect can be achieved by the addition of 1% lignocaine to 10% dextran and 1 in 250 000 adrenaline.

Overdosage. The effects are over-stimulation of the cerebral cortex and depression of the cardiovascular and respiratory systems. Various combinations may occur, symptoms varying from excitement, with or without convulsions, to collapse and unconsciousness. A personal account of lignocaine overdosage has been reported. Following the administration of 700 mg of 2% lignocaine subcutaneously, the subject felt sleepy and drunk, with a fullness in the head and numbness in the arms. This 'wonderful feeling' gave way to a feeling of faintness, with increasing depth of respiration, twitching and diplopia. The observer noticed the euphoria of his patient, which very rapidly became associated with jactitations.

As has been outlined above, prevention is the better part of cure. Particular care should be taken when administering these agents to the old or cachectic patient, as the injection of local anaesthetic solutions into highly vascular areas predisposes to rapid absorption. Should convulsions occur, the airway should be secured, 100% oxygen delivered and diazepam (10–20 mg) and/or suxamethonium injected either intravenously or intramuscularly. The intravenous injection of thiopentone, as treatment, carries with it the risk of inadvertent extravenous injection, together with the possibility of overdosage and resultant cardio-vascular depression. There is no strong evidence to support the view that premedication with barbiturates has a specific effect in reducing the toxicity of the agent.

Hyaluronidase: by the use of a spreading factor the distribution of the local anaesthetic agent is enhanced and the time it takes to act reduced: the addition of 1000 International Units of hyaluronidase to 20 ml of solution provides a satisfactory degree of spread.

Intravenous local anaesthesia

Intravenous local anaesthesia was first described by Bier in 1908 and fairly recently reintroduced into practice. It is an extremely valuable technique which enables minor surgery to take place on the limbs without the necessity of general anaesthesia (e.g. casualty surgery). The dangers associated with supraclavicular plexus block, such as pneumothorax, are avoided and good analgesia and relaxation occur. 0.5% lignocaine *without* adrenaline may be employed, using up to 40 ml (200 mg) for the adult arm, and up to 100 ml (500 mg) for the leg. Prilocaine has been used in 0.5%, 1.0% and 2.0% solutions, with a dose range of 75 mg to 800 mg in patients from 6 years to 60 years. It is probably better to give a large volume of weak solution rather than a small volume of concentrated.

Procedure: orthopaedic wool is wound round the upper arm and around this is placed a sphygmomanometer cuff, which is inflated to just over the diastolic blood pressure, and either a scalp vein needle, or a Mitchell needle inserted into a vein in the dorsum of the hand. The cuff is released and the arm elevated and exsanguinated by winding on an Esmarch bandage; in the case of a painful lesion of the arm such as a Colles' fracture, a Biscard bandage may be used. The sphygmomanometer cuff is now inflated to well above the systolic pressure, the Esmarch bandage removed and an injection of the local anaesthetic made into the vein through the in-dwelling needle. A second sphygmomanometer is now placed just below the first; this is inflated to above the systolic pressure and the first one removed.

Dose: doses of lignocaine varying by as much as from 1.5 mg to 4 mg/kg have been recommended, using 0.5% solution, the maximal doses varying from 200–350 mg: despite this, it is potentially dangerous to exceed 200 mg i.v. in a healthy, 70 kg adult male. If the tourniquet is released intermittently at the end of the injection, the entry of solution into the circulation can be delayed. Clenching the fist after injection helps to hasten the spread of the analgesic solution. Many workers have had a high degree of success with this technique, but not all have been equally enthusiastic.

Complications: venous thrombosis and cardiac arrest have been reported. Convulsions have occurred associated with the slipping of the tourniquet and after its release dizziness or even unconsciousness has supervened.

Continuous intravenous analgesia. Procaine and lignocaine have been given in the form of continuous 'drips'. 125–250 ml of 0.1% procaine may be administered in 10 minutes, and then the infusion slowed to 40–80 drops per minute. Consciousness is sometimes lost but a pharyngeal airway is not always necessary. Intravenous lignocaine may be given as a supplement to thiopentone and gallamine; 2 ml of 2% lignocaine may be administered every five minutes during the first hour of anaesthesia and 1 ml 2% every 5 minutes during the second hour. The intravenous administration of procaine and lignocaine increases the duration of apnoea with succinyl choline.

Intramuscular lignocaine may also be used as an adjuvant to nitrous oxide and oxygen anaesthesia. An initial dose of 250 mg may be given with half the normal amount of premedication and, immediately following induction, a further 250 mg administered intramuscularly and the dose repeated hourly.

Intra-arterial injection distal to the sphygmomanometer cuff has been employed; it is claimed that less exsanguination is needed than for intravenous analgesia.

Spinal anaesthesia

The administration of local anaesthetic solution into either the subarachnoid or extradural space (see Table 14.4) has been practised for many years. Corning, in 1885, injected cocaine into the subarachnoid space of a dog and, in 1898, produced spinal subarachnoid anaesthesia in man. Extradural (epidural) block was also introduced by Corning and employed in surgery by Pages in 1921.

The subarachnoid space lies between the pia mater and the arachnoid mater, is occupied by cerebro-spinal fluid and terminates at its lowest limit at the level of the second sacral vertebra. The extradural space lies between the periosteum lining the vertebral canal (continuous with the outer layer of the cerebral dura) and the spinal dura mater (which is continuous with the meningeal layer of the dura mater covering the brain). Prolongations of the dura surround the spinal nerve roots as they traverse the intervertebral foramina.

Spinal subarachnoid block has experienced fluctuations in its popularity over the years. Neurological catastrophies, associated with the toxicity of the agents used, and meningitis, associated with the introduction of infection into the subarachnoid space, have led to lack of enthusiasm for its use. In the days when general anaesthesia had distinct imperfections, it held pride of place for surgery involving the trunk and lower limbs. Today, with advances in general anaesthesia and the introduction of neuromuscular blocking agents, its widespread use has fallen off. It still holds, however, an undoubted place amongst the techniques available to the anaesthetist, and in some circumstances it may be the method of choice, in particular in situations where skilled anaesthetists are not available and where equipment and drugs are limited.

Extradural anaesthesia has gained popularity because, in theory, there is less danger of meningitis and of post-operative headache, a most disturbing complication of subarachnoid block both to the patient and the administrator. It used to be thought that the fall in blood pressure was more pronounced with subarachnoid than extradural block. Recent work suggests that a fall in blood pressure is just as likely in both and that the degree is more a function of the height of block than the particular space into which the anaesthetic solution is placed.

Preparation. An explanation of the nature of the procedure and reassurance about the technique should be given to all patients. Adequate sedation should be administered where necessary, the patient brought to the anaesthetic room, placed in the position for injection and made as comfortable as possible. He should not be allowed to witness preparations for the surgical procedure. Some administrators prefer to carry out the injection with the patient asleep, in which case a sleep dose of thiopentone may be necessary, with supplementation by inhalational agents. If this procedure is adopted, it will be necessary to have a second trained individual supervising the general anaesthetic. Table 14.4 gives the solutions employed for both techniques.

Table 14.4 *Solutions employed in spinal subarachnoid and epidural anaesthesia*

Spinal subarachnoid block	
'Heavy solutions':	
amethocaine	1 in 200 in 6% dextrose (0·5–2·0 ml) Or as 1% solution with or without 10% glucose according to height of analgesia required
nupercaine	1 in 200 in 6% dextrose (0·5–2 ml)
lignocaine	5% solution in 3·0% dextrose (0·5–2 ml)
procaine	5% solution (rarely used because of short duration of action). (0·5–2 ml)
'Light solutions':	
nupercaine	1 in 1500 in 0·5% sodium chloride solution (7–20 ml). This solution is hypobaric
Spinal epidural block	
lignocaine	1·0–1·5% with adrenaline (15–50 ml)
prilocaine	1·5% without adrenaline (15–25 ml)
bupivacaine	0·5% with adrenaline (8–14 ml) 0·25% with adrenaline (12–20 ml) 0·25% without adrenaline } 0·375% without adrenaline } (6–16 ml) 0·5% without adrenaline }

Volume of solutions is determined by site of injection and level of anaesthesia required

Asepsis. Regardless of whether the injection is to be made into the subarachnoid space or the extradural space, full aseptic technique is necessary. The administrator should be gowned and wear gloves and mask; the skin should be thoroughly cleaned, using a no-touch technique – iodine in spirit is not only a reasonably satisfactory solution for cleansing the skin, but helps to delineate the area which has been cleaned and the site for injection. (This site should be determined by palpation with the finger, separated from the skin by a gauze swab.) All needles, syringes and solutions should be autoclaved but on no account sterilized by boiling or immersion in sterilizing liquids. Cotton wool should not be used for packing because of the danger of introducing small particles of charred foreign matter into the subarachnoid space.

Subarachnoid block

Very many techniques have been described over the years and it is beyond the scope of this book to deal with them in detail. The two techniques employing hypobaric solutions (Howard Jones Technique and Etherington-Wilson Technique), are now less commonly employed. Techniques using 'heavy' solutions (hyperbaric) rely on gravity, and the quantity of solution injected, for the level at which anaesthesia is reached. For operations on the perineum and for bladder neck procedures, the sitting position is usually adopted. For abdominal operations, lumbar puncture is usually carried out with the patient lying in the lateral position, with the knees and chin in close proximity.

Perineal operations: the patient is sat up with the arms folded and the back flexed as much as possible, the arms either resting on the thighs or placed on a 'bed table': additional support should be provided by a nurse. The L4–5 interspace should be chosen for lumbar puncture, and 1.0 ml of heavy solution injected under full aseptic conditions. The patient should remain in the sitting position for five minutes.

Lower abdominal operations: inguinal herniorrhaphy; caesarean section; prostatectomy. Injections should be made with the patient in the lateral position and the table in a 5° head down tilt. They should be made at L3–4 interspace and 1.4–1.8 ml of heavy solution injected, followed by the immediate turning of the patient into the supine posture.

Upper abdominal operations: the lateral position of the patient should be adopted, the injection of 2 ml of heavy solution being made at L3–4 interspace.

The Howard Jones type of needle, of the narrowest possible diameter, is suitable for subarachnoid puncture. The skin should be punctured prior to the introduction of the spinal needle with either a Size introducer or another needle; then the spinal needle should be inserted so that the bevel is at right angles to the long axis of the body.

'Light' subarachnoid block: the injection is made in the lateral position, using nupercaine 1 in 1500 in a dose varying from 7–20 ml, depending on the height to which it is desired to ascend. The patient is immediately placed prone, with the head, shoulders and the lower part of the trunk lowered, so that the level to which the anaesthetic is desired is at the highest point. This position is maintained for four minutes, to allow the anaesthetic to become 'fixed', after which the subject is carefully and gently rolled supine with the table in a 5° head-down tilt.

Precautions: the higher the spinal subarachnoid block, the more likelihood of a fall in blood pressure, so the blood pressure should be continuously monitored, using a phygmomanometer. A catheter should always be placed in a vein so that fluids can be rapidly administered. Although depression of respiration is unlikely when using the techniques described here for adults, ventilatory inadequacy may develop with a high abdominal spinal anaesthetic, if the diaphragm is splinted by an abdominal tumour, such as the gravid uterus or an ovarian cyst.

Contraindications: spinal subarachnoid block is contraindicated in the presence of skin sepsis in the region of the possible site of injection; in association with disease of the spine; with neurological disease; or in the hypertensive, where a sympathetic blockade is likely to produce a significant fall of the blood pressure, possibly leading to the blood supply of vital organs being impaired.

Management of patients following spinal anaesthesia: a patient who has had a spinal (subarachnoid) anaesthetic will have anaesthesia and paralysis below the level of the block. Therefore all positioning and movement must be done with this very much in mind, or serious injuries to ligaments or even vertebrae may result. In order to minimize 'spinal headache' the practice was, after removal from the operating table, to nurse the patient flat, or on only one pillow for 24 hours. This seems, however, rather a long period, and twelve hours is probably sufficient. It is, in any case, doubtful whether this is the means of preventing the headache, which is probably due to leakage of CSF through the puncture site. If this is small enough, i.e. a fine needle (s.w.g. 24) has been used, and the plane of the bevel has not been at right angles to the long axis of the body during puncture, headaches will be unlikely. If the bevel was at right angles to the long axis of the body, the fibres of the dura will have been cut rather than separated, causing a large hole. Should a headache develop it is relieved by the head-down position, 'forcing' fluids (on the assumption that it is a low pressure headache), and analgesics. Ergotamine is of no value in relief of this headache, but an epidural injection of the patient's own blood has recently been stated to be efficacious.

Epidural anaesthesia

The success of this technique depends on the precise location of the epidural space. Many methods have been developed, in order to establish that the tip of the needle lies within this space, of which there are two main ones:

1. The existence of a negative pressure within the space has been recognized for many years. Various techniques have been devised to recognize this feature, such as the Gutierrez Hanging Drop sign. With a drop of saline hanging within the hub, the spinal needle is advanced and, as the tip of it enters the epidural space, the drop is noticed to be drawn into the needle. This principle is also applied to Odom's indicator. A short capillary tube containing a small quantity of sterile saline is attached to the needle, which is advanced into the epidural space, where the vacuum causes the saline to be drawn inwards. Brooks has modified the Odom's indicator so that it contains a small bulb which can be warmed with the hand; this leads to a positive pressure which is released when the epidural space is entered, thus permitting the small quantity of saline in the capillary tube to move.

2. Other methods of detection have relied upon the loss of resistance

experienced when the epidural space is entered (Dogliotti). Macintosh has devised a small balloon which, when attached to the needle, can be filled with air under slight pressure; advancement of the needle into the epidural spacc leads to collapse of the balloon. Macintosh has also devised a spring loaded stylet which, when the epidural space is entered by the needle, allows movement of the stylet. Loss of resistance can also be detected by attaching a mechanically perfect syringe containing air on to the needle and advancing the needle while the finger presses gently on the plunger. Prior to use the syringe should be tested by attempting to compress the air within the barrel by occluding the nozzle with the finger: when used the entry into the epidural space is heralded by movement of the plunger. Mechanical devices using this principle have also been developed (Iklé syringe). Zelenka described a U-shaped capillary tube closed by a tap at one end and having a small balloon attached to the other: the balloon is inflated with air plus a little water, to make a froth in the capillary tube, and the tap is then closed; when the tip of the epidural needle is judged to lie in the ligamentum flavum, the device is plugged into the hub of the needle and the tap opened; as soon as the needle enters the epidural space, the balloon discharges down the capillary tube and this movement reinforces the movement of the froth in the capillary tube which occurs if a negative pressure is present. Thus by the use of both techniques combined in one device, recognition of the space is made easy. Dawkins, who has devised a simple modification of the Odom indicator to produce an instrument similar in principle to Zelenka's device, has also suggested the use of a rubber band on a syringe, thus replacing the somewhat cumbersome Iklé syringe, and has also employed a drop indicator.

Needles: An 18 s.w.g. needle preferably rather blunt and with a short bevel is suitable for epidural analgesia. Lee has advised a marked needle for this purpose, which has alternate black and silver zones, each measuring 1 cm, there being 4 cm to the first black zone.

Site of injection: the site varies considerably, and is influenced largely by the level of the surgical procedure. Hyaluronidase has been used to extend the spread.

Techniques: suggested techniques are set out in Table 14.5.

Caution: particular care should be taken with elderly and parturient patients as excessive spread may occur. Inadvertent puncture of the subarachnoid space is a potentially hazardous situation, as total respiratory and circulatory paralysis may occur if the solution is injected intrathecally: should such a mishap occur, the proposed procedure should be terminated or a purposeful subarachnoid injection made, using the appropriate spinal solution in place of the epidural one.

Continuous epidural. One of the disadvantages of the single injection

Table 14.5 *Suggested techniques for epidural analgesia*

Operation	*Dose*	*Site and posture*
Perineal; and transurethral resection	15 ml of 1·5% lignocaine with 1/200 000 or 1/400 000 adrenaline	L_2–L_3 sitting up
Lower abdominal	20 ml of 1·5% lignocaine with adrenaline	L_1–L_2 10° Trendelenberg tilt
Upper abdominal	30 ml of 1·5% lignocaine with adrenaline	L_1–L_2 15° Trendelenberg tilt

technique is that anaesthesia may prove to be inadequate for prolonged operations. The introduction of a catheter (under full aseptic technique) into the epidural space allows anaesthesia to be maintained continuously. The Tuohy needle with a blunt Huber tip, allows the passage of a 1 mm bore catheter.

Technique: the needle should be advanced into the epidural space with the bevel directed along the long axis of the body, in an upwards or downwards direction. (Catheters with markings calibrated at 5, 10 and 15 cm from the tip have been described, which facilitate the final position of the catheter tip during the withdrawal of the needle). Puncture should be made at the T_{12}–L_1 interspace. For upper abdominal surgery, the tip of the catheter should be gently advanced until it comes to lie at the level T_8–T_9, and for lower abdominal surgery at T_{10}–T_{11}. Doses of 1.5% lignocaine with adrenaline should be administered, of the order of 10–20 ml for prostatectomy, 25–40 ml for lower abdominal surgery and 35–50 ml for upper abdominal surgery.

Great care should be taken to avoid contamination of the epidural space during intermittent injections, so the use of a sterile bladder syringe, within a sterile plastic bag is suggested. (A specific disposable syringe has been described: alternatively a Millipore filter should be used.) This bladder syringe should be charged with 50–60 ml of 1.5% lignocaine with adrenaline. The catheter must be firmly secured with sticking plaster to the long axis of the back. The use of a continuous 'drip' is potentially dangerous; should the clip inadvertently become loose, a disastrous overdose of the drug might follow.

Post-operative continuous epidural anaesthesia: the use of continuous epidural analgesia for the relief of post-operative pain has been advocated (Simpson *et al.*, 1961). Catheters have been introduced into the mid-thoracic region, injecting up to 14 ml at a time of analgesic solution, with the dose repeated as required. Using relatively small doses in a selective area, hypotension is not a serious problem. Evidence suggests that there is no serious degree of respiratory paralysis associated with epidural block and it is of particular value therefore in patients with poor pulmonary function and injury to the chest wall.

Technique: with the patient either sitting up or lying on his side, and with the spine flexed, a skin weal is made 1 cm lateral to the lower edge of the spinous process marking the upper limit of the chosen space (5th to the 8th thoracic spine). Underlying subcutaneous tissue and muscle are infiltrated with local analgesic solution and the skin and muscle sheath are punctured with a Size introducer or wide-bore needle, the skin being held firmly stretched between the fingers of the left hand. The Size introducer is then withdrawn and a Tuohy needle is inserted through the puncture hole at right angles to the skin, until the vertebral lamina is reached; the needle is then withdrawn as far as the muscle sheath and re-introduced, aiming inwards at about 10 degrees towards the patient's head. When the needle point lies at a depth at which contact was made with the lamina, the stilette is withdrawn and a 10 ml syringe, filled with saline, attached to the hub; by slowly advancing the syringe and needle, the extradural space can be located by 'loss-of-resistance'. After a little practice with this method, extradural puncture in the mid-thoracic region proves to be no more difficult than in the lumbar region.

With the bevel of the Tuohy needle pointing upward, a catheter marked at 10 cm intervals is inserted until its tip lies 4 cm beyond the point of the needle; the needle is then withdrawn and the site of skin puncture sprayed with Nobecutane. The distal end of the catheter is fitted on to the syringe containing the local analgesic solution, via a Millipore filter. A rolled 3 × 3 inch (7.5 × 7.5 cm) gauze bandage is placed between the catheter and the skin to avoid a right-angled bend which might cause kinking of the catheter. The catheter is then strapped in position, its distal end being passed over the patient's shoulder with the syringe fixed below the clavicle.

The blood pressure should be measured and sufficient local anaesthetic administered to provide pain relief. Approximately 8–9 ml of 1.5% lignocaine with adrenaline may be administered at about 90 minute intervals; alternatively, to overcome frequent injections bupivacaine may be employed. (Attention must be drawn to the need for scrupulous asepsis during the establishment of the block and when 'top-up' doses are required.) The blood pressure should be checked at frequent and regular intervals, and the patient's ability to cough also checked by getting him to breathe deeply. After lying down for about 15 minutes and provided the blood pressure remains stable the patient may then get out of bed.

Caudal anaesthesia. The patient is requested to lie in the prone position, with two pillows under the hips. After cleaning the skin, the tip of the coccyx is identified, and the sacral hiatus palpated about 4–5 cm above this. After a skin weal is raised, a needle marked 4 cm from the tip is advanced until the sacrococcygeal ligament is punctured; the hub of the needle is then depressed until the needle lies at an angle of 30° to the surface, when it is advanced in the mid-line up the sacral canal, for not more than 4 cm (special care is required in obstetric cases). Following an aspiration test for blood or cerebro-spinal fluid, a few ml of air are injected and the loss of resistance tested together with palpation over the sacrum for crepitus. 8 ml of 1.5% lignocaine and adrenaline are then injected. If, after 5 minutes, the patient has no analgesia or paralysis of the feet (i.e. the injection is not in the subarachnoid space), further injections may be given according to the height to which anaesthesia is desired. 30 ml of solution are satisfactory for perineal operations, but for upper abdominal operations, it may be necessary to inject volumes up to 90 ml, in which case a less toxic agent such as prilocaine should be employed.

Continuous caudal anaesthesia: this technique has definite application in the field of obstetric pain relief. Using the technique described above, but using a wide bore needle, a catheter can be passed up the sacral canal and, after a test dose of analgesic solution (8 ml), a further dose of 22 ml is given, which is repeated approximately every 90 minutes. As adrenaline should be avoided in obstetric work, there is a very real danger of toxic overdosage; therefore, a relatively less toxic agent than lignocaine should be used, e.g. prilocaine, administered not by a drip but by a sterile enclosed syringe, as described above. The continuous administration should be commenced once the presenting part is engaged and when contractions are occurring at five minute intervals or less: by adding hyaluronidase to the anaesthetic solution, the latent period can be reduced. Provided that such administration is not started too early, good pain relief can be achieved without delaying the course of labour.

Stellate ganglion block

Anatomy: this ganglion is formed by coalescence of the inferior cervical ganglion and the first thoracic ganglion, situated opposite the interval between the base of the transverse process of the last cervical vertebra and the neck of the first rib, behind the origin of the vertebral artery. As well as having communications with the heart, the ganglion is linked to a plexus of nerves around the subclavian artery and its branches.

Indications: stellate ganglion block has been employed in the treatment of cerebro-vascular disease, cardiac pain, vascular disease of the arm, and ophthalmic disorders.

Anterior or paratracheal approach: this approach is relatively free from complications, although it passes important structures. The patient is placed in the dorsal recumbent position, without a pillow and the neck maximally extended to straighten the oesophagus. A skin weal is raised two fingers' breadth lateral to the jugular notch of the sternum and two fingers above the clavicle – this position corresponds to the level of the seventh transverse process, and should be 1 cm below the cricoid. The sternomastoid and the carotid sheath are displaced laterally, a needle advanced about 3 cm until it hits the seventh transverse process and then withdrawn about 0.3 cm, and 5–10 ml of 1% lignocaine are injected after aspiration to be sure a vessel has not been entered. Within 5–10 minutes, if the block is effective, Horner's syndrome (meiosis, narrowing of the palpebral fissure, injection of the sclera and unilateral flushing of the face accompanied by dryness and warmth of the hand) will develop. This approach carries the disadvantage that the vertebral artery can be accidentally injected.

Antero-lateral and lateral approach: these techniques differ in the degree to which they are lateral to and above the clavicle. The stellate ganglion is approached by passing postero-laterally to the carotid sheath and above the subclavian artery and the apex of the lung. Accidental spinal block or pneumothorax is a risk common to all.

Posterior or para-vertebral approach: this technique approaches the stellate ganglion by passing through the posterior vertebral muscle between the transverse processes and following the side of the body of the vertebra to the region of the head of the rib. Complications include pneumothorax, puncture of the subclavian artery or oesophagus, and block of the recurrent laryngeal or phrenic nerve or the brachial plexus.

Brachial plexus block

Anatomy: the brachial plexus is formed by the union of the anterior primary rami of the lower four cervical nerves with the greater part of the anterior primary ramus of the first thoracic nerve. These nerves constitute the roots of the plexus, which divide and re-unite to form the trunks lying above the clavicle, the trunks further dividing as they pass towards the axilla to form the cords. In the lower part of the axilla these cords split up to form the nerves of the arm.

Indications: brachial plexus block is extremely valuable for operations on the distal part of the arm and it has been applied for the relief of vascular disorders in the upper extremities.

Brachial plexus block by the supraclavicular route. This was first described by Kulenkamff in 1911: the sitting position was chosen with the point of the needle introduced just above the midpoint of the clavicle and the needle passed in the direction of the spinous processes of the first and second dorsal vertebrae. Nowadays, it is customary to settle the patient in the supine position with the head on a shallow pillow; the head is then rotated towards the opposite side and the pillow pushed under the shoulder. The patient is requested to reach, with the tips of his fingers, down the lateral aspect of the leg on the side of the injection, thereby depressing the shoulder. Standing by the side of the patient facing towards his head the administrator raises a skin weal 1.0 cm above the midpoint of the clavicle (this point can readily be determined by requesting the patient to carry out the Valsalva manoeuvre, when the point at which the external jugular vein disappears through the deep fascia marks the point of injection). The subclavian artery is palpated with the forefinger of the left hand, retracted downwards and medially and a 5 cm needle is advanced downwards, inwards and backwards, aiming towards the upper surface of the first rib, with the needle lying in between the subclavian artery and the trunks of the brachial plexus. The point of the needle will then come to lie on the upper surface of the first rib, but no attempt should be made to elicit paraesthesia: one injection only is made of 25 ml of 1.5% lignocaine with adrenaline. The supraclavicular approach to the brachial plexus carries with it the danger producing a pneumothorax.

Axillary block. Over recent years the axillary approach to the brachial plexus block, originally described by Hirshel, has been re-introduced.

The pre-vertebral fascia envelops the brachial plexus from the cervical vertebrae to the distal axilla, forming a subclavian peri-vascular space that is continuous with the axillary peri-vascular space. Just as with epidural techniques, once the space has been entered only a single injection is necessary; the extent of the anaesthesia will depend on the volume of the anaesthetic and the level at which it is injected. Since the median, ulnar and radial nerves are lying in close proximity to the axillary artery in the neurovascular compartment of the axilla, all three nerves are easily and completely blocked by the axillary approach, with the injection of a moderate volume of anaesthetic agent. Because of its more proximal origin, however, complete motor and sensory block of the musculocutaneous nerve can be obtained only by the injection of a relatively large volume of local anaesthetic into the axillary neuro-vascular compartment. Block of the distal sensory portion of the musculocutaneous nerve (the lateral forearm, wrist and hand) may be obtained with a smaller volume and thus with a lower total dose of local anaesthetic: de Jong (1965) has therefore modified the technique. With the arm abducted and supinated, the axillary artery is palpated at the level of the insertion of the lower border of the pectoralis major muscle. This is the site for the injection. The neuro-vascular compartment is then compressed digitally, distal to the site of the injection, a short needle is passed into the neurovascular sheath and the click of the needle, as it passes into the sheath, and the subsequent production of paraesthesiae signify that the space has been entered. A volume of 20–30 ml of local anaesthetic solution is injected, followed by a supplementary injection of the lateral antebrachial cutaneous nerve, which is made at the point where it emerges from the lateral cleft between the biceps and the brachialis muscle at the elbow.

Local anaesthesia for abdominal surgery

In certain circumstances, particularly in some countries where a surgeon may be forced to work single handed, it may be necessary to perform a laparatomy under local anaesthesia and Farman (1962) has described a technique of intercostal block for this purpose. Using lignocaine (2% with 1 in 80 000 adrenaline), 2 ml of solution are injected into each requisite intercostal space. The nerves are all blocked posterior to the mid-auxiliary line so that the lateral cutaneous branches are included; in order to facilitate this procedure the arms are placed above the head and five segments are injected on each side. For the upper abdomen spaces 6–10 are injected, for the mid-abdomen 7–11, and for the lower abdomen 8–12. If the procedure is expected to be lengthy, Marcain is to be preferred. The injection should be made by striking the rib above the nerve to be blocked and then advancing the needle 3 mm below the rib, always with the syringe attached to avoid pneumothorax. (If a bleb occurs under the skin the injection can be assumed to be not deep enough.) In view of the large quantities of anaesthetic agent required, prilocaine, which is less toxic, may be chosen.

Defalque and Stoelting (1964) have devised a method for giving continuous intercostal block. A Tuohy needle is advanced in the mid-axillary line under the rib into the space between the external and internal intercostal muscles; with the bevel turned in a dorsal direction a vinyl catheter is advanced 2–3 cm beyond the tip, through which the initial and subsequent topping up injection may be given.

Abdominal field block. 0.25% lignocaine or 0.5% prilocaine with 1/200 000 adrenaline should be used. Raise cutaneous weals at the lateral border of rectus abdominis muscle, on each side, at the following levels:

1. Just above the pubis.
2. 5 cm above this.
3. 1 cm below the level of the umbilicus.
4. 5 cm above the previous weal.
5. At the level of the 9th costal cartilage, if the incision is to supra-umbilical.

A needle is inserted through each weal and, as it penetrates the anterior layer of the rectus sheath, a distinct 'snap' will be felt. Insert the needle a further 0.5 cm, taking care not to penetrate the posterior layer of the sheath or the peritoneum will be entered, and inject 10 ml of local anaesthetic solution.

Before each injection, aspirate to be sure that a blood vessel has not been inadvertantly entered: finally, join the weals on each side by subcutaneous infiltration of solution and then wait at least 15 minutes before the incision is commenced. This technique is for median or paramedian incisions and not more than 150 ml solution should be necessary in a 70 kg adult.

Local block for repair of inginal or femoral hernia. Using 0.5% lignocaine or 0.5% prilocaine, with 1/200 000 adrenaline, block the ilioinguinal and iliohypogastric nerves by injecting 30 ml solution through a weal 1 cm medial to the anterior superior iliac spine, just beneath the aponeurosis of the external oblique muscle. A small snap will be felt as it is penetrated. As the needle is withdrawn to the skin, a further 5 ml solution should be deposited en route; then, through a weal 1 cm above the midpoint of the inguinal ligament, a needle is inserted again through the aponeurosis and 20 ml solution are injected. (Aspiration, to ensure that no vessel is penetrated, is important before these injections.)

Using 0.25% lignocaine or 0.5% prilocaine, in adrenaline 1/200 000, infiltrate subcutaneously along the line of the incision and also about 6 cm from the symphysis pubis upwards towards the umbilicus and around the neck of the sac. Only about 35 ml will be necessary for these. Wait at least 15 minutes before commencing the incision: later, the surgeon may infiltrate deeper tissues with the weaker solution, should this become necessary during the course of the operation.

Lumbar sympathetic block. This procedure is sometimes indicated as a diagnostic aid in assessing the feasibility of a surgical sympathectomy and sometimes as a therapeutic measure.

Diagnostic procedure: Bryce-Smith (1951) suggests the introduction of a 12 cm needle three fingers' breadth lateral to the spine of L3: with the needle pointing anteriorly and medially at an angle of 60° to the plane of the back, it is advanced until it strikes the lateral aspect of the vertebral body. After aspiration, 15 ml of local anaesthetic solution are injected.

Therapeutic procedure: (this method can be used for diagnostic procedures using local anaesthetic). Phenol block of the lumbar sympathetic ganglia is an extremely useful procedure in certain ischaemic states, of which the principle indication is pre-gangrene or incipient gangrene – patients with intolerable rest pain in their feet, who are unsuitable for either lumbar sympathectomy or reconstructive arterial surgery (grafts or disobliteration), by reason of their age or general condition.

The patient lies on his side, as for a lumbar puncture, except that it is unnecessary to flex the hips and knees more than is required to keep him comfortable lying on his side. It is important to keep the patient's back at right angles to the couch or bed – the tendency to tilt over towards the prone position must be avoided. Head pillows, except for one small flattish one, should be removed. After the legs from the knees downwards have been exposed to room temperature for ten minutes or so before the injection, an intradermal weal of lignocaine is raised just within the outer border of the erector spinae muscle (3–4 fingers breadth from the midline), at the level of L2. A very fine bore 14 cm needle, fitted with rubber marker, is inserted and passed so as to strike the antero-lateral aspect of the lumbar vertebra: the tip of the needle is aimed at the umbilicus. At about 10–11 cm it strikes bone. (With the lateral site of entry through the skin it is likely that a transverse process will not be encountered). If the needle passes in front of the vertebral body there is a danger of striking the aorta or vena cava in which case the blood is likely to flow back through the needle. Having struck bone at about 10–11 cm, the needle should be slightly withdrawn, the marker moved to lie about 1.5 cm from the skin and the tip of the needle manipulated to pass tangentially past the body of the vertebra and traverse the psoas muscle so that the marker comes to lie against the skin. Having satisfied oneself that the needle is not in a blood vessel, 1 ml of 2% lignocaine should be injected: if the positioning of the needle is very accurate, some increase in temperature and change in colour of the foot will be noted within a minute or two; if the point of the needle is a little further from the chain it may take 10 minutes before there is any temperature change. (Temperature changes are best detected in the skin on the side of the heel.) 10 ml of 5% phenol in water are now injected slowly down the needle.

The patient is left lying on his side for about twenty minutes, after which time he is turned on to his back, keeping his head on a small pillow. If there is no immediate effect this does not necessarily mean the block has failed as it may take 12–24 hours to show evidence of sympathetic block.

Provided the needle is inserted some distance from the midline there is no danger of piercing the dura: nevertheless, though safe, this procedure should not be carried out in young people or where there is any likelihood of surgical sympathectomy or graft procedure, as phenol leads to a very dense fibrosis between the psoas and peritoneum, making access to the major vessels quite impossible. Other similar procedures for chemical sympathectomy have been described.

15 *Pain Relief*

Post-operative pain relief

Many different sensations and pains confront the patient in the post-operative period. The mental make-up of the patient will influence the degree of this discomfort, and fear of disrupting a surgical wound by movement may lead to muscle rigidity, which in itself may intensify pain : the presence of pain on breathing may make the patient reluctant to cough in order to void retained bronchial secretions: pain which arises from peritoneal irritation or involvement of nerves may be particularly severe.

Some patients derive benefit from reassurance and tactful 'psychotherapy' on the part of the medical and nursing staff. Most require supplementation by drugs: a proportion of them derive benefit from placebos such as saline – the 'placebo reactors'. Masson (1964) demonstrated that it was impossible to distinguish by simple enquiry the degree of relief achieved by saline or 100 mg pethidine. Unless the natural history of post-operative pain is understood, large numbers of patients will receive unnecessary drugs while others will develop complications because drugs are withheld. To give larger doses by no means always brings more relief because, as the dosage increases, so does the incidence and intensity of side effects: attempts to eliminate such side effects by a combination with 'analeptics' has produced unconvincing evidence of success. Conduction analgesia, intravenous analgesia and inhalational analgesia have all been used to produce post-operative pain relief.

Antanalgesia. Thiopentone, methohexitone, and some drugs commonly used in premedication, exhibit antanalgesic effects (see page 11), so medication with such agents may have a considerable bearing on the degree of restlessness and pain in the post-operative period. Geffin (1964), in a study related to the use of thiopentone, points out that this agent in narcotic doses raises the pain threshold, whereas subnarcotic doses lower the pain threshold: subnarcotic doses can, therefore, antagonize any analgesic effect of the premedication. Clutton-Brock (1960) has shown that the dose of thiopentone normally used for induction produces a plasma concentration post-operatively that may fall within the range of antanalgesia, while Dundee (Dundee *et al.*, 1960) has shown that with doses of 4–5 mg/kg of thiopentone antanalgesia is present for 2 hours.

Site of pain. Certain operations are associated with more pain than others; upper abdominal wounds are particularly painful and the pain following haemorrhoidectomy can also be very intense.

Certain post-operative pain arises as a result of spasm, e.g. the intense pain sometimes arising in relation to haemorrhoidectomy. Stretching of the sphincter at operation can greatly contribute to a reduction in this pain; the injection of 20 ml of 6% butylaminbenzoate in oily base (Proctocaine) has been employed and, more recently, 1% lignocaine in 10% dextraven injected prior to haemorrhoidectomy has been suggested. Spasm may also arise in the wall of the bile duct, following an operation, and may be accentuated by the administration of morphine. As there is no universal agreement on the treatment of post-operative pain because no one method or drug is ideal, a review of present methods of practice will be in place.

Analgesics (see Table 15.1). Morphine has long held pride of place amongst drugs available for pain relief in the post-operative period. Unfortunately it is not devoid of side effects, producing a drowsy, immobile individual, with a depressed cough reflex, which may lead to sputum retention; it also depresses the respiratory centre and may produce considerable discomfort in susceptible individuals by provoking nausea and vomiting. Many other agents have been used for pain relief, none being free from side effects. Phenazocine produces no significant difference from morphine in the degree of duration of pain relief following abdominal surgery; it is an effective analgesic in 1–2 mg doses (0.5–1.5 mg being the average post-operative intramuscular dose). Circulatory and respiratory side effects have, however, been observed, though phenazocine has been found to be associated with a pleasant absence of other side effects. In patients after abdominal surgery, oxymorphone (0.02 mg/kg), phenazocine (0.03 mg/kg), dextromoramide (0.08 mg/kg), and morphine (0.15 mg/kg) exhibit no significant difference in the degree of duration of relief of pain. Conaghan *et al.* (1966) in a double blind comparison of the two benzomorphan derivatives, pentazocine and phenazocine, found that both drugs were efficient for the relief of post-operative pain and they did not cause nausea or vomiting, 38 mg of pentazocine being equivalent in analgesic effect to 2–6 mg phenazocine. Pentazocine is said to be non-addictive and is not subject to the restrictions applicable to morphine. Piritramide (Dipidolor) is a potent analgesic recently introduced into clinical practice – its true place has

Table 15.1 *Some of the more potent drugs used for analgesia*

All may at times cause undesirable side effects such as nausea, vomiting, dizziness, respiratory depression or hypotension

Drug	*Administration*	*Dose (for adult unless otherwise stated)*
diamorphine (heroin)	subcut. or i.m.	5–10 mg
dihydrocodeine (DF 118)	oral	30–60 mg
	deep subcut. or i.m.	50 mg
levorphanol (Dromoran)	oral	1·5–4·5 mg
	i.m.	2 mg
methadone (Physeptone)	oral	5–10 mg
	i.m.	10 mg
morphine	subcut. or i.m.	10–20 mg Children over 1 month 0·2 mg/kg body wt.
papaveretum (Omnopon)	subcut. or i.m.	10–20 mg Children over 1 month 0·2 mg/kg body wt.
pentazocine (Fortral)	i.m.	30–60 mg Children 1 mg/kg body wt.
	oral	25–100 mg
	rectal suppos.	Adult, or child over 12, 50 mg
pethidine	oral or i.m.	50–100 mg Children 1·5 mg/kg body wt.
phenazocine (Narphen)	oral	5 mg
	i.m.	0·5–3 mg Children weighing 25 kg or less – 0·02 mg/kg Children over 25 kg – 0·015 mg/kg
piritramide (Dipidolor)	i.m.	20 mg may be repeated 6-hourly to total of 80 mg maximum
dextro-propoxyphene (Doloxene)	oral	65 mg 3–4 times/day
dextro-moramide (Palfium)	oral or i.m.	5–10 mg
*dihydromorphinone (Dilaudid; Dimorphone)	oral or i.m.	1·2–2·5 mg
*oxymorphone (Numorphan)	oral	10–40 mg/day
	i.m.	0·5–2·0 mg
*alphaprodine (Nisentil)	i.m.	30–60 mg
*anileridine (Alidine, Leritine)	oral or i.m.	10–60 mg

* not available in UK.

yet to be fully evaluated. A dose of 20 mg may be given intramuscularly and repeated 6 hourly.

Combination with analeptics (see page 384). One of the common side effects of powerful analgesics is the marked respiratory depressant effect. The *n*-allyl derivatives of morphine have the property of antagonizing the respiratory depressant effects of morphine without reducing the analgesic action: however, the clinical evidence for this antagonism is, in many instances, unconvincing and the vasomotor effects of analgesics may be augmented rather than antagonized. 1.25 mg levallorphan (Lorfan) has been employed in combination with 100 mg pethidine (Pethilorphan). This is said to abolish the respiratory depressant effects, while maintaining the analgesia, but workers disagree on these points. Amiphenazole (Daptazole) in very big doses in combination with morphine largely eliminates respiratory depression and makes the patients alert and co-operative in a certain number of cases. Tetra-hydroaminacrine (Tacrine) is more effective in eliminating respiratory depression. Patients are more alert with Tacrine but pain relief even after twice the dose of morphine is no greater. There is no real evidence that Tacrine modifies respiratory depression, but here again writers disagree.

Intravenous analgesia. Intravenous analgesia has been advocated for post-operative pain relief, but the results have been somewhat disappointing when using local analgesic agents, which have the added disadvantage of their toxicity. Alcohol and ether have had their advocates; alcohol is completely metabolized to carbon dioxide and water and has a wider margin of safety than ether, but the action of these two agents appears to be unpredictable when used intravenously.

Intramuscular local analgesia. As with intravenous local anaesthesia, this technique is limited by the toxicity of the agents used. It has also been employed, in conjunction with nitrous oxide, for general anaesthetic purposes.

Conduction analgesia. The use of 'long acting' mixtures of local analgesic agents has been tried. Efocaine fell into disrepute on account of sloughing and neuritis which occurred as a result of its use. Loder (1960) has advocated the addition of dextran to local analgesics, while Massey Dawkins (1964) introduced a continuous epidural drip for the relief of upper and lower abdominal pain. Simpson *et al.* (1962) and Green and Dawkins (1966) have further developed this technique, which has the disadvantage of producing hypotension, if the solution is introduced at too high a level in the thoracic region. Simpson *et al.* (1962) suggest entry to the mid-thoracic region, using the loss of resistance technique, intermittent rather than continuous administration being preferred. The volume of solution injected varies from 6–14 ml of 1.5% lignocaine: vinyl catheters were used. Though complete analgesia can be obtained if injections are so timed as to precede the return of pain, the method is time consuming and requires careful and constant supervision. Continuous intercostal nerve block for post-operative pain relief has been advocated by Ablondi *et al.* (1966), who have inserted plastic catheters into the intercostal space to allow continuous therapy.

Inhalational agents

Nitrous oxide, trichloroethylene and methoxyflurane, have been used for the relief of post-operative pain, particularly when physiotherapy and lung drainage are carried out.

Nitrous oxide. Parbrook *et al.* (1964) compared 25% nitrous oxide and 75% oxygen with morphine given on the basis of 0.16 mg/kg. Using vital capacity and peak expiratory flow rate as objective measurements, they found a significant degree of pain relief, lasting for a few minutes after cessation of the administration of nitrous oxide, and this pain relief was better than that with morphine. The combination of morphine and nitrous oxide produces even better pain relief. When 25% nitrous oxide was combined with Physeptone, there was no increase in undesirable side effects and the combination was twice as potent as a similar concentration of nitrous oxide with morphine. More recently Entonox (premixed nitrous oxide/oxygen 50:50) has been found to be of great value.

Trichloroethylene. Ellis and Bryce-Smith (1965), studying patients who had undergone thoracic surgery, administered 0.5% trichloroethylene in air to provide post-operative analgesia for physiotherapy. The results were encouraging, the physiotherapist being enabled to perform duties with a minimal waste of time.

Methoxyflurane. Methoxyflurane is worthy of a trial for this purpose. 0.2% methoxyflurane in oxygen raises the pain threshold; there is no nausea or vomiting, but some double vision and slight slurring of the speech occurs, though it remains clear and rational. An inhaler delivering 0.35% in air has been produced. As halothane has no analgesic effect the administration of halothane/trichloroethylene mixture has been advocated for use during surgery as post-operative pain is kept away for longer.

Hypnosis. Mason (1958) has reported that the deep trance state required for complete analgesia can be produced only in about 15% of cases. The routine use of such a technique, though valuable in that side effects such as respiratory depression are absent, involves the use of an experienced hypnotist with ample time available.

Neuroleptanalgesia

Two butyrophenone derivatives, haloperidol and droperidol, have been used in combination with potent analgesic narcotics, such as phenoperidine, fentanyl and piritramide. These combinations give the subject a feeling of dissociation from his surroundings (neuroleptanalgesia).

Phenoperidine is a potent analgesic, chemically related to pethidine, and it has found wide application in the field of anaesthesia and surgery. It has been used alone to produce analgesia with complete respiratory depression, in patients requiring prolonged artificial respiration, e.g. crush injury of the chest. In anaesthesia it has been used in conjunction with a neuroleptic in techniques of neuroleptanalgesia, thereby permitting procedures such as pneumoencephalography with an anxiety free, co-operative patient. When used alone to produce a high degree of analgesia without marked respiratory depression, a dose of 1 mg may be given intravenously; in doses higher than this respiratory depression will result and where this is desirable, the dose may be increased up to 5 mg.

Fentanyl 0.1–0.2 mg i.v. may be given alone where spontaneous respiration is required and 0.2–0.6 mg i.v. for controlled ventilation, instead of phenoperidine. The action of both these drugs is reversible with nalorphine (5–10 mg).

Droperidol may be given as a premedication, either alone or with a barbiturate or analgesic. The mixture of 50 : 1 of droperidol and fentanyl (Thalamonal) provides a useful premedication mixture and 5 mg droperidol may be given intravenously combined with 0.1 mg fentanyl (or 1.0 mg phenoperidine), or on its own.

A suggested technique with droperidol and fentanyl for anaesthesia is as follows:

15–45 minutes pre-operatively—
droperidol 2.5 –5.0 mg i.m.
fentanyl 0.05–0.1 mg i.m.
and standard dose of anticholinergic

Induction
droperidol 10.0–15.0 mg i.v.
fentanyl 0.4– 0.6 mg i.v. (assisted ventilation)
or 0.2 mg i.v. (spontaneous ventilation)
and nitrous oxide/oxygen 3/1
and muscle relaxant to facilitate intubation

Maintenance
fentanyl 0.05–0.2 mg i.v. (assisted ventilation)
0.05 mg i.v. (spontaneous ventilation)
Additional doses of fentanyl are administered, when signs of lighten-

ing of analgesic are observed, and unconsciousness maintained by nitrous oxide/oxygen 3/1

Recovery

Reversal of respiratory depression due to fentanyl can be achieved by administering 5–10 mg nalorphine i.v.

Intractable pain

Intractable pain can prove extremely distressing, not only to the patient but also to the medical attendant, who may often feel powerless to help. In many cases this pain is associated with the terminal stages of some irreversible condition and it is the doctor's duty to make sure that the patient's last days are made as comfortable as possible. Much can be done towards this end. In the first place, attention should be paid to the patient's underlying anxieties, reassurance given where required and the environment made as cheerful as possible, with kind, sympathetic nursing. The reader is referred to writings which have dealt with this matter, in particular to a series of excellent articles by Saunders (1967). She stresses the importance of dealing with the many other factors, apart from pain, which add up to produce physical discomfort; such factors include nausea, vomiting, bowel disturbances, dyspnoea, weakness and anorexia, many of which are made worse by the pain relieving drugs that may be prescribed by the physician. Saunders stresses that constant pain calls for constant control and that drugs should be used to prevent pain from occurring, rather than to control it once it occurs; consequently, the analgesic should be given regularly, in a dose assessed to cover a little longer than the chosen period. This regimen will call for constant attention and the assessment of any change in the intensity of the pain. Very many pain relieving agents are available, from the mild analgesics such as aspirin and codeine to the potent analgesics with their undesirable side effects. In order to overcome such unpleasant side effects the combination of these agents with analeptics or phenothiazines not only potentiates their effect, but also brings into play their antiemetic properties. Prolonged administration of some analgesics may result in renal lesions. Where physical dependance on a drug has become a problem, amiphenazole (Daptazole) has been found of value. However, before starting pain relief with drugs, every effort should be made to reduce the intensity of pain by removing any sepsis and by immobilization of pathological fractures and secondary deposits in the spine.

The Brompton cocktail. This mixture, containing morphine or diamorphine, cocaine and gin, when given regularly not only relieves pain, but also alleviates the depression associated with these conditions. The mixture may be modified by the addition of phenothiazines.

Further, reduction of the patient's dependence on drugs can be achieved by chemical nerve block, a procedure which is of particular value in certain sites. The pain associated with carcinoma of the cervix and rectum can be abolished in some cases by the intrathecal injection of phenol (see below); pain in the trigeminal area can often be relieved by block of the trigeminal ganglion; and one of the writers (J.A.T.) has successfully relieved pain in the shoulder joint and chest by the extra-dural injection of phenol at cervical level (see below).

Irradication of trigeminal pain in cancer: by using Harris' route (Harris, 1937) over the sigmoid notch of the mandible, and inverting the head so that the orbit is higher than the mastoid, 1–2 ml of 5% aqueous phenol will flow towards the foramen ovale at a needle depth of 4.4 cm: the foramen ovale should not be penetrated. This injection may be repeated if necessary.

For pain in the distribution of the cervical nerves epidural injection of phenol in Myodil 1 in 20 is often of value. The injection should be made under full X-ray control, using, if possible, an image intensifier, with the patient lying in the lateral position, the head resting on a pillow and the affected side, if possible, lying dependent. An 18 gauge Howard Jones needle, with a short bevel, should be advanced through a skin bleb raised in the midline between the cervical spines, passing at an oblique angle to the long axis of the body, so that the needle lies between the cervical spines. The actual site of injection is governed by the distribution of the pain. The needle is advanced under X-ray control and should be repeatedly aspirated for CSF until the tip is seen to lie in the correct position; if no CSF flows a small quantity of 2 ml phenol in Myodil should be cautiously injected, still under X-ray observation. When the solution is deposited in the correct layer, a characteristic distribution of the radio opaque dye will be noted, running bilaterally both cephalically and caudally and tending to divide into portions opposite the root exits. We have found it necessary to inject up to 9 ml on occasion to produce adequate pain relief. Repeat injections are often most difficult as it may not be easy to relocate the epidural space. Great care should be taken to avoid subarachnoid block and if appreciable quantities are injected into the subarachnoid space the head should be elevated: epidural injection may be made at other levels of the body when appropriate.

For pain in the rectum and the bottom of the coccyx. A subarachnoid puncture is done at L4–L5 with the patient vertical; he then lies on the side of greatest pain, with the trunk elevated to 20° with the horizontal. 0.7 ml of 1 in 20 phenol in glycerin is allowed to flow gently down the lateral dura to the end of the dural sac and the patient is gradually raised to the vertical.

For lumbar and high sacral injections. The patient is laid on the painful side in the lateral lumbar-puncture position and rotated slightly backwards, with a very slight downward slope of the spine towards the sacrum. To reach roots at the lumbar level the injection is made at the L1–2 or L4–5 interspace, 1 ml of phenol (1 in 20 in glycerin) being the standard dose. The first 0.5 ml is injected, the pain should diminish, and then the remaining 0.5 ml is immediately injected. The slope of the spine is increased as much as is necessary to relieve all pain.

Solution used: 1 in 20 phenol in glycerin will keep for approximately 2 weeks: 0.75 mg of silver nitrate may be occasionally added to a 1 in 25 solution of phenol in glycerin solution, where previous injection with phenol has proved unsatisfactory. The immediate sensory symptoms induced by intrathecal phenol can be matched against the final result and are seen in this order of events: first, instantaneous relief is commonly followed by tingling and parasthesia at the appropriate site; there follows diminished sensation to pinprick and scratch, compared with the opposite side and, after further doses, pinprick and scratch sensation may vanish, but light touch is unaffected. Later, light touch diminishes compared with the opposite side and, finally, light touch sensation may cease and the limb become awkward. If this is permanent, movement of the limb may be impaired.

The nervous mechanism of micturition may become impaired if phenol covers the lowest part of the cord, but disturbance of micturition is normally transient, unless there is a previous history of bladder disturbance, when the symptoms may be made far worse and permanent.

Hypothermia. It has been suggested that hypothermic subarachnoid irrigation is of value for the management of intractable pain, the evidence suggesting that the good results obtained may be due to the hypertonicity of the solution employed. In view of the severe autonomic reaction to this treatment, general anaesthesia is usually employed to render it acceptable to the patient.

Hyperthermia. The technique of deliberately elevating the patient's temperature by submergence in a paraffin wax bath whilst under general anaesthesia has recently been claimed to be of value.

Drug antagonists

A variety of pharmacological agents is available to counter the effects of drugs used in association with general anaesthesia. Certain of the neuromuscular blocking agents (the non-depolarizing blockers) can have their action reversed by the administration of neostigmine; some other antagonists are also specific in their action, in the same way as neostigmine is specific for curare, gallamine and similar agents.

However, some agents, such as the barbiturates and the narcotic analgesics, can produce profound side effects upon the body when administered in an uncontrolled manner – prolonged recovery time and respiratory depression are two undesirable side effects of these drugs. Alveolar hypoventilation leading to hypoxia and retention of carbon dioxide arising from drug action should, in the first place, be treated by artificial ventilation (IPPV), but there are some schools of thought who feel that rapid termination of the respiratory depressant effect, and reversal of unconsciousness, can be more readily achieved by the administration of drug antagonists or analeptics. These agents have not only been employed to facilitate recovery in the treatment of intoxications with drugs, but also in relation to outpatient anaesthesia. In conjunction with narcotics and analgesics, they are also used to lessen the side effects of these agents when they are employed for obstetric or post-operative pain relief, and for the relief of pain associated with inoperable cancer and other conditions.

Provided facilities exist for respiratory and cardio-vascular support, analeptics probably have very little place in the treatment of drug intoxications, as it is wiser to await detoxication and elimination of the drug causing over-dosage. It should also be remembered that the effect of many of the analeptics is transient in nature and the drug for which it is given may outlast its effect; for this reason it would appear unwise to use analeptics for outpatient anaesthesia.

It is our opinion that narcotic antagonists have a very limited place and, even then, should be given only if it is absolutely certain that the patient's condition is associated with overaction of a particular narcotic analgesic. For instance, levallorphan can itself produce respiratory depression if given in situations where the depression is not due either to morphine or pethidine. Narcotic antagonists should, therefore, never be given where there may be a mixed drug effect. Analeptics may be given in association with powerful narcotic analgesics, in order to lessen their side effects, but they are rarely indicated in other circumstances: they should never be employed at the termination of a general anaesthetic, as they tend to complicate the picture, particularly if the patient is apnoeic. (The possible exceptions are the use of carbon dioxide or nikethamide.)

Tetrahydroaminacrine (THA, Tacrine, 1, 2, 3, 4-tetra-hydro-amino-acridine hydrochloride). This substance is a stimulant both of the central nervous system and the respiratory system: also it has anticholinesterase activity. Clinical trials have shown that THA will counteract the narcotic and respiratory depressant effects of morphine, whilst there is some evidence that it may enhance its analgesic action. 10–30 mg may be administered intravenously as a respiratory and central nervous system stimulant.

Doxopram hydrochloride (Dopram). A single intravenous injection in a dose of 0.5–1.0 mg/kg has been shown to be an effective respiratory stimulant and to produce abrupt arousal in patients recovering from anaesthesia. A continuous intravenous infusion at a rate of 1–3 mg/min for 30–45 minutes (total dose 200 mg) causes a significant rise in oxygen tension, with a similar fall in carbon dioxide tension. Analgesics are, however, required at an earlier stage of the post-operative period. In the United Kingdom doxopram is available for infusion as a clear, colourless 0.2% aqeous solution with a pH of 2.5–5.0. Doxopram is thought to work by stimulating carotid and aortic bodies and the medullary respiratory centres.

Amiphenazole (Daptazole). This agent is a non-specific central nervous system stimulant, and has been used in conjunction with morphine in the treatment of intractable pain. The combination of large doses of morphine with 25 mg amiphenazone counters the side effects of morphine such as respiratory depression, vomiting and constipation, without apparently interfering with the analgesia. It has also been employed in the treatment of morphine addiction.

Bemegride (Megimide). Although introduced initially as a specific antagonist to the barbiturates, bemegride is regarded today as an analeptic. 25–30 mg may be given intravenously; it can lighten the degree of unconsciousness but does not shorten the duration of it, nor can it be relied upon to awaken a patient after barbiturate anaesthesia.

Nikethamide (Coramine). A non-specific central nervous system stimulant of brief action, 1–2 ml of the 25% solution may be given intravenously and even larger quantities for the treatment of carbon dioxide narcosis, associated with respiratory failure in patients with chronic lung disease.

Vanillic acid diethylamide (Vandid, Ethamivan). This agent is similar in action to nikethamide. 5–10 ml of the 5% solution may be given intravenously.

Crotethamide (Micoren). This compound is a central nervous system stimulant and has been successfully employed in the treatment of chronic respiratory failure, morphine overdose, hypnotic intoxication and post-operative respiratory depression. It has a low toxicity. 225–450 mg (1–2 ampoules) may be given slowly over a period of not less than 4 minutes, or as an infusion of 2700 mg diluted in saline over 45–90 minutes, at a rate of 20–30 mg per minute. 45–75 mg in 5 ml saline has been injected into the umbilical vein in the treatment of asphyxia neonatorum (see page 260).

Leptazol, picrotoxin, strychnine, lobeline : in the writers' opinion these four agents no longer have a place in anaesthetic practice.

Specific narcotic antagonists

Levallorphan tartrate (Lorfan). It is said that this substance will counter the respiratory depression of morphine, without reducing the analgesia. Where it is definitely known that respiratory depression is caused by narcotic intoxication, 1–3 mg of levallorphan may be administered; non-narcotic depression, however, is intensified by levallorphan. 0.25 mg may be given into the umbilical vein in neonatal asphyxia due to narcotic depression and levallorphan may be combined with morphine or pethidine for the relief of intractable pain and for obstetric pain relief. Levallorphan is of no value in countering the effects of barbiturates.

Nalorphine (Lethidrone). When given with morphine or other powerful narcotic analgesics, this will counter any respiratory depression that may occur; 5–10 mg may be given intravenously. If given in the absence of a previous dose of morphine or pethidine, however, it may itself cause respiratory depression.

Both levallorphan and nalorphine may be given to the mother prior to delivery of the baby, if morphine or pethidine have been given as sole agents during delivery. Such administration may counter respiratory depression in the baby.

Naloxone (Narcan) is an opiate antagonist with little or no agonist activity. It may be given in an intravenous dose of 0.4 mg to counter the respiratory depressant effect of morphine or pethidine.

16 *Respiratory Intensive Therapy*

Progressive patient care, in hospital practice, involves the segregation of patients according to the degree of illness into self care, intermediate care and intensive care. One facet of intensive care is respiratory intensive therapy, mainly involving the management of prolonged intermittent positive pressure ventilation (IPPV), the care of tracheostomy and prolonged endotracheal intubation. Patients requiring intensive respiratory therapy usually suffer from acute or incipient respiratory failure. There are two broad groups of respiratory failure.

1. Low output respiratory failure: inadequate ventilation, associated with reduced tidal volume. Caused by drug overdose, myasthenia, poliomyelitis, polyneuritis etc.: characterized by a high carbon dioxide tension and a low oxygen tension.
2. High output respiratory failure: patient unable to breathe fast enough to satisfy oxygen demands; associated with high minute volume. Seen in tetanus, status epilepticus, septicaemia, pancreatitis, fat embolism, etc.: characterized by low or normal carbon dioxide tension and low oxygen tension.

When therapy with artificial ventilation is considered these conditions can be further regrouped into patients:

with normal lungs – tetanus, status epilepticus, myasthenia, etc.

with pathological lungs – pneumonia, fat embolism, asthma, chronic lung disease, post traumatic lung syndrome.

Choice of ventilator

This division into two broad groups is of importance when the choice of ventilation arises. In cases with normal lungs the choice of ventilator for IPPV is not critical, but when dealing with pathological lungs the underlying disease and the characteristics of the ventilator must be taken into consideration. There is no such entity as a universal ventilator for intensive therapy. Even with normal lungs, it must be remembered that there is associated with IPPV, a 50% decrease in compliance, an increase in the ratio of physiological dead space to tidal volume (VD/VT ratio) and sometimes a decrease in cardiac output, with resulting drop in blood pressure. Ventilators can be further classified according to the character of the inspiratory phase, i.e. the wave form.

Flow generators. In these the ventilator determines the pattern of flow in the lungs, the pressure being the result of this flow and the physical characteristics of the patient's lung.

Pressure generators. In these the ventilator determines the pressure pattern and this pressure pattern, acting on the lung fields fixes the flow pattern and volume.

Constant flow generators. Examples include the Blease, Cyclator, Howells ventilator, and Bird (without air entrainment). These ventilators produce a steadily rising alveolar pressure. If the change to the expiratory phase is followed by an abrupt fall of pressure to atmospheric, then a Cournard Type III wave form is produced. This wave form produces the lowest mean intrathoracic pressure compatible with adequate ventilation and, because the intrathoracic pressure is kept to a minimum, there is little interference with venous return and, consequently, no fall in cardiac output, or reduction in blood pressure. This wave form is, therefore, the choice for the shocked state, often associated with cor pulmonale, bronchopneumonia and myocardial infarction. If a subatmospheric or negative phase is applied during the expiratory cycle, there should be no resultant drop in cardiac output, even if venomotor tone is impaired.

(Medical respiratory failure is sometimes associated with cardiovascular collapse. These patients require a central venous pressure line and infusion of 5% dextrose at the same time as IPPV, to maintain a steady cardiovascular state.)

Sine wave flow generators. Examples include the Cape and the Engstrom. The Cape ventilator produces a flow rising to a maximum in the middle of the inspiratory phase and then slowly falling off.

The Engstrom ventilator acts indirectly on the patient's airway, through a 'bag in a bottle'; it produces a small initial flow, with gradual increase, followed by a final plateau, before rapidly falling off to atmospheric pressure. Owing to these characteristics, the tidal volume is distributed in the optimal way to the lung fields. These are ventilators appropriate for asthma and obstructive lung disease.

Constant pressure generators. Barnett, Radcliffe, Bennett, Harlow and Bird (with air entrainment): these constant pressure generators produce an almost square wave form, the length of the plateau depending on the inspiratory time setting. This wave form is valuable in lung collapse, as it pulls the viscous lung surfaces apart and keeps them apart, and also in the crushed chest syndrome for re-expanding the underlying lungs and for splinting fractured ribs.

Cycling mechanism: ventilators also vary according to their cycling mechanism, i.e. the change-over from inspiration to expiration. Pressure cycling ventilators are not suitable for obstructive lung disease, nor for increased airway resistance, as the cycling pressure is reached too soon and ventilation is reduced. Pressure cycling ventilators need frequent adjustment of pressure, if used for obstructive disease.

Volume cycling is advantageous in obstructive disease, as the pressure will vary according to airway resistance: time cycling is a disadvantage in pressure generators, if the compliance is reduced, as, when the time is fixed, the tidal volume drops.

Evidence based on animal experiments would suggest that variation of inspiratory flow wave form, in hypervolaemic, normovolaemic and hypovolaemic animals, does not produce any significant changes in cardiorespiratory function. When commencing IPPV in any patient, care must be taken regarding the cardiovascular side effects of IPPV and active measures taken to minimize them by providing the lowest mean intrapulmonary pressure for the shortest time. An inspiratory/expiratory ration of 1 :2 is advisable, an inspiratory time of 1 second to 1.25 seconds and a reasonably high tidal volume.

It is important to remember that IPPV allows temporary control of the respiration during the acute phase of illness and until the patient is once again able to cope for himself. The original disease is treated by the usual methods, whilst the patient is on IPPV. The treatment of respiratory failure is directed at the maintenance of adequate levels of oxygen in the patient's arterial blood and adequate carbon dioxide elimination whilst the cause of the respiratory failure is being treated.

All ventilators used for intensive respiratory therapy must possess efficient humidifiers on the inspiratory circuit of the ventilator. The ventilator chosen should be the simplest possible that will perform the task required and, above all, must be nurse acceptable; the nurse is with the patient and the ventilator 24 hours of the day and has many other jobs to do as well as observing and understanding the ventilator.

Careful recording is necessary during ventilator treatment and includes the following:

minute volume or tidal volume
respiratory rate
peak airway pressure

These other factors are frequently recorded:

blood pressure. Central venous pressure

pulse rate and ECG monitoring
temperature
cuff deflation: ml of air in cuff and cuff pressure
suction: with comments on quality and quantity. Presence of blood
eye toilet
mouth toilet: cleaning teeth
2 hourly turning, recording side. Physiotherapy
volumes and frequency of gastric aspirate and gastric feeds
volume of bladder drainage
intravenous fluid intake chart

Endotracheal tube or tracheostomy

Patients suffering from respiratory failure and requiring ventilatory support, may need it for hours, days or weeks. In almost all cases an artificial airway will be necessary; in many cases, an artificial airway will become necessary even if intermittent positive pressure ventilation is not immediately indicated. The common choice of an artificial airway lies between an endotracheal tube and a tracheostomy tube.

Endotracheal intubation is indicated, in order to maintain a clear artificial airway in an unconscious patient; to lessen the dead space – emphysema, cor pulmonale etc.; to allow removal of secretions – sputum retention, pneumonia, etc.; to permit IPPV.

The current practice is to commence treatment using an oral, or often a nasal, endotracheal tube. When the duration of therapy is known to be short, e.g. in poisonings, endotracheal intubation is to be preferred, though there is an increasing tendency to leave endotracheal tubes in situ for longer periods and ten to twelve days' intubation is now common. When prolonged endotracheal intubation is planned, careful atraumatic insertion of the tube is necessary; a local anaesthetic and diazepam sedation may be used for this purpose. In order to minimize any tendency to local irritation, a plastic or 'neoprene' tube should be employed in preference to the red rubber variety. The tube should be changed at regular intervals of two or three days and an opportunity at that time taken to make a visual inspection of the glottis. Any gross tendency to local laryngeal trauma is a direct indication to convert to a tracheostomy. Great care must be taken to ensure that the endotracheal tube is not placed in the right main bronchus, thus causing complete left lung underventilation and collapse. A misplaced tube can also occlude the right upper lobe bronchus, but careful auscultation of the chest areas after insertion of the tube will allow this complication to be immediately recognized. When the patient is turned during treatment, the endotracheal tube may ride into the right main bronchus, so the habit of auscultating the left lung after each patient turn must be encouraged. All other complications, such as kinking, over-inflation of the cuff, etc. must be actively avoided. If an oral endotracheal tube is used, it is current practice to place a London Hospital pattern mouth prop around the endotracheal tube before insertion, to protect the tube from being bitten through by the patient.

Advantages of endotracheal intubation over tracheostomy are the decreased local morbidity, the lack of a skin scar and easy removal of the tube. Disadvantages are discomfort for the patient, interference with swallowing, local laryngeal trauma (oedema, granulations, ulceration, abrasions, fibromata) the development of subglottic oedema, subglottic slough formation, ulceration and subglottic stenosis. Choanal ulceration and stenosis have occurred following prolonged nasal intubation.

When the time comes for extubation, great care must be taken as, during the first few hours following it, hoarseness, loss of voice and inco-ordinate action with inability to protect the larynx from saliva or swallowed liquids may occur; harsh breathing, developing into full respiratory stridor, may follow. Constant humidification and inhalations are necessary over this period and topical steroid insufflations may help control the resulting tendency to oedema. Increasing or persistent stridor are direct indications for immediate laryngoscopy and re-inspection of the glottis: increasing laryngeal oedema, subglottic oedema, or subglottic slough formation at this stage are indications for tracheostomy.

Insufficient humidification over the immediate post-extubation period may lead to cumulative drying of secretions over subglottic abrasions, leading to incipient laryngeal occlusion over 24 to 48 hours. Any increase in respiratory rate over this period should be treated with suspicion. Serial recordings of $FEV_{1.0}$ can be a diagnostic aid, as any tendency to glottic or airway occlusion would lead to a gradual deterioration in $FEV_{1.0}$, remembering that almost complete subglottic occlusion may occur before there is any audible inspiratory stridor. The commonest cause of subglottic oedema is the use of too large an endotracheal tube.

Although complications of prolonged endotracheal intubation do occasionally occur, strict attention to correct management enables endotracheal intubation to be continued for periods up to 11 or 12 days without undue complication. Personal experience has shown the incidence of subglottic slough formation with laryngeal obstruction to be 0.04%.

Tracheostomy is indicated in order to maintain a clear airway, or decrease the dead space (this alone is seldom an indication today); to bypass a blocked larynx; and to deal with certain cases known to require prolonged IPPV – crushed chest, tetanus, polyneuritis, etc.

Tracheostomies have a higher morbidity rate than endotracheal intubation. There is more tendency to infection of both the wound and the tracheostome; there is always a permanent scar; there may be tracheal dilatation, tracheomalacia, erosion into the great vessels or oesophagus. Surgical emphysema occurs and may be extensive.

A tracheostomy tube should not be removed for at least four days, to allow adequate sealing of the wound edges. The wound will take a further four or five days after this to heal completely, i.e. there is a potential of at least 9 days morbidity, which would be excessive in a case that only needed 48 hours' artificial airway. Tracheal stenosis may occur at the level of the stoma, at the level of the inflated cuff, or at the level of the tip of the tracheostomy tube. Tracheal stenosis has been reported following the use of both endotracheal tubes and tracheostomy tubes.

Management of tubes and tracheostomies

A note must always be made on the patient's chart of the time of insertion of tube, the type and the size; these details should be charted each time the tube is changed.

Securing tapes: the method of securing the tube varies with the variety used. Endotracheal tubes are best secured with tapes within plastic tube protective sleeves. The James and Portex plastic tracheostomy tubes have flanges, to which tape can be attached: the Oxford tracheostomy tube has no flange, and the tape has therefore to be attached around the firm expanded end of the tube. All these tapes are secured at the side of the patient's neck by a bow and should be changed regularly, as dirty tapes lead to infection and are uncomfortable to the patient, especially when wet. A tracheostomy tube must be tied in firmly and checked frequently. If the tapes are allowed to become slack, the tube may become displaced, especially if heavy ventilator tubing is attached to it. This may prove catastrophic to the patient, as during the first few hours in particular it may not be easy to replace. If the tube does come out, dilators should be inserted into the trachea to facilitate replacement.

Care of the tracheostomy wound

(1) In the first few days the skin edges are cleaned with chlorhexidine (Hibitane) and a Nusan dressing applied, which is covered by sterile gauze.

(2) 'Polybactrin' spray is used – which not only helps to prevent infection but is also soothing and cool for the patient.

(3) 'Hibitane' or Eusol dressings, dipped in solution and squeezed dry, are soothing to the patient especially after suction.

(4) After the fifth day, Nystatin powder may be indicated to prevent monilia infection.

(5) After the tenth day – a local application of carbenicillin can be used to prevent pyocyaneus infection.

(6) After the wound is fully healed, dry dressings or Hibitane dressings should be used.

Infection of the wound leads to infection of the trachea and, in turn, to chest infection, which can become serious. All tracheostomies should have swabs taken from the wound and the tube on the first day, for culture and sensitivity, and thereafter on each third day. If infection occurs, daily swabs are taken.

Suction to tracheostomy or endotracheal tube: a tracheostomy is an open surgical wound and therefore, sterile treatment is essential in the active prevention of infection; sterile disposable suction catheters should be used.

Aspiration of the trachea should be carried on the following occasions:

to remove secretions as necessary
before the cuff is released; (the pharynx should also be aspirated before release of the cuff)
if the tidal volume drops, or ventilation pressure rises
before and after altering the patient's position
if sputum is required for culture (a sterile sputum trap should be used for this purpose)
in association with physiotherapy, and accompanying manual inflation of the lungs using a reservoir bag

Technique of suction

(1) Wash hands and wear a disposable sterile glove on the hand holding the suction catheter or, alternatively, use the full 'no touch' technique, with disposable or sterile forceps.

(2) Never use a suction catheter that is too thick, i.e. it should be not more than half the internal diameter of the tube. If the diameter of the suction catheter exceeds half the diameter, a temporary vacuum may be created inside the lungs which will certainly be uncomfortable for the patient and may cause lung collapse, promote pulmonary oedema or even cause cardiac arrest.

(3) A 'T' or 'Y' connection should be used, the thumb occluding the 'T' or 'Y' piece only during rotation and removal of the catheter, so that the active suction is applied only during withdrawal.

(4) The catheter should only be inserted once, rotated to and fro, removed and then discarded.

(5) Suction is unpleasant to the patient and should not be prolonged; the whole operation must be completed in the time that the nurse can hold her own breath, if the patient is paralysed. The patient's colour should be watched and not allowed to become cyanosed during suction. The patient should be ventilated for a few breaths

before reintroducing a catheter. Prolonged suction may cause reflex bradycardia.

(6) It is important when aspirating, that the suction catheter is introduced beyond the end of the tracheostomy tube; more than 6in.–7in. must be inserted and 9in.–12in. through an endotracheal tube.

(7) If the patient can cough, then encourage coughing to raise the secretions to carinal level before suction commences, especially during physiotherapy.

(8) It is easy to aspirate the right bronchus with a straight suction catheter, but the left bronchus is not so easily accessible, as it is at an angle to the trachea. Consequently suction should be associated with physiotherapy, with the patient lying on the right side. Alternatively a coudé tipped catheter may be introduced into the left main bronchus.

(9) Stethoscope – you can listen with a stethoscope to ascertain (a) which side you are aspirating, and (b) whether you have cleared secretions, or improved air entry over various parts of the lung. Simple physiotherapy can be applied by nursing staff.

Inflation of cuffed tracheostomy tube or endotracheal tube: there are two reasons for inflating cuffs: (1) To facilitate IPPV by avoiding leaks. (2) To prevent soiling of the lower respiratory tract in patients who cannot swallow (from disease or paralysis by drugs). The amount of air that is put into the cuff should be just enough to inflate the cuff to an extent that prevents leaks, i.e. the minimum amount of air should be used. By listening to the leak in a patient being ventilated, or asking a spontaneously breathing patient to speak, the correct amount may be ascertained. Any forceps used for clamping inflating tubes should have rubber covers over the jaws.

It is important that the amount of air needed to reinflate the cuff be charted each time, so that a tendency to tracheal dilatation, or the presencc of oesophageal fistula, may be suspected; both complications are suggested by an increasing amount of air being necessary over a period of time. Over-inflation of the cuff will encourage these complications as well as being uncomfortable for the patient, so a cuff which is inflated should be released intermittently to allow circulation to recur in the tracheal mucosa, which may otherwise undergo ischaemic necrosis. In the average case, five minutes release every two hours is adequate, but in cases that cannot swallow or are hypotensive this may be modified to five minutes deflation every hour. If the patient cannot swallow adequately, it is important also to use a head-down tilt and to perform pharyngeal suction before releasing the cuff, to prevent soiling the trachea with saliva, etc. To obviate these difficulties some workers use a double cuffed tracheostomy tube, a tube having two cuffs, which are inflated and released alternatively.

The cuffs of tracheostomy tubes and endotracheal tubes can be deflated and reinflated at much less frequent intervals, e.g. every 12 hours, or 24 hours. If this latter practice is adopted, 'cuff inflation pressure' should be measured, recorded, and not allowed to exceed the prevailing systolic blood pressure in millimetres of mercury.

Changing tracheostomy tubes: once a 'track' has been established, i.e. after three or four days, changing a tracheostomy tube is a simple procedure and does not normally necessitate the introduction of tracheal dilating forceps. Under normal circumstances a tube should not be changed before the 7th day, but indications for changing the tube before this are : (1) Crusting of lumen by secretions, blood clot, etc. (2) Obstruction of the lumen by foreign debris. (3) Burst cuff. Endotracheal tubes should be changed every third day.

Dysphagia : if there is difficulty in swallowing, this must be overcome before a tracheostomy can be closed. Tests for the ability to swallow include the following : (1) Give the patient fluid to drink, with cuff deflated, and listen with stethoscope on chest; it can be heard to go down the oesophagus, or if it pools in the throat, to gurgle. (2) Give the patient coloured fluid to drink then aspirate the trachea; the tracheal secretions will be 'stained' if there is dysphagia and tracheal soiling.

Closure of a tracheostome can follow removal of the tube, or can be encouraged gradually by inserting tubes of a smaller size over a few days. In some instances tracheostomy tubes may be occluded, allowing patients to breathe around them.

Remove the tube, clean with Hibitane, apply suction, clean with Hibitane, apply dressing of vaseline gauze or Nusan over tracheostome, then plain gauze, and seal using a Sleek strapping, making it as airtight as possible. Change the dressing daily, re-seal and continue with dressings until the tracheostome allows no air leak on coughing. If not closed at the end of 7–8 days, then plastic surgery should be considered.

The commonest complication of a tracheostomy is infection : the commonest infective organisms are *staphylococcus albus, B. coli, B. pyocyaneus* and *monilia.* The commonest sources of infection are from hands, urine and faeces. In order to reduce the incidence of infection strict attention to sterility should be paid when handling the tracheostome.

A tracheostomy tube is painful and uncomfortable and this discomfort is exaggerated if the ventilator tubes are allowed to pull on tracheostomy tubes. It is of vital importance to the comfort of the patient that the tracheostomy tube be allowed to sit neatly and comfortably in the neck (like a man's necktie). Flexible endotracheal mount connections and swivel mounts allow greater comfort to the patient.

A patient with a tracheostomy or endotracheal tube cannot speak and therefore feels a lack of communication. The patient should be encouraged to communicate by writing on paper, a pen and paper should be at hand and tolerance shown while he writes his wishes down: patient-request indicator charts are very helpful. Time should be taken to reassure and explain to the patients anything they may want to know.

Complications of tracheostomy and endotracheal tubes

crusting, with resultant infection – pneumonia ,abscess, etc.
obstruction of lumen and consequent asphyxia; this may be due to over-inflation of the cuff, blood clot, secretions, etc.
tracheal ulceration and ischaemic necrosis – also due to over-inflation of the cuff, or excessive movement of the tube
ulceration leading to tracheo-oesophageal fistula – again due to over-inflation of the cuff, especially when associated with infection
tracheal dilatation and erosion of major arterial vessels
tracheomalacia and collapse of trachea on extubation
tracheal stenosis

Humidification. When the normal humidifying apparatus, the nose, is bypassed, either by an endotracheal tube or tracheostomy, the inspired air must be artificially humidified. If this is omitted secretions dry, crusts form on mucosa, and ciliary action is depressed and may even be completely obliterated. The removal of secretions from the bronchial tract, either by coughing or suction, is an essential part of any respiratory therapy. Loose secretions are easier to cough up, or remove by suction, and the easiest way to reduce the viscosity of a liquid is to dilute it by water. Well timed humidification can prevent total respiratory failure from viscid sputum retention.

As ill patients do not drink adequate fluids, they may become dehydrated, especially if on diuretics and consequently produce viscid sputum which is difficult to remove. The starvation usually associated with severe illness weakens them further, making their cough mechanism less effective. 'Local humidification' helps loosen secretions, making sometimes even a weak cough capable of removing them from the bronchial tract. 'Superhumidification' may be necessary to liquefy secretions – i.e. the water content of the inspired air being higher than that present when fully saturated for that temperature. The particle size of the mist produced is also important, i.e. the smaller the particle size the further along the bronchial tract will it travel in suspension. Over vigorous therapy with superhumidification may 'drown' the patient and therefore caution should be observed.

Hot water humidifiers: cannot produce this super humidity and must be reinforced by frequent instillation of sterile normal saline, or by the use of mucolytic agents.

Cold air nebulizers: produce efficient super-saturated mist and disperse it through the bronchial tract.

Ultrasonic nebulizers: are very efficient and can produce more than 44 g water, per cubic metre in a small particle mist.

'Artificial nose': the condenser humidifier acts by reducing water loss from the tracheobronchial tree .

Humidifiers can be attached to tracheostomies or endotracheal tubes via 'cages' or a T-piece, or be so placed as to blow humidified air towards them. Plastic attachments should be changed frequently and washed in Hibitane solution, otherwise they become a great source of infection. In some cases humidifiers are not used and, as an alternative, sterile normal saline is instilled directly into the trachea, after each aspiration. The dose commonly used is 2–10 ml every hour.

Position of patients

Patients are turned frequently to avoid pressure sores, and to prevent secretions from accumulating in any one part of the lung, with resultant hypostatic infection.

Unconscious patients are nursed in lateral positions and are turned from side to side every two hours, day and night. The lateral position is maintained by supporting pillows, the limbs being maintained in a natural position to avoid joint strain and the lower leg drawn up slightly to prevent pressure from the upper leg. Unconscious or paralysed patients cannot complain, so make sure that the ears are not folded back under the head or the arms squashed under the patient.

When turning the patient, disconnect him from the ventilator or humidifier, aspirate the trachea and pharynx and turn the patient on to his back. Reconnect the ventilator for two minutes. Aspirate, then disconnect again, turn the patient onto the opposite side, once again aspirate and reconnect to the ventilator. Physiotherapy may be associated with turning. Speed is essential, because a paralysed patient cannot breathe when not connected to the ventilator : work within the time you can hold your breath.

Treatment of pressure areas. Provided the patient is kept clean and dry, turning every two hours is enough to prevent the development of pressure sores. Occasionally the condition of the patient demands that he be nursed supine, or in the sitting position. 'Ripple' beds are of assistance in preventing pressure sores in patients nursed in the supine position and nursing on sheepskins is also valuable. In the sitting position the patient is inclined from side to side every two hours to lessen the pressure on each buttock in turn. Pressure areas are treated with silicone barrier cream. Patients who suffer from diarrhoea may find the application of arachis oil to the skin quite soothing. Frequent washing of these skin areas, with soft soap, followed by a soothing cream, will prevent deterioration of the skin surface. Patients who are on ventilators can have bed baths. Zinc or castor oil cream can be applied over bony prominences or reddened areas to keep the skin supple: bed accessories such as foam cushions, foam heel pads, and leg cradles are also useful.

Physiotherapy. Chest physiotherapy is an essential part of respiratory intensive care and is needed frequently and regularly, ideally at least four times per day. It should coincide with turning the patient as it encourages the movement of secretions from the peripheral lung areas into the more accessible parts of the bronchial tract, from whence they can be removed by suction. Chest percussion, vibration, clapping, postural draining, simulated coughing and lower chest cage compression are all necessary.

Manual ventilation is a technique used by doctor and physiotherapist to simulate a cough mechanism. A maximal inflation, by squeezing a reservoir bag of at least 4 litres capacity, is performed, in order to fully inflate all alveoli and encourage air to get behind the contained secretions; then the pressure on the manual inflating bag is released to coincide with maximal lower chest cage compression by the physiotherapist, with the resultant effect that a cough is simulated and secretions are projected into the main bronchi. The procedure is repeated, as necessary, after placing the patient for maximal postural drainage for the main affected lung areas. The procedure may cause a Valsalva effect in the patient and should be avoided, or undertaken with extreme caution, in patients with unstable cardiovascular function. Vigorous chest physiotherapy has been shown to be responsible for marked decrease in cardiac output.

Physiotherapy to limbs by passive movement must be carried out while any patient is on IPPV as venous thrombosis of the lower limbs is a hazard. Active measures must be taken to prevent this and its associated embolic pulmonary complications. Nurses and doctors should observe and learn simple physiotherapy, i.e. chest vibration and percussion, so that treatment can be given at any time during the night or day, when physiotherapists may not be readily available. In cases where chest physiotherapy may be considered painful, analgesia can be provided during treatment by using Entonox (50% nitrous oxide, 50% oxygen) inhalations, or alternatively trichloroethylene or methoxyflurane inhalations in air or oxygen.

Care of eyes. Unconscious or paralyzed patients cannot blink, therefore the cornea dries: if this is untreated, corneal ulceration progressing to blindness may result. Eyes should be irrigated with normal sterile saline to remove any crusts or discharge, and then one drop of 1% methylcellulose, sterile liquid paraffin or alternatively, antibiotic ointment is placed in the conjunctival sac. This is repeated four hourly. If the eyes are not closed, then the upper lid must be gently held down with strapping, or both the eyes covered with vaseline gauze. In extreme cases more drastic measures such as lid suture may be necessary.

Mouth. A thorough oral toilet is essential, even though it may be difficult if an endotracheal tube is in place. Four hourly oral toilet and cleaning of the teeth should be carried out with glycerine or glycothymol solution. It is often necessary to moisten the lips with glycerine or vaseline to prevent cracks and sores.

Bowels. In a short term patient no treatment is required. However, in a long term patient, suppositories or enemas may be necessary. A low residue diet may be of value.

Nutrition. (Peaston, 1968; Jones *et al.*, 1966). By the very nature of their condition it is unlikely that certain patients will be able to swallow, so nutrition must be given either by means of a stomach tube or by intravenous drip. All patients receiving prolonged IPPV, suffer from weight loss, which may be due to a combination of four factors; immobilization, infection, stress and reduction of input. In addition to this weight loss patients suffer from sodium retention and, despite all efforts, they may develop a negative nitrogen balance.

The sodium retention, associated with IPPV, usually commences within the first few days of the therapy and can precipitate pulmonary oedema. This is readily reversed by diuretic therapy, e.g. frusemide, which causes a rapid natriuresis and reduction in pulmonary oedema, even though the physiological mechanisms by which IPPV causes sodium retention and pulmonary oedema are not known. (Gett *et al.*, 1971). Alimentation through an intragastric tube is clearly the ideal method of administering nourishment. However, there are very real dangers of regurgitation of stomach contents and aspiration of this acid material, despite the presence of an inflated cuff on the tracheostomy tube. If the patient is breathing against the ventilator, dilatation of the trachea can occur and this allows the passage of material down between the cuff and the tracheal wall. Particular care should therefore be taken to nurse patients receiving enteral therapy in the upright position and the pharynx should also be frequently aspirated.

Patients receiving IPPV have a high energy requirement and many types of fluid diets have been devised to meet their needs. A useful diet which, given at the rate of 3 1/day or 125 ml/h, provides 2.580 calories is shown in Table 16.1 : but because of its constituents, also shown in the table, and hypertonicity, diarrhoea may occur though only in about 5% of cases.

Table 16.1 *A fluid diet for patients receiving IPPV*

Mixture	*Quantity*
Complan	100 g
glucose	100 g
methyl cellulose	3 g
water	1 l
Constituents	*Quantity*
protein	93 g
carbohydrate	432 g
fat	48 g
calories	2580
nitrogen	14 g
sodium	64 mEq
potassium	84 mEq
chloride	63 mEq
calcium	123 mEq
magnesium	31 mEq
phosphate	76 mEq

The sodium constituent can be cut down to 20–30 mEq/day but the potassium must not be allowed to fall below 50 mEq. Some authorities use Prosparol lg/kg with milk (70 g/2.51). This fluid diet, and its constituents, are shown in Table 16.2; it provides 2017 calories.

However a proportion of the population, varying from 35% (McMichael *et al.*, 1965) to 55% (Cuatrecasas *et al.*, 1965), are unable to metabolize lactose, the reason for this being a deficiency of jejunal B galactosidase from prolonged milk or lactose deprivation. Liquidized normal ward diet can be used for intragastric feeding, to complement or replace Complan diet, aiming to provide 40 cal/kg body weight per day. In certain cases, such as hypercatabolic illnesses, the daily intake may need to be increased to 60 cal/kg body weight to maintain positive nitrogen balance.

Carnation Instant Breakfast is one ready way of increasing the calorie intake; alcohol is another and may even be given intravenously.

More recent additions in this field are Caloreen and Gastrocaloreen. Caloreen is a glucose-polymer mixture, virtually electrolyte free, palatable, much less sweet than glucose and can be added to any other food preparation; it provides 4 cal/g and patients will easily tolerate 250–

Table 16.2 *Fluid diet for patients receiving IPPV: Prosparol with milk*

Constituents	*Quantity*
cow's whole milk	2 l
Prosparol	50 ml
glucose	100 g
sodium chloride	3 g
water	500 ml
This mixture contains	
carbohydrate	200 g (40%)
fat	105 g
protein	68 g (13%)
(nitrogen)	(10·9 g)
sodium	100 mEq
potassium	82 mEq
total volume	2550 ml
Total calories	2017
Total water	2265 ml

500 g per day, without diarrhoea. Gastrocaloreen is essentially similar, but contains sodium and potassium in small quantity. Another oral preparation suitable for intragastric feeding is Trisorbin: this is a well balanced, complete nutritional supplement providing 500 kcal, and 3 g nitrogen per 100 g, the protein content being a mixture of egg albumin and milk protein. It should be completely absorbed in the gut and leave no residue, reducing the tendency to any osmotic diarrhoea.

However, it must not be forgotten that simple egg, milk, alcohol and added sugar is very rich in protein and calories and is easily prepared and administered.

Many patients develop a pseudo-ileus when first placed on IPPV, especially if muscle relaxants or narcotic sedatives are used for control. Gastric feeding must therefore cautiously be introduced over the first 48 hours, commencing with 30 ml water hourly, and increasing in quantity and quality of food, according to the pattern of the four hourly gastric aspirate. Until intragastric feeding is established, the intravenous route of feeding remains the method of choice.

If the intravenous route is to be employed a combination of :

aminosol–fructose–ethanol	1500 ml	(1310 cal)
intralipid 20%	1000 ml	(2000 cal)
aminosol 10%	500 ml	(165 cal)

provides 3 l of water per day, 225 g of carbohydrate, 200 g of fat, and 3475 cal. These substitutes may occasionally cause allergy and, in order to cut down the high incidence of venous thrombosis, the peripheral veins should not be used but the liquid given through a central venous catheter instead. It is important that vitamins are added to the enteral or parenteral diet. Intravenous 30% sorbitol, which provides 4 cal/g, is broken down to fructose in the liver and further metabolized to glucose. Sorbitol is of value in getting adequate input of carbohydrate; 10% (410 cal/1) or 20% (820 cal/1). Frucotose may also be used to provide carbohydrate. Optimal utilization by mouth follows if the main constituents are given in the ratio 50–55% carbohydrate, 35% fat, and 10–15% protein. At least 200 cal should be provided for every gram of nitrogen.

Despite the provision of adequate calories to these patients, it is still extremely difficult to avoid negative nitrogen balance and more work requires to be carried out into means of artificial nutrition in patients receiving IPPV. Gamma-hydroxy-butyric acid has been employed in an effort to overcome this negative nitrogen balance and it is worthy of further study.

The problem of cross infection

(Robinson, 1966; Gibson, 1967; Harris *et al.*, 1969). Patients needing IPPV are prone to cross infection, as their tissues are very susceptible to invading organisms; such patients are commonly in a state of low resistance to disease.

It is preferable for the patient to be isolated, either in a single room, or by provision of adequate space, 300 square feet of floor space per patient. As the patient's urine, skin and faeces are sources of infection, the urine should be collected by closed, sterile drainage, and the skin should be frequently cleaned.

Other patients: isolation and segregation will prevent this route. Nurse assignation to each individual patient is necessary, with no transfer of nurses, staff, or equipment, between patients. Barrier nursing can be employed and air conditioning and bacterial air infiltration is advisable.

The elimination of infective sources among staff and visitors is carried out by routine throat and nose swabs and by the wearing of masks, gowns and overshoes.

Floors, walls and shelves should be cleaned thoroughly; the furniture should be minimal and washable, and the cotton sheets regularly changed. Frequent air changes and ventilation are important.

As much disposable presterilized equipment should be used as is practical and possible; if not disposable then it should be capable of being sterilized easily, preferably autoclaving. Anaesthetic masks, metal suction catheters, suction jars and suction tubing should be autoclaved, at least daily whilst in use.

Humidifiers should be chemically sterilized in or out of use, with

Hibitane solution, changed daily. Humidifier tubing should be autoclaved; the ventilator tubing should also be autoclaved daily and stored in sterile drums when not in use. Plastic tracheostomy attachments should be chemically cleaned with Hibitane. Sink drainage sumps, a common source of *B. pyocyaneus,* should be cleaned with Lysol and ventilators should be sterilized frequently. Preferably only ventilators with removable autoclavable patient inserts should be used.

All procedures concerning the patient should be treated as highly sterile and, throughout this period on IPPV, methods should be orientated towards the active prevention of infection or cross infection. Respiratory intensive therapy is a highly complicated technique, where scrupulous attention to detail is essential if management is to be successful and complications are to be avoided.

Ethical problems. The increasing use of intensive therapy units in the modern hospital, has placed the clinician in charge in the unenviable position of having to face decisions previously inconceivable. Modern advances have made us very adept at keeping human beings physically alive in biological circumstances that would have proved inevitably fatal not so long ago. The question of whom and when to resuscitate presents itself, together with the related questions – having started should one ever stop and if so, when? Further, should a lung ventilator be switched off in a case with irretrievable brain damage?

The decision to undertake treatment by IPPV should never be undertaken lightly, and then only in the belief that the patient will benefit and fully recover. There are mistaken decisions regrettably, and occasional patients will become machine dependent, without hope of recovery. Medicine is in danger of becoming officious in its efforts at all costs to prolong life. There should in future be some serious consideration of the selection of cases to undergo intensive therapy, and an attempt made to limit the effort to those patients who will benefit maximally.

Post-operative respiratory problems

Patients who fail to breathe adequately following anaesthesia may have the following characteristics:

1. Primary carbon dioxide retention produced by lung pathology or inadequate ventilation during anaesthesia.
2. Central nervous system depression, often associated with hypotension and hypoventilation.
3. Abnormal reaction to muscle relaxants, (latent myasthenia, suxamethonium apnoea).
4. Paralysis associated with antibiotic therapy.
5. Chest injuries.

In all these instances, the correct treatment is intermittent positive pressure ventilation until the problem is resolved; in the case of antibiotics, the response to intravenous calcium salts is often dramatic. Associated metabolic acidosis and hypokalaemia must be corrected.

Acute chest infections

These are usually cases of fulminating bronchopneumonia. The picture is of respiratory failure in toxic, often 'medically shocked' patients with acute sputum retention: the common associated conditions are prerenal uraemia (as a result of dehydration, due to low fluid intake with heavy insensible loss from hypermetabolism and pyrexia) and metabolic acidosis due to starvation.

The immediate treatment is to oxygenate the patient and aspirate the retained secretions via endotracheal intubation or bronchoscopy. Once secretions are removed, oxygen should be administered if necessary by intermittent positive pressure ventilation, a central venous pressure line is advisable, and the infusion of 5% dextrose or Hartmann's solution should be given to achieve a positive central venous pressure. Adequate pain relief is essential. Humidification of inspired gases, adequate fluid and calorie intake are also essential in the management of these cases. Bronchial lavage, using repeated (10–12 ml) quantities of sterile saline, immediately re-aspirated, is useful for the initial removal of thick viscid sputum.

Patients should be gradually 'weaned off' intermittent positive pressure ventilation and oxygen therapy. When the collapse of any lobe is present, re-expansion by the use of a 'square wave form' ventilator for intermittent positive pressure ventilation is recommended: bronchoscopy with suction alone is usually not sufficient. Suitable antibiotic therapy must be given intravenously if necessary.

'Acute on chronic' chest disease

Acute exacerbations occur in patients with existing chronic chest disease, usually emphysema, chronic bronchitis or cor pulmonale. These patients usually have chronic respiratory inadequacy, which is precipitated into sub-acute respiratory failure by an infective episode.

Respiratory failure is considered to be present in these patients when the arterial oxygen tension falls below 50 mmHg, or the arterial carbon dioxide tension rises above 50 mmHg. Acute exacerbations alter the values even further. The essential in treatment is to maintain adequate oxygenation to support life, but often unless oxygen therapy is rigidly controlled, this itself may endanger the patient by causing increasing hypercarbia, leading to carbon dioxide narcosis.

It must be remembered that an arterial oxygen tension below 30 mmHg, can cause irreversible cerebral damage unless corrected within minutes. Such severe degrees of hypoxia must thus be avoided, the aim in this type of patient being to achieve the highest arterial oxygen tension possible, without causing excessive rise in the arterial carbon doxide tension. If it is impossible to achieve a reasonable arterial oxygen tension without hypercarbia, intensive respiratory therapy and intermittent positive pressure ventilation should be considered.

Patients with hypoxic lung disease are treated medically with controlled oxygen therapy (24%–35% oxygen) and sometimes respiratory stimulant drugs. If, during this therapy, the arterial carbon dioxide tension continues to rise over a period of hours, or a higher oxygen percentage in the inspired air is indicated by an arterial oxygen tension below 40 mmHg, intermittent positive pressure ventilation is indicated (Finnegan and Jones, 1969). Alveolar ventilation and perfusion can be improved by removal of secretions from the bronchial tract.

Patients presenting with 'acute on chronic' chest infections have a tendency to dehydration and prerenal uraemia. This is often aggravated by a low oral fluid intake in a critically ill patient, who may be on diuretics for cor pulmonale. Dehydration produces viscid thick sputum which is difficult to remove : an absent or low calorie intake will lead to starvation, weakness and metabolic acidosis and, with the respiratory acidosis present, this produces the blood gas picture of a mixed lesion. Metabolic acidosis must be corrected by infusion of sodium bicarbonate or THAM. Removal of secretions is a prime aspect of treatment, accomplished by intensive humidification and physiotherapy.

Treatment by IPPV

If physiotherapy and humidification are not effective in clearing the chest of secretions, then endotracheal intubation, bronchoscopy, or mild bronchial lavage (with sterile saline or 1% bicarbonate) and mechanical removal of secretions by suction, is indicated. This may necessitate intermittent positive pressure ventilation for a period of 12 to 24 hours during which intensive physiotherapy, endotracheal toilet, lavage and suction are continued. The patient is sedated, if necessary, with chlordiazepoxide, phenoperidine, or droperidol; occasionally pancuronium is indicated. A central venous pressure line is introduced and the central venous pressure maintained at + 5 cmH_2O, by infusion of 5% dextrose or Hartmann's solution, and continuous ECG monitoring is instituted. A nasogastric tube is passed and either intragastric alimentation or parenteral feeding commenced. After 24–48 hours the patient is weaned off intermittent positive pressure ventilation with careful control and monitoring of blood gases. It is not uncommon to have periods of 'rest' on IPPV, a common regime being spontaneous ventilation by day, and a rest on IPPV overnight, the period of rest being diminished as rapidly as the patient can tolerate.

All patients are nursed with endotracheal tubes, as tracheostomies are actively avoided in this type of case; oro- or naso-endotracheal tubes are well tolerated, especially if the patient is sedated with a small background dose of chlordiazepoxide. Although some subjects manage to eat and drink quite normally with endotracheal tubes *in situ*, the tube is removed as soon as is practical (as indicated by the blood gas analysis, the return of an effective cough, and the ability to clear the respiratory tract of secretions). Antibiotic treatment is determined as a result of bacteriological sensitivity tests.

The essence of management is to try to wean the patient off IPPV after 24 hours or less. Attention to nutrition is very important, as a weak patient has neither the strength nor the inclination to breathe, and the cough reflex is not strong enough to remove secretions. During this weaning off period, frequent estimations of arterial blood gases are necessary to estimate progress. Oxygen therapy must be continued, as must physiotherapy, endotracheal suction and intense humidification. Useful guide lines can be achieved by frequent recording of tidal volume, respiratory rate and minute volume, at half hourly intervals, using a Wright respirometer. Cessation of IPPV is followed by a gradual reduction of oxygen therapy and patients must be observed and monitored closely during this critical phase.

The type of ventilator used for these patients should be capable of high inflation pressures and low inspiratory flow rates, in order to cope with the high airway resistance and low dynamic compliance. Recommended ventilators are the Cape and Engstrom. A rate below 20 respirations per minute should be chosen, to give a minute volume of 10–12 litres: an inspiratory-expiratory ratio of 1:2 is acceptable. Respiratory stimulant drugs such as nikethamide, amiphenazole, daranide and prethcamide are useful in the latter stages, as is the temporary use of a patient trigger ventilator, such as the Bird.

Mucolytic drugs have been used, but it is debatable whether these have any great advantage over the intensive humidification and bronchial lavage. If bronchospasm is a feature of the acute disease, bronchodilator drugs are indicated. Endotracheal lignocaine is useful, as is the continuous intravenous infusion of aminophylline, or etophyllate. Local insufflation of isoetherine, orciprenaline and hydrocortisone has also been carried out in some cases. The treatment must be directed at the control and cure of the precipitating infection.

A certain proportion of chronic respiratory failure patients will be impossible to wean off IPPV. These are severe respiratory cripples with poor respiratory reserve, the likelihood of continued reliance on the ventilator being dependent on the respiratory reserve power. IPPV is not curative – at best one can end up with the lungs slightly less adequate than before the episode. It is debatable whether IPPV treatment should be commenced in the severe respiratory cripple with no respiratory reserves in terminal respiratory failure, unless facilities exist for long term IPPV, or even a 'home on ventilator' programme is considered, along with permanent tracheostomy.

Ideally, an assessment of the patient's respiratory function prior to the acute infective episode should be available, so that an estimate of the potential outcome can be made. Nevertheless, it should be remembered that for these patients 'normal' blood gas levels may be quite bizarre, and a compromise made when an arterial oxygen tension of 60–80 mmHg, or a carbon dioxide tension of 50–60 mmHg is reached during treatment. It may be utterly impossible to improve on these results, and the patient may well be accustomed to life at these levels.

Status asthmaticus

Status asthmaticus is defined as persistent bronchospasm that does not respond to medical treatment. Patients develop progressive hypoxia, due to viscid 'plug' and sputum retention. Respiratory acidosis and occasionally metabolic acidosis occur, leading to myocardial depression and peripheral circulatory failure, the patient eventually dying from exhaustion and respiratory failure. The condition is a serious medical emergency.

In asthma, there is hypoxaemia during paroxysms, which is not due to alveolar hypoventilation but to uneven ventilation/perfusion ratios. When status asthmaticus supervenes, a rising arterial carbon dioxide tension is superimposed as a result of hypoventilation and the hypoxaemia is markedly increased; the secretions are viscid, dry and difficult to remove and the patients also, are dehydrated.

Cyanosis is invariably present when arterial oxygen saturation is below 85% and is usually associated with restlessness. Oxygen must be administered, but uncontrolled oxygen therapy may aggravate respiratory acidosis and cause carbon dioxide narcosis: should hypoxia continue, despite controlled oxygen therapy, IPPV must be undertaken. Respiratory control must be achieved by anaesthesia following pre-oxygenation, and propanidid and suxamethonium are recommended for this, the lungs being oxygenated by manual pressure on a reservoir bag. High pressure may be necessary to overcome airway resistance and both the inspiratory and expiratory phase may need to be prolonged. Ether or halothane may be added in an attempt to break the bronchospasm, and if neuromuscular blockade becomes necessary, then pancuronium or alcuronium should be used. (Tubocurarine should be avoided, because of its tendency to release histamine.) At this stage bronchial lavage should be considered as, by removing bronchial debris, it helps to correct any ventilation/perfusion imbalance. Early attention to direct humidification, using an ultrasonic nebulizer, combined with medical treatment, oxygen therapy and careful physiotherapy, will prevent the occurrence of status asthmaticus in a large proportion of cases.

Following bronchial lavage, IPPV may be necessary and neuromuscular blockade will be needed to maintain control. Sodium bicarbonate or THAM should be given for any metabolic acidosis present, a central venous pressure line inserted and 5% dextrose infused intravenously to reconstitute a positive central venous pressure, if this is low. Intravenous aminophylline and hydrocortisone may be required and intrabronchial isoprenaline or isoetherine given with caution.

When considering IPPV for status asthmaticus the choice of ventilator is important. Flow generators which are volume cycled, such as the Cape, or an accelerated flow generator such as the Engstrom, improve distribution of gases within the bronchial tract. Pressure cycled machines will cycle too frequently and are ineffective; if set to a high pressure, then the 'airways resistance' may suddenly decrease and pneumothoraces result from gross distension. The Cape ventilator will show high pressure at first, but when the bronchospasm is relieved the volume cycled ventilator will compensate with lower airway pressures.

If prolonged IPPV proves necessary, a tracheostomy should be considered, as indwelling endotracheal tubes can promote further bronchospasm in conscious patients. Careful blood gas measurement is essential throughout the management of status asthmaticus and hypoxaemia must be avoided. Viscid plugs and 'spirals' of secretions interfere with adequate ventilation and must be removed, if necessary by bronchoscopy and bronchial lavage. Steroid therapy should be continued throughout resuscitation. The appropriate antibiotics should be administered as many cases of status asthmaticus have an infective origin.

Bronchial lavage. The technique of bronchial lavage is receiving widespread acceptance as a treatment for the removal of bronchial debris in the severe 'respiratory cripple'. Several methods are in present use. 1. Bronchoscopic technique: the main advantage of this technique is that the operator can visualize the respiratory tract and accurately place the lavaging fluid. 2. Endobronchial technique: using a Robertshaw left endobronchial tube with cuffs adequately inflated, any spill of surplus lavage fluid into the ventilated lung can be prevented.

Preanaesthetic preparation: as most of the patients will be receiving bronchodilator drugs and steroids, these should be given approximately four hours pre-operatively, in their usual dosage. Half an hour pre-operatively the patient receives intramuscular atropine 0.6 mg and hydrocortisone 100 mg. An intravenous infusion of aminophylline 1.0 g and hydrocortisone 100 mg in 500 ml of 5% dextrose is commenced immediately prior to the induction of anaesthesia. Where possible, the patients should be pre-oxygenated by the inhalation of 100% oxygen for at least three minutes.

Anaesthesia. This is induced with a sleep dose of propanidid, followed by 50 mg of suxamethonium, and the vocal cords are sprayed with 4% prilocaine. The patient is intubated with as large an endotracheal tube as is practicable and the cuff inflated. Using a 50 : 50 mixture of nitrous oxide/oxygen and a gradually increasing concentration of diethyl ether or halothane/ether azeotrope, the patient is inflated vigorously, until spontaneous ventilation occurs and approximately the third plane of the third stage of general anaesthesia is achieved. During this time, the bronchospasm is gradually felt to relax. A very careful watch must be kept upon the pulse and blood pressure in order not to tax the already labouring heart.

When the pupils are fixed centrally and moderately dilated, the ether is switched off and the patient allowed to inspire 1.5–2% halothane for five minutes by the clock. This is to ensure that there is no explosive ether mixture in the air passages. The endotracheal tube is now removed, the bronchoscope inserted and oxygen with 2% halothane is insufflated into the side tube of the bronchoscope. A total of 800–1500 ml of lavage fluid is introduced down the various bronchi on either side in doses of 30–50 ml, each dose is immediately aspirated, but only 25–30% is recovered.

The general anaesthetic technique. This is the same as for the bronchoscopic technique, but instead of an endotracheal tube, a Robertshaw left endobronchial tube is inserted and anaesthesia is maintained with either diethyl ether or halothane, or the azeotropic mixture, using 100% oxygen. When the lungs have been denitrogenated by breathing the oxygen for 10 minutes, one of the lumina is clamped in expiration, and also the corresponding catheter mount, which is then disconnected from the Cobb's type connector. Next, the lung selected for lavage is partially degassed for 5 minutes. During this time oxygen is absorbed, the lung collapses into about two-thirds of its original size and the trachea is drawn over to the degassed side. Negative pressures of about 12 cmH_2O have been measured at the end of degassing, remembering that it is most important that the time for degassing should not exceed five minutes. Meanwhile the clamped tube is connected, via the Cobb's connector, to a length of plastic tubing into which is inserted a funnel. This tubing is filled with lavage fluid : at the end of degassing the clamp is released and the lavage fluid poured in continuously, care being taken not to raise the funnel higher than 30 cm above the mid-chest. The patient breathes spontaneously and the fluid oscillates in the tubing with respiration. Casts and sputum are seen in the funnel and aspiration begins immediately fluid has been instilled. The lung having been brought into the anaesthetic circuit and ventilated, intermittent suction of it is carried out over the next 10–20 minutes: the total volume aspirated is about one third of that instilled. Only one side should be lavaged on each occasion.

Fluids. The following fluids may be used for lavage: 1 Isotonic saline. 2 Isotonic saline, buffered by the addition of sodium bicarbonate to pH of 7.2, with 100 mg of hydrocortisone hemissuccinate added to every litre. 3 Buffered hypertonic saline, with an osmolality of approximately 520 milliosmol per litre. 4 1% sodium bicarbonate. During instillation, posture should be frequently changed, and chest percussion carried out by a physiotherapist to facilitate removal of debris.

Post-operative. Adequate oxygenation must be maintained and artificial ventilation may be required: coughing is encouraged and physiotherapy is essential. If artificial ventilation is necessary, neuromuscular blockade is best achieved using either alcuronium or pancuronium bromide. Full hydration of the patient must be maintained by oral and/or intravenous fluids.

Fat embolism

Fat embolism can be defined as the blockage of the smaller blood vessels by globules of fat. Classically, fat embolism occurs after single or multiple large bony injury, particularly pelvic or long limb bones: it can also complicate crush or blast injury. However, fat embolism has been reported in other diseases – diabetes, epilepsy, after external cardiac massage, following burns and during orthopaedic procedures under general anaesthetic, particularly during and following replacement arthroplasty.

Pathogenesis. The origin of the embolic fat globules may be from two possible main sites, the bone marrow and the depot fat, the most common source being the bone marrow. In cases where bony injury is not a feature, then the depot fat is probably the source of emboli. The effects of the fat emboli seem to be caused by blockage of pulmonary vessels initially, with smaller emboli escaping through into the systemic circulation leading to intra-pulmonary alveolar haemorrhage. The most likely sequence is initial blockage, followed by local irritation from the hydrolyzed unsaturated fat contained in the embolus, causing intra-alveolar and other haemorrhages in the body tissues.

Clinical features. There are three types: (1) Fulminating fat embolism – rapidly fatal and rarely diagnosed in time for treatment to be successful. (2) The classical presentation – showing pulmonary and systematic symptoms. Pulmonary fat embolism may occur alone, but systemic or cerebral fat embolism is always accompanied by the pulmonary type. (3) Incomplete fat embolism – not usually identified unless the possibility is actively considered: it is then diagnosed on the lowered arterial oxygen tension level.

The classical presentation follows a traumatic injury, after which there is a lucid interval, followed by increasing tachycardia, restlessness and rising respiration rate proceeding to gross hyperventilation with loss of consciousness. Pulmonary compliance is increased and pulmonary oedema may be present, or can be readily precipitated by intravenous infusions. Petechial may appear on the skin of the trunk or limbs. Subconjunctival haemorrhages may occur, as may retinal exudates and fat globules in the retinal vessels. Fat may be found in the sputum and urine and a period of oliguria or anuria is not uncommon. The ECG may show evidence of right heart strain, right bundle branch block and generalized ischaemic changes, with a tendency to develop runs of sustained dysrhythmia of the supraventricular variety. More rarely ventricular dysrhythmias, or even cardiac arrest may be precipitated.

A chest examination reveals audible râles. Radiographic examination shows a typical snowstorm appearance – widespread loss of pulmonary translucency, obliteration of peripheral vascular markings, and diffuse parenchymal exudate, almost indistinguishable from the X-ray appearances of pulmonary oedema. These radiographic changes may not appear for the first 24 hours and may persist for as long as 20 days. Confusion disorientation, acute restlessness, irritability, headache, coma and convulsions can be caused by cerebral fat embolism or the hypoxaemia of pulmonary fat embolism. The latter is due to maldistribution of ventilation and perfusion within the lungs, with arterial oxygen tensions commonly reduced to 50 mmHg or even below. Hypoxaemia is an early sign and can suggest the diagnosis, even before clinical hypoxia is appreciated. The arterial desaturation may not be clinically diagnosed, until blood gas analysis is undertaken as the raised cardiac output and increase in skin perfusion that occurs may allow no visible cyanosis, even at arterial oxygen tensions below 50 mmHg.

Treatment

The fall in arterial oxygen tension promotes an increasing hyperventilation which, although commonly leading to hypocarbia, can never completely correct the hypoxaemia because of the large venous admixture. These patients need oxygen therapy. In the less severe cases, oxygen added to inspired air during spontaneous respiration may be adequate, but the more severely hypoxic patients need more intense treatment. This will necessitate IPPV, with a high oxygen saturation in the inspired air, to bring oxygen tension up to adequate levels (above 70 mmHg): it may be required for as long as 16 to 20 days. The response to serial diminution of inspired oxygen tension on the arterial oxygen tension can be taken as a reasonable assessment of progress. Similarly, serial blood gas monitoring is an essential part of the management of fat embolism. Great care must be taken to prevent secondary chest infection, as the multiple infarcted lung is an excellent breeding ground for bacteria, particularly pyocaneus. Cerebral oedema and pulmonary oedema are often present; therefore, suitable dehydration therapy using mannitol or large doses of frusemide, should be considered. System hydrocortisone or dexamethazone are also useful to prevent both cerebral and pulmonary oedema.

Hypothermia has been recommended for the coma of fat embolism and is useful if commenced early in the treatment. The body temperature should be maintained at 31 °C, shivering being controlled by chlorpromazine, methyl phenidate, or muscle relaxants if the patient is also receiving IPPV. Patients treated with hypothermia often regain consciousness when the body temperature is lowered. IPPV and hypothermia, commonly used together, may need to be maintained for up to 13 or more days. Low molecular weight dextrans have been suggested to improve blood flow and prevent red cell aggregation; heparin has been recommended for its lipase activation; in addition, the use of clofibrate (Atromid) in the prevention of fat embolism has been suggested but its use is not yet clearly defined. More recently produced evidence suggests that when Trasylol (Aprotinin – the kallikrein-trypsin inactivator with associated other multiple anti-enzymatic activity) is given to patients with fat embolism and low arterial oxygen tensions around 40 mmHg, there tends to be a dramatic improvement of their arterial oxygen tensions up to 80 and 90 mmHg over a period of 24 hours, associated with a slower but positive clearance of the lung pathology and radiological appearances. The current dose recommended for this treatment is two or three million units per day. More work is needed on the use of Trasylol in fat embolism, and other associated hypoxaemic states to assess its true value. Care should be exercised when using suxamethonium as prolonged apnoea has been reported in patients receiving both drugs.

Myasthenia gravis

Types of myasthenia gravis

Neonatal myasthenia, in infants of affected mothers is a self-limiting disease.

Juvenile myasthenia. This is true childhood myasthenia; it is severe, rapidly progressive and responds poorly to treatment.

Adult myasthenia gravis. This may be divided into the following groups:

(1) localized, non progressive form, which responds well to treatment, (2) generalized myasthenia with a gradual onset and long remissions, (3) acute fulminating myasthenia with early and frequent crises and poor response to therapy. Early myositis may be present, (4) late severe myasthenia – the end result of groups 1 and 2, (5) myasthenic myopathy – a rapid wasting over six months, with a very poor prognosis.

The slow progression to myasthenic myopathy can produce a 'brittle' state where response to therapy is exceedingly poor and sensitivity to anticholinesterase overdose is markedly increased. These patients alternate rapidly between myasthenic and cholinergic crises.

Pathogenesis of myasthenia gravis. Myasthenia gravis is considered to be an autoimmune disease. The cause is unknown, but the lesions can be explained on the hypothesis that these patients have an abnormal immune response to their own tissues. Microelectrodes inserted into single neural end plates have shown that the only abnormality that can be detected in the myasthenic neuromuscular function is the size of the quanta of acetylcholine formed in the presynaptic vesicles. They are about one-fifth normal size. The thymus secretes a hormone, thymin, which can reduce the size of acetylcholine quanta and in myasthenics this hormone (probably a polypeptide of small size) is present in excess: the theory is that an antibody is produced that stimulates the thymus to produce excess thymin. These concepts on pathogenesis explain the role of the thymus, the overlap with thyrotoxicosis, and the spontaneous exacerbations and remissions typical of this disease. An incomplete cure following thymectomy is due to associated myositis and to permanent loss of neuromuscular fibres.

Myasthenic myositis leads to degeneration of the receptor sites at the neuromuscular end plate and a consequent failure of acetylcholine to act at these sites, the response to acetycholine at any phase in the disease being dependent on the percentage of end plate receptors available. Neostigmine overdosage, therefore, will tend to produce a toxic cholinergism, if the optimum stimulation of available receptive neuromuscular end plates is exceeded. The increasing tendency to gradual myositic degeneration, leads into the myopathic phase seen later in the progression of the disease and, as the patient becomes more myositic and myopathic, the response to anticholinesterase drugs will deteriorate. Myositic and myopathic degeneration may be of variable degree in different muscle groups; for instance, the muscle mechanism of swallowing may be less severely affected than respiratory or limb muscles. The logical conclusion is that the dose of anticholinesterase needed to achieve swallowing is a toxic cholinergic dose for respiratory muscles and leads to respiratory failure.

Throughout the treatment of myasthenia with anticholinesterase drugs, the muscarinic side effects must be suitably controlled by the administration of atropine, hyoscine or hyoscyamine. There is no standard dose of anticholinesterase for the myasthenic, as there is no standard dose of insulin for the diabetic. The dose of anticholinesterase to produce optimal muscle function must be carefully controlled by frequent assessment and the use of suitable combinations of neostigmine and pyridostigmine. (1 mg of intramuscular neostigmine can be taken as approximately equal to 15 mg neostigmine given by mouth.) This drug may be needed as often as two hourly with possible booster doses before meals: pyridostigmine has a much longer action of about 8 hours, but is less predictable in its effect.

Myocardial muscle degeneration may also occur in myasthenia, particularly in the myositic and myopathic phases of the disease. In addition, cardiomyopathic ECG changes may develop, with associated cardiac dysrhythmia, cardiac failure or sudden unexpected cardiac arrest.

Myasthenic crisis. This is an acute exacerbation of the myasthenic symptoms, progressing to respiratory inadequacy. There is a response to anticholinesterase therapy up to an optimal point but, if this point is exceeded, an overdosage of anticholinesterase will produce a 'cholinergic crisis', with excessive salivation, rapid deterioration of muscle function and marked respiratory insufficiency. The critical margin between the suboptimal dose of anticholinesterase drugs and the toxic dose, may be very narrow indeed. At particular risk of cholinergic crises are the myositic and myopathics.

When a cholinergic crises is imminent, or precipitated, the elective treatment should be to withdraw all anticholinesterase therapy and ventilate the patient artificially through an endotracheal tube for 48–72 hours. Following this an edrophonium test (10–20 mg) will indicate whether a predictable response to anticholinergic drug therapy is returning.

Reliable indications of returning muscle power in the myasthenic are:

returning strength of grip
ability to clench the jaw against observer counter-pressure
ability to lift the head and place the chin on the chest
ability to tightly close the eyes and prevent the lids being opened by an observer
the return of swallowing, this may be the most difficult function to

regain and persistent attempts to improve swallowing may easily re-precipitate cholinergic crisis.

It should be remembered that semi-solids such as ice cream, jelly, etc., are much easier to swallow than clear liquids when a patient has incoordination of swallowing, weak muscle function and an extended latent period between 'sip' and 'swallow'.

If there is improvement of muscle activity, cautious re-introduction of anticholinesterase therapy should begin. It is wise, initially, to rely on intramuscular doses, to avoid the pitfall of erratic and uncontrolled absorption from the gastro-intestinal tract. If there is no improvement of muscle activity following an edrophonium test, then it is wise to continue IPPV for a few more days and repeat the test. If the patient is in the brittle state, then even minimal neostigmine will produce a cholinergic crisis: these patients will need IPPV until the response to anticholinesterase therapy returns, which may take days, weeks, months or years. An attempt to break the auto-immune cycle may be made. ACTH and hydrocortisone have been used, but with mixed results, some are improved, some show no change and others deteriorate. Thymectomy has a place in treatment and occasionally thymectomy in 'crisis' has been successful: occasionally, however, there is a post-thymectomy deterioration after a latent interval of some improvement, usually due to myasthenic myositic myopathy. Such a myopathic cannot respond to anticholinesterase and is easily precipitated into cholinergic crisis.

Because myasthenic women usually improve their myasthenic state during the first trimester of pregnancy, oestrogen/progesterone mixtures have been used with success in some cases to produce remission. Potassium-conserving diuretics have been recommended, such as triamterine and spironolactone as well as insulin and potassium.

In the myopathic and myositic myasthenic it may be necessary to perform a permanent gastrostomy. Patients on minimal anticholinesterase therapy can breathe spontaneously, but any higher dosage, given in order to allow swallowing, precipitates immediate cholinergic crisis. A permanent tracheostomy may help respiration. Intermittent positive pressure ventilation is probably the treatment of choice on these occasions, while awaiting a spontaneous remission.

In long term management of myasthenic crisis by intermittent positive pressure ventilation, early gastrostomy should be considered, because the presence of an indwelling feeding tube in conjunction with a cuffed tracheostomy tube may lead to tracheo-oesophageal ulceration with fistula. It is essential to maintain adequate caloric intake in myasthenics, who otherwise show weakness from starvation as well as from their original disease.

Myasthenic crisis is usually triggered off by emotional stress or infection. Antibiotics such as streptomycin, neomycin and kanamycin, polymixin and bacitracin can exacerbate myasthenia. Deterioration can be precipitated by drugs which reduce the excitability of the muscle membrane, e.g. quinine and quinidine, and also by drugs that depress respiration (the narcotic analgesics or the barbiturates).

The recent availability of antilymphocytic serum, as a result of immunologic studies of organ transplantation, has led to the cautious trial of antilymphocytic serum and other immunosuppressive drugs, in the attempt to break the auto-immune cycle of myasthenia gravis. It remains to be seen whether their use will be of significant value.

Tetanus

Tetanus remains one of the ten principle causes of death in many countries, neonatal and puerperal tetanus accounting for 50% of the incidence in India. In England, tetanus has a low annual incidence, mainly in agricultural areas. Efficient treatment has reduced the mortality from tetanus from 70% 20 years ago, to under 4% in Leeds more recently. The overall mortality for the United Kingdom is about 30%. An unusually high incidence of tetanus in drug addicts has been reported.

Classification of general tetanus is difficult – local tetanus is rare in humans – and many simple classifications have been suggested, see Table 16.3. In view of the varying way in which tetanus presents, the patients are commonly classified retrospectively, especially where the severe grades are concerned.

Table 16.3 *Classification of general tetanus*

Class	*Severity*	*Characteristics*
Grade 1	Mild	Mild to moderate trismus; no dysphagia, no convulsions and no respiratory difficulty
Grade 2	Moderate	Moderate to gross trismus, spasticity and dysphagia: some respiratory embarrassment and 'fleeting' muscle spasms
Grade 3a	Severe	Grade 2 plus spontaneous spasms or convulsions
Grade 3b	Very severe	With rapid onset of severe extensor spasms Central effects of toxin on brain stem

In order to avoid tetanus, in all cases of severe injury, previous history of antitoxin therapy or of severe reaction should be noted. The common practice should be that all wounds receive adequate toilet, debridement, and antibiotic cover with penicillin, erythromycin or tetracycline. Toxoid is used in both immunized and unimmunized patients. In the latter, additional prophylaxis can be provided by using antitoxin. Local treatment should be aimed at removing the source by a wide excision, followed by antitoxin 250 units of human tetanus immunoglobulin intramuscularly. A course of antibiotics (e.g. penicillin in high doses) is given for 5 to 7 days.

Treatment should be aimed at the active avoidance of any cyanotic or apnoeic attacks. The shorter the interval between the onset of the first symptoms and the onset of full generalized spasm, the worse is the prognosis: patients developing severe spasms in 48 hours usually have a stormy course. Hyperpyrexia (above 40°C), persistent tachycardia and hypotension due to a labile cardiovascular state, are signs of medullary tetanus and have a poor prognosis. Increased catecholamine release with multiple cardiac arrhythmia may also cause problems.

Mild case: these cases are treated in quiet surroundings, with careful surveillance and sedation. Many drugs have been used to produce tranquillity, e.g. chlorpromazine, promazine, chlordiazepoxide, pethidine, levorphan (Dromoron), phenoperidine, Omnopon, diazepam, meprobamate, sodium amylobarbitone, chloral hydrate, mephenesin and heminevrin. Close attention must be paid to nutrition, as treatment may have to be continued for many weeks: it is wise to feed only intravenously for the first few days, until the pattern of the disease is clearly defined.

Moderate case: when the patient shows impairment of the airway, or any tendency to dysphagia, an early tracheostomy is a recommended precaution.

Severe case: when 'spontaneous' spasms occur, despite reasonable sedation, then full and early curarization should be instituted, as a precaution, and IPPV therapy commenced. Tubocurarine or pancuronium may be used to achieve this, initially by large doses. Secondary pulmonary infection, unexplained persistant tachycardia, labile blood pressure and hyperpyrexia are also indications for immediate curarization and IPPV. Full curarization is necessary to inhibit all clonic spasms. Heavy sedation should be continued and the addition of analgesics may be necessary, such as:

50–100 mg chlorpromazine 4 to 6 hourly in adults
10– 20 mg diazepam 4 to 6 hourly in adults
15– 20 mg/kg per day of chlordiazepoxide.

Physiotherapy and other highly disturbing procedures should be performed under nitrous oxide/oxygen amnalgesia, while hypertensive crisis should be treated by α- and β-adrenergic blockade, along the same lines as for phaeochromocytoma. Cardiac dysrhythmias may be controlled by adrenergic β-blockade.

Complications: cardiovascular lability, systolic murmurs, persistent tachycardia and ECG changes may occur. Occasionally, 'stocking glove' peripheral cyanosis, with increasing peripheral circulatory failure may be witnessed. Paralytic ileus, gastric dilation, acute gastric ulceration, gastrointestinal haemorrhage bulbar palsies, facial palsy, and strabismus may occur. Profuse salivation and excessive sweating may lead to fluid depletion.

Neonatal tetanus. This occurs mainly in India and Africa. The importance of a clean dressing to the umbilical stump cannot be overlooked, in countries where tetanus is prevalent. Two spaced doses of aluminium adjuvant toxoid should be given to all pregnant women where this problem exists. Neonatal tetanus is rarely, if ever, seen in the United Kingdom. Death from tetanus in the neonatal period is a very real problem in underdeveloped countries. A significant contribution to the reduction of mortality has been achieved by introduction of intubation and positive pressure ventilation. Following aspiration of the pharynx, and preoxygenation, 20 mg suxamethonium are administered and the patient intubated and artificially ventilated, apnoea being maintained by incremental doses of 3 mg tubocurarine. Tracheostomy is preferred by some as prolonged perlaryngeal intubation may be harmful. Particular attention should be paid to humidification of the inspired gases, meticulous bronchial toilet, and to care both of the tracheostomy tube and of the gastric feeding tube. Deaths from infection via the tracheostomy and likewise pneumonia, have been strikingly reduced by instilling 0.25 ml of a mixture of penicillin and Colistin (500 units of each per ml in distilled water freshly prepared every day) and by giving routine antibiotics. Particular care is taken to ensure that the tracheostomy tube does not rotate and unduly impinge upon the trachea, that the patient is nursed in a well humidified atmosphere and that the secretions are removed. Where secretions are a problem, direct aspiration, using an auroscope via the tracheostome, may be useful. Because of these regimes, the major cause of death is no longer infection.

Crush injury of the chest

The increasing incidence of road traffic accidents has resulted in a greater number of patients with crush injury of the chest wall. The degree of injury may vary very considerably, from mild contusion or fracture of one or two ribs, to a completely flail chest, moving paradoxically on respiration. In addition, haemothorax, lung perforation with pneumothorax and surgical emphysema, pneumopericardium, or gross lung contusion with red cell extravasation into the alveoli with accumulation of blood and secretions in the air passages may all occur.

There may be associated multiple injuries, e.g. fractures of the skull, jaw, limbs and pelvis, or haemoperitoneum from a ruptured intra-abdominal viscus such as the liver or spleen. Electrocardiographic evidence shows that cardiac damage of a mild nature is usually present, but occasionally severe cardiac tamponade from haemopericardium or massive intrathoracic haemorrhage from ruptured aorta may be seen. Tension pneumothorax may also be a presenting feature, demanding emergency treatment.

In crush injury of the chest there is gross ventilatory disturbance due to ventilation/perfusion abnormalities, with right to left shunting of pulmonary blood flow and intermittent atelectatic collapse of lung segments beneath any flail segment. Lung contusion can further embarrass oxygenation and acute blood loss can lead to oligaemic shock. Pulmonary fat embolism may further complicate the picture.

The disturbed ventilatory mechanics lead to increased respiratory work, with a respiratory rate of 30 to 40 per minute and a minute volume approaching 20 litres: this leads to increased oxygen consumption, while coexistant oligaemic shock increases physiological dead space and all these factors promote hypoxaemia. Less severe chest injuries may produce problems of acute traumatic lung failure in patients with pre-existing chronic chest disease.

Aims of emergency treatment. Emergency treatment must be directed at the management of oligaemic shock by the transfusion of blood, plasma, or plasma expanders. Central venous pressure monitoring is extremely valuable in the assessment of blood volume replacement and should be part of the routine treatment. Equally important is the maintenance of a clear airway, if necessary by endotracheal intubation, the removal of blood and secretions from the respiratory tract by aspiration, the provision of adequate ventilation and stabilization of the chest wall. Tension pneumothorax necessitates emergency treatment by prompt insertion of a needle through the chest wall on the affected side. Similarly, pneumothorax or haemothorax should be controlled by the insertion of intercostal drains with an underwater seal, if necessary into both pleural cavities. Positive pressure ventilation should be undertaken with caution, unless intercostal drains are *in situ*, because of the danger of producing rapid tension pneumothorax with sudden death.

Haemopericardium should be suspected in the presence of a persistently raised central venous pressure and relieved by percutaneous puncture of the pericardial sac, through the sixth left intercostal space. The possibility of a ruptured intra-abdominal viscus should be considered at this stage, and exploratory laporotomy planned if necessary. Thoractomy may be indicated for the treatment of ruptured trachea or bronchus (persisting pneumothorax), ruptured aorta (continued intrathoracic haemorrhage) or a ruptured diaphragm. A leaking aortic arch will produce, on X-ray examination, evidence of an increasingly widening mediastinum. Intravenous sodium bicarbonate will be necessary to counteract the metabolic acidosis subsequent to the prolonged hypoxia.

Assessment and ventilation. After these emergency measures have been completed, the patient should be assessed according to the respiratory state. In mild cases, involving only one or two rib fractures with an effective cough reflex and no frank ventilatory impairment, pain relief and oxygen therapy is all that is needed. Moderate cases, having mild ventilatory inadequacy, which is improved by adequate pain relief, but with an ineffective cough and a tendency to secretion retention, will need endotracheal intubation or tracheostomy, and mechanical removal of secretions by repeated aspiration, associated with intensive humidification and physiotherapy.

More severe cases will have a flail segment, an ineffective cough reflex and obvious clinical evidence of inadequate ventilation. These patients will require intermittent positive pressure ventilation for a varying number of days. Arterial carbon dioxide tension is a poor guide of overall respiratory impairment in these cases, the arterial oxygen tension being much more reliable. This is due to extra respiratory work, additional oxygen demand with increased peripheral extraction and 'shunting' of blood past damaged and underventilated alveoli. Although blood gas analysis is a guide to efficient treatment, emergency measures should not be delayed to await these results.

All cases with ventilatory impairment should be intubated and intermittent positive pressure ventilation carried out, with 100% oxygen in the acute phase, then serially reduced according to arterial oxygen tension results. If adequate tracheobronchial toilet cannot be achieved by aspiration through an endotracheal tube, bronchoscopy is indicated. (Intermittent postive pressure ventilation for crushed chest can be managed with an indwelling endotracheal tube, but there are also strong grounds for early tracheostomy.)

For severe injuries prolonged intermittent postive pressure ventilation will be necessary, and in view of the atelectatic lung underlying the flail portion of chest, a constant pressure generator type ventilator with a square wave form, should be chosen, e.g. Barnet or Radcliffe. This type of wave form will re-expand the viscous surfaces of collapsed lung areas and also serves the secondary purpose of preventing over-riding of the ribs, keeping the edges closely apposed to encourage early fixation. Care must be taken to adjust the peak airway pressures so that the rib ends are neatly apposed. Ventilation should restore the blood gases to normal values, but in the presence of lung contusion, hypoxaemia may persist for some 4–8 days, or longer with fat embolism.

Initially, to prevent straining against the ventilator, 'patient triggering' is useful, but smooth acceptance of ventilation is usually facilitated by adequate pain relief. Opiates, neuroleptics, tranquillizers, and continuous thoracic epidural analgesia have been used for this purpose. It is also practicable to use muscle relaxants, to help settle the patient to intermittent positive pressure ventilation during the first few hours: mild hyperventilation helps to achieve this.

Intermittent positive pressure ventilation should be continued until the flail segment is fixed and ventilation is adequate, usually in 8–21 days. However, fat embolism may complicate multiple injuries and acute renal failure requiring peritoneal dialysis or haemodialysis may become a problem. Further management should be as directed for patients on long term intermittent positive pressure ventilation therapy. Though surgical mechanical direct fixation of the chest has its advocates, this is generally unnecessary. Associated severe head injury will increase the mortality of crush injury of the chest.

Traumatic lung syndrome. Respiratory failure may occur following multiple peripheral injury, although there is no actual bony trauma to the thoracic cage, or even to any other bone. Such pulmonary effects are commonly delayed until twenty-four or more hours after the original injury and are clinically presented by increased respiration rate, tachycardia, restlessness and hypoxaemia on arterial blood gas analysis. The lung picture is clinically that of pulmonary oedema, with decreased lung compliance and lung pathology showing intra-alveolar haemorrhage and haemorrhagic consolidation. This syndrome is essentially similar to fat embolism and should be treated in a similar fashion.

Poisoning

Although the barbiturates and salicylates are still the commonest form of suicidal poisoning in this country, poisoning with tranquillizing and psychotropic drugs is increasing annually. In addition accidental poisoning occurs, especially in children, where any tablet within reach may be taken and consumed.

Emergency treatment of poisoning. It is beyond the scope of this book to deal with this matter in detail, but general emergency measures should always be instituted. (1) remove the patient from the source of poison, i.e. fumes or carbon monoxide, (2) if a corrosive has been swallowed and the patient is conscious, give several pints of milk to drink.

General conservative intensive supportive treatment. The treatment of any case of self-poisoning is best treated in general terms, attention being directed to three main features: (1) supportive therapy, (2) the elimination and excretion of the poison, (3) specific antidote therapy – only very rarely can this be utilized.

Attention to airway and ventilation. The airway should be cleared, and artifiicial ventilation commenced if necessary, with the patient placed in the lateral position and the head lowered. If he has an active cough reflex and is pink on breathing air (except in carbon monoxide or cyanide poisoning) he is relatively safe in this position.

If the patient is unconscious and has no cough reflex, a cuffed oro-endotracheal tube should be passed: if respiration is depressed, oxygen can be administered and intermittent positive pressure ventilation commenced. Respiratory depression is diagnosed on clinical evidence, in the first instance, but should be confirmed as soon as practical by direct measurement of respiratory function, or by blood gas analysis. There is evidence that positional protection of the airway in an unconscious patient is unreliable, any patient with a depressed cough reflex being unable to protect completely the tracheobronchial tract from aspiration of stomach contents.

Attention to cardiovascular state. The blood pressure, heart rate and state of peripheral circulation should be observed repeatedly. If hypotension is a feature, then an intravenous infusion should be commenced and plasma, or some other plasma expander, used to increase the blood volume, using the central venous pressure level as a monitoring guide. If infusion to a central venous pressure of + 10 cmH_2O fails to raise the systolic blood pressure, myocardial depression should be suspected and the use of intravenous hydrocortisone or a vasopressor (such as methylamphetamine) should be considered. Cardiac irregularities, if they occur, should be treated with the appropriate anti-dysrhythmic drug: cardiac arrest if present, must be treated promptly and congestive cardiac failure should be treated with digitalis and diuretics (e.g. frusemide). Pulmonary oedema should be treated with diuretics, IPPV, or venesection, but if the pulmonary oedema is due to irritant contamination of the lungs, bronchial lavage should be performed.

Attention to removal of poison. Except where a corrosive has been swallowed, the first item is the attempted removal of the poison from the stomach. If the patient is conscious active vomiting should be stimulated with syrup of ipecacuanha (10–15 ml), strong salt solution, or by placing the fingers in the back of the throat. This is very useful in children. If the patient is semi-conscious with a poor cough reflex, or unconscious with no cough reflex, then a cuffed endotracheal tube must be introduced before gastric emptying by lavage is considered. This may entail giving the subject a light anaesthetic to facilitate endotracheal intubation, prior to gastric lavage.

Gastric lavage is not very effective if more than 8 hours have elapsed since the ingestion of the toxic agent. Warm water should be used and the washings retained for analysis. Gastric aspiration and lavage should always be performed in: (1) patients with barbiturate poisoning, who have ingested the drug within four hours, unless it is known that less than 10 tablets have been taken, (2) an unconscious patient, with time of ingestion unkown, (3) all cases of salicylate overdosage, regardless of the time of ingestion.

Attention to fluid balance and excretion of poison. Fluid and electrolyte balance is an important aspect of the general management of acute poisoning, as is the correction of any degree of metabolic acidosis. An adequate renal output should be maintained, (about 3–4 litres of urine per day) to encourage excretion of the drug or any associated metabolites. Electrolyte imbalance must be watched for, as this can occur as a result of vomiting, diarrhoea, excessive sweating, or renal malfunction. If oliguria occurs, in the presence of adequate rehydration and a positive central venous pressure, a test dose of intravenous mannitol should be tried, before accepting a diagnosis of acute renal failure and instituting the appropriate treatment.

Elimination of the poison can be attempted by forced diuresis, peritoneal dialysis or haemodialysis, if it is known that the poison taken can be removed in this way. In small children exchange transfusion may be a more feasible treatment than acute haemodialysis. Diuresis may be commenced by using frusemide or intravenous mannitol.

Attention to convulsions. If the patient is convulsing, this must be controlled. Anoxic convulsions will respond to oxygen therapy and artificial ventilation, but other convulsions are best dealt with by administering a muscle relaxant and instituting positive pressure ventilation. Diazepam is effective in some cases.

Attention to temperature control. Acute poisoning is often accompanied by hyperthermia, which increases metabolism by 10% for each 1°C rise, or by hypothermia, which lowers metabolism, but also slows excretion and detoxication of drugs. Temperature of above 40°C must be treated by induction of active cooling: temperature below 35°C must be treated by controlled warming, using electric blankets or space blankets.

Barbiturate poisoning

The minimal lethal dose of most barbiturates is between 1500–1800 mg and the principal manifestations are coma with depression of respiration. Adequate ventilation is the first essential, and treatment of inadequate ventilation should include endotracheal intubation and IPPV. The blood gases should be routinely monitored as additional oxygen is usually required. Hypotension should be treated with plasma expanders using a central venous pressure line as a guide. There is little use for analeptic drugs.

With careful ventilatory support, tracheobronchial toilet, antibiotics and systemic cardiovascular support, the subject will be in a position to detoxicate and excrete the ingested drug. A reasonable intravenous fluid intake, 2–3 litres per day and the use of diuretics, such as frusemide, will encourage urine flow and will maintain a free channel of excretion of the drug. Serial serum barbiturate levels are useful in deciding treatment and assessment of the situation: for instance, a blood level of 2 mg/100 ml of short acting barbiturate, or 3–5 mg/100 ml of medium acting barbiturate will cause deep coma for 24–72 hours; a blood level of 6–8 mg/100 ml of long acting barbiturate will cause a deep coma for 4–5 days; higher levels will be associated with coma of longer duration. Hastening the elimination of the drug can be justified in the more severe cases, because of the associated cardiovascular depression. Forced diuresis, peritoneal dialysis and haemodialysis can be used for this purpose, being most effective with the longer acting barbiturate drugs (which are less protein bound than shorter acting drugs). Haemodialysis should be considered at a blood level of 10 mg/100 ml of butobarbitone, or 15 mg/100 ml of phenobarbitone.

Patients with barbiturate poisoning have a tendency to hypothermia and therefore steps should be taken to maintain the body temperature of 37°C: conversely, reactive pyrexia is not uncommon and occasionally hyperpyrexia, necessitating active cooling, may be encountered. These patients can be managed with an indwelling endotracheal tube, until full consciousness returns, usually within five days: resort to tracheostomy should be a rare occurrence.

Salicylate poisoning

Here the problem is predominantly an acute disturbance of the acid-base balance of the body. The reaction to the ingestion of fixed acid is by hyperventilation and increased carbon dioxide elimination, due to direct stimulation of the respiratory centre: the kidneys excrete base and a sodium deficiency arises; loss of base by vomiting, sweating and disturbed kidney function combined with ketosis from disturbed carbohydrate metabolism, then leads to a marked acidosis. The blood pH should be monitored as soon as possible.

The patient with salicylate overdosage is usually conscious, therefore vomiting should be induced, or gastric lavage carried out, regardless of the time elapsed since the ingestion of the drug. Aspirin clings to the gastric mucosa and may cause acute ulceration with gastro-intestinal haemorrhage, and low prothrombin level produced by interference with vitamin K metabolism in the liver may aggravate this situation: consequently, intravenous vitamin K should be given as part of the treatment. As the method of disposal of salicylates by the body is almost entirely renal, the treatment should be directed at maintaining an adequate output of urine; an intravenous infusion should be commenced and the acidosis corrected by the administration of sodium bicarbonate. THAM has also been used in salicylate poisoning and greatly increases the rate of elimination and salicylates, by alkalinization of the urine. Forced alkaline diuresis has been recommended, employing at the same time central venous pressure monitoring.

Winters (1967) uses alkali only when the blood pH is below 7.15, because potentiation of the first stage of alkalosis may precipitate tetany and convulsions. Indeed, in the presence of advanced keto-acidosis it is difficult to alkalinize the urine with sodium bicarbonate and hypernatraemia may result: in the presence of good renal function the use of additional potassium, in the form of potassium acetate, may be more likely to alkalinize the urine. Hypokalaemia is a problem, and additional potassium will be required in the intravenous fluids. In the presence of adequate renal function, 50% of the ingested dose of salicylate will be excreted in the first 24 hours, excretion being three times as rapid, if the urine is alkaline.

Serum levels of salicylate are essential guides to treatment and can be performed easily on the ward. A level of over 100 mg/100 ml is indicative of severe poisoning and necessitates haemodialysis: levels below this can be managed with forced diuresis, and levels below 60 mg/100 ml need only a forced oral intake of fluids. Mannitol or frusemide can be used to stimulate diuresis. If the renal function is impaired, haemodialysis or exchange transfusion is indicated: if peritoneal dialysis is used, 5% human albumin should be added to the dialysate. Neuromuscular block and IPPV have been recommended in severe cases and, where hyperpyrexia occurs, it must be treated promptly by active cooling.

Carbon monoxide poisoning

It is essential that patients with carbon monoxide poisoning should have an adequate alveolar ventilation with 100% oxygen. The addition of carbon dioxide as a respiratory stimulant is of doubtful value, especially in a patient who has been hypoxic with an associated metabolic acidosis, or in a patient with frank respiratory acidosis. Metabolic acidosis should be corrected by the administration of sodium bicarbonate, and respiratory acidosis by artificial ventilation. Hyperbaric oxygen is possibly of more value than intermittent positive pressure ventilation using 100% oxygen in carbon monoxide poisoning, but obvious difficulties arise because of the lack of ready availability.

If ventilation is inadequate, then artificial ventilation is indicated. Hypothermia and partial exchange transfusion have also been used in the treatment of carbon monoxide poisoning and intravenous mannitol should be given if cerebral oedema is suspected. Cardiovascular stability should be maintained with supportive measures.

Iron salts

This type of poisoning is becoming more common among children, due to the attractive colour of tablets. The principal manifestations are vomiting, diarrhoea and peripheral circulatory collapse. Wash out the stomach and immediately instil 5 g–7 g desferoxamine (Desferal) in 50–100 ml water into the stomach: give intravenous desferoxamine in a dose of 10–15 mg/kg body weight/per hour, up to a maximum dose of 80 mg/kg in the first 24 hours and 50 mg/kg/day thereafter. Maintain blood pressure by intravenous transfusion of blood or plasma expander and treat any tendency to metabolic acidosis with intravenous sodium bicarbonate. If the patient is asymptomatic at the end of 48 hours, recovery is likely.

Organophosphorus poisoning

In agricultural communities accidental poisoning with organophosphorous pesticide may occur. As these can be ingested, inhaled or absorbed through the skin, skin decontamination by washing must be part of the treatment as well as routine gastric lavage. The drugs act as permanent anticholinesterases, by permanently phosphorylating cholinesterase. The principal manifestations are respiratory inadequacy, secretory hyperactivity and convulsions. The emergency treatment is atropine in large doses (2 mg) given intravenously, repeated as 10 minute intervals until secretions are completely controlled and full atropinization is achieved: any lapse in atropine therapy may lead to fatal pulmonary oedema. Aspiration, endotracheal intubation and intermittent positive pressure ventilation may be necessary and, as soon as possible one of the aldoxime 'cholinesterase rejuvenator' drugs should be given (Pralidoxime 1 g in 5 ml water) intravenously and repeated at 3 hour intervals according to the response. If convulsions occur they are best treated with diazepam, given intravenously.

Morphine and other narcotic analgesics

The principal manifestations are severe respiratory depression and coma with pin-point pupils; convulsions are not uncommon. Emergency treatment begins with artificial ventilation, followed by an appropriate antidote. Nalorphine (5–10 mg) can be given intravenously, but this drug can cause respiratory depression itself in conditions other than opiate poisoning: a safer and more effective drug is levallorphan tartrate (Lorfan), 0.3 to 1.2 mg intravenously every 15 minutes, until respiration returns and the patient responds to stimuli. If depression returns repeat the levallorphan administration.

Mushroom poisoning

Poisoning following ingestion of *Amanita phalloides* or *Amanita muscaria,* may result in liver or renal damage with jaundice, convulsions and coma, but cases have been successfully treated. Remove by repeated gastric lavage and treat muscarinic symptoms by large intravenous doses of atropine (2 mg) repeated every 30 minutes, until full atropinization is achieved. Repeated haemodialysis has been successful; also, for liver protection, intravenous carbohydrate infusion is advised (about 4 to 5 litres 5% dextrose per day) if renal function is adequate. Convulsions are controlled with muscle relaxants and intermittent positive pressure ventilation, and hyperpyrexia treated by induced hypothermia.

Tranquillizers and selective depressants

This group of drugs includes promethazine, chlorpromazine, diazepam, chlordiazepoxide, oxazepam, meprobamate, etc., and the manifestation of over-dosage is drowsiness, progressing to coma with respiratory depression. Treat by gastric lavage, ensuring a moderate urine output to allow for urinary excretion of the drugs and with general ventilation and cardiovascular support.

Psychotropic drugs

Nortriptyline, amitriptyline, imipramine and desipramine are drugs which block the parasympathetic responses; their effects are potentiated by the monoamine oxidase inhibitors. The principal manifestations of overdosage are coma, clonic movements or convulsions, respiratory depression and marked cardiac dysrhythmias, such as ventricular flutter and tachycardia, atrio-ventricular or intraventricular block.

Emergency treatment is aimed at the removal of ingested material by gastric lavage: (osmotic diuresis has also been used to encourage removal of the drug). Artificial ventilation is indicated if respiration is depressed. Control convulsions with diazepam, or muscle relaxants and intermittent positive pressure ventilation. The cardiac irregularities should be treated, where necessary, with appropriate cardiac dysrhythmic agents.

Monoamine oxidase inhibitors

These include isocarboxazide, phenelzine, nialamide, tranylcypromine, and ipromiazid. The main manifestations are drowsiness, clonic movements and hyperreflexia, hyperpyrexia and convulsions. Death is associated with respiratory failure and vascular collapse, jaundice and liver necrosis.

Treatment: artificial ventilation, gastric lavage or emesis, intravenous plasma expanders to support blood pressure, induced hypothermia for hyperpyrexia. Control convulsions with chlorpromazine, or muscle relaxants and intermittent positive pressure ventilation, repeated as necessary: protect against liver damage by dextrose infusion containing vitamins, especially vitamin K.

Forced diuresis

The technique of forced diuresis is commonly employed in the treatment of acute poisoning, differing from simple diuresis only in the quantity of urine passed. A simple diuresis means an output of 3–4 litres of urine in 24 hours, while a forced diuresis means 10–20 litres of urine in the same period of time. The patient must be catheterized and it is advised that a central venous pressure monitoring line be introduced.

Commence an infusion with 500 ml normal saline, followed by 200 ml 20% mannitol or 80 mg frusemide intravenously. When diuresis commences infuse:

(1) 1 litre normal saline in the first hour;
(2) 1 litre 5% dextrose in the second hour;
(3) 500 ml M/6 sodium lactate in the third hour;
(4) 500 ml 5% dextrose with $1\frac{1}{2}$ g potassium chloride in the fourth hour;
(5) 500 ml isotonic saline in the fifth hour; and then repeat 3, 4 and 5 at hourly intervals, or shorter intervals if the diuresis is well maintained.

Diuresis should achieve 500 ml–1000 ml urine per hour, but the patient should never be transfused above a central venous pressure of + 8 cmH_2O, or be more than 1 litre in advance of urinary output. If urinary output falls behind the volume of infused fluid, then repeat frusemide 40 mg intravenously.

Serum electrolytes must be checked frequently and the necessary alteration made to the infused fluids: similarly, urine pH should be checked frequently and appropriate measures taken. If hypotension is present and does not respond to transfusion, the cautious intravenous injection of 5–10 ml methylamphetamine may help to promote a diuresis. The patient must be carefully watched for any signs of pulmonary oedema and a strict hourly input and output fluid balance chart maintained.

Peritoneal dialysis

This is basically the use of the peritoneum as a semipermeable membrane – i.e. by the introduction of a strong solution into the peritoneal cavity, various salts, drugs and fluid are withdrawn from the body. The urinary bladder is emptied. A sterile trocar and cannula is then inserted under local anaesthesia into the peritoneal cavity, through the midline of the abdominal wall, one third of the way from the umbilicus to the pubis. A sterile plastic catheter is next inserted through the cannula, into the left iliac fossa and the catheter connected to the dialysing fluid, by a transfusion set. (Two dialysis fluids are available, a weak one containing 1.36% dextrose, and a strong one containing 6.36% dextrose.)

One litre bag of dialysis fluid is run into the peritoneal cavity, as fast as possible, (this should take less than 10 minutes). When the bag is empty, allow it to drop to a level below the patient's abdomen, and to refill from the abdominal catheter over the next 30 minutes to 1 hour; remove the bag with strict aseptic technique, and repeat the process with a new bag of dialysis fluid, and so on. A special input and output dialysis chart should be maintained throughout the procedure, with the patient's oral or intravenous fluid intake charted separately. More frequent changes can be carried out if desired, or even two litres per hour can be infused using a 'Y' connection.

The patient should be observed and weighed frequently during the procedure if possible, in an effort to gauge any fluid retention that is occurring and to note complications. These may be failure to get return of fluid (usually due to a blocked catheter), leaks round the catheter, hypokalaemia, hypotension and perforation of abdominal viscus (rare). The splinting of the diaphragm that usually occurs, due to the temporary presence of fluid in the abdomen, may encourage basal pulmonary atelectasis with subsequent chest infections. This must be avoided by physiotherapy and deep breathing exercises, or by intermittent positive pressure ventilation.

Intensive therapy units

The importance of treating patients suffering from acute poisoning in specially designed Poisons Treatment Centres cannot be over-emphasized. Mathew and Lawson (1966) showed a death rate of 0.8% for 766 patients with barbiturate poisoning treated in a Poisons Unit, whereas in the general wards of provincial teaching hospitals the death rate was 2.1%. Designated Regional Poisons Treatment Centres should possess facilities for intensive therapy and haemodialysis and should have immediate access to an established Poisons Information Centre (see page 456). Complicated therapy such as exchange transfusion, induced hypothermia, elective intermittent positive pressure ventilation, etc. can only be safely attempted in units specially equipped for the purpose. (Ellis *et al.*, 1965).

Status epilepticus

Status epilepticus is a rare complication of epilepsy, that may either occur in a known epileptic, or following trauma or infection in a previously normal patient. It is defined as frequent epileptiform attacks, not adequately controlled by anti-convulsive therapy. If allowed to continue unchecked, severe anoxic cerebral and other damage will occur and the patient will remain comatose, eventually dying from anoxia and exhaustion, due to the excessive metabolic demands resultant from convulsions. However, if the status is brought under control for 24–48 hours, treatment can usually be discontinued without fear of an immediate recurrence.

Patients presenting in status, that have already been heavily sedated with anticonvulsive drugs such as phenobarbitone and paraldeyhyde, may be unconscious because of either the status or the drugs. In fact, excessively heavy sedation, which is ineffective, can actually endanger the patient, who may inhale vomit, etc., or even succumb to the therapy.

Methods of controlling status epilepticus include the following.

Intravenous lignocaine: this is given in doses of 2–6 mg/kg/h, associated with background barbiturate antiepileptic therapy, the dose of lignocaine being reduced as control is gained.

Intravenous phenytoin sodium: in doses up to 250 mg, this generally suppresses fits. The dose may be repeated after an hour.

IPPV and paralysis regime: full paralysis, using a D-tubocurarine or pancuronium for 24 to 48 hours on a background of barbiturate and phenytoin sodium therapy, has been advocated.

Intravenous thiopentone: a very small dose of sodium thiopentone is effective, the patient remaining awake during therapy and free from fits. The suppressing dose of thiopentone is far smaller than the sleep dose and must be administered as a continuous infusion of 0.25%. An initial dose of 20 to 50 mg is followed by 2 mg per minute, and the rate controlled according to the incidence of 'fits', a fine intravenous catheter avoiding inadvertent overdosage. The patient should be awake: a lapse into unconsciousness is a signal of a 'fit' and indicates more thiopentone, not less.

Intravenous diazepam (Valium): almost immediate suppression is seen with doses of 10 mg either intravenously or intramuscularly, followed by an intravenous infusion of 100 mg in 500 ml normal saline. It may also be necessary to control respiration by IPPV.

The treatment of choice is probably intravenous thiopentone, proceeding to full paralysis with muscle relaxants and IPPV, if it does not completely control the status alone. IPPV, if necessary, can be performed through an endotracheal tube; tracheostomy is not usually required. Status epilepticus has also been treated with methohexitone as an intravenous infusion, and with heminevrin, the latter being given in a dose of 40–100 ml 0.8% solution in 5–10 minutes. Cerebral oedema is a common finding in status epilepticus and intravenous glucose (30%), mannitol, urea, or frusemide are effective in controlling it.

Cardiac dysrhythmias in myocardial infarction

Cardiac dysrhythmias associated with acute myocardial infarction can be supraventricular, ventricular, or associated with some disconductive form of A.V. block. In coronary care, attention must be paid to the early diagnosis and treatment of dysrhythmias.

Supraventricular dysrhythmias

Supraventricular ectopic beats: these commonly herald a significant dysrhythmia such as atrial fibrillation or flutter. They are distinguished from ventricular ectopics by the abnormal P wave, which can be inverted, distorted or biphasic, or which, in nodal ectopics, can follow the QRS complex.

Supraventricular tachycardia: in most cases complexes are normal, but in paroxysmal atrial tachycardia with bundle branch block, the trace can simulate ventricular tachycardia. Treatment of either of the above is by digoxin, propranolol, practolol, or d.c. shock. Quinidine is useful and intravenous lignocaine is also effective, though not always predictably so.

Atrial flutter: this may be paroxysmal or established. There is often a degree of regular or varying block (e.g. '2 in 1' flutter) and pressure on the carotid sinus may halve the pulse rate by increasing the degree of block. The treatment of choice is d.c. counter shock, but digoxin is of value in some cases: lignocaine and quinidine are contraindicated for treatment of the acute attack.

Atrial fibrillation: this may be established or paroxysmal and should be treated by digoxin. d.c. shock is often necessary for established atrial fibrillation and both propranolol and practalol are useful.

Ventricular dysrhythmias

Ventricular ectopic beats: these usually indicate an irritable ventricle and can proceed to ventricular fibrillation. Intravenous lignocaine, oral procaine amide, or quinidine constitute the treatment of choice, in that order.

Ventricular tachycardia: this can happen in bursts or become continuous. The treatment of choice is d.c. counter shock, followed by procaine amide, intravenous lignocaine or propanolol to prevent further occurrences; oral lignocaine can be used for maintenance. Intravenous diazepam 0.3 mg/kg is a valuable sedative agent as well as an amnesic.

Ventricular fibrillation: the treatment is d.c. counter shock, combined with full resuscitative measures for treatment of circulatory arrest. Intravenous lignocaine is usually commenced after restoration of a heart beat. A loading dose of 70–100 mg is given, followed by an hourly dose, 100 mg per hour being usual, though doses of up to 300 mg per hour have been recorded. The main side effects of lignocaine are convulsions, or twitching with marked hallucinations, but these can be controlled by diazepam and by reducing the dose of lignocaine. Under these circumstances, it might be necessary to combine lignocaine infusion with oral procaine amide or quinidine.

Heart Block

This may be partial or complete. Atropine, ephedrine or isoprenaline may be used in treatment and steroids are extremely effective. Complete block with syncope or convulsions is treated in the short term, by passing a temporary transvenous cardiac pacemaker catheter, either down the jugular vein or up the cubital vein. In the long term, a permanent indwelling internal pacemaker needs to be inserted by elective surgery.

Appendix I Administrative forms

Consent forms recommended by the Medical Defence Union

FORM I. CONSENT BY PATIENT

.... Hospital.

I.. of...

hereby consent to undergo the operation of..
the nature and effect of which have been explained to me by
Dr/Mr..

I also consent to such further or alternative operative measures as may be found to be necessary during the course of the operation and to the administration of a general, local or other anaesthetic for any of these purposes.

No assurance has been given to me that the operation will be performed by any particular surgeon.

Date.................................... (*Signed*)..
(*Patient*)

I confirm that I have explained to the patient the nature and effect of this operation.

Date.................................... (*Signed*)..
(*Physician/Surgeon*)

FORM II. CONSENT BY PARENT OR GUARDIAN

....Hospital.

Patient's name ....

I.. of..,

the...of the above named, hereby

consent to the submission of my...

to the operation of..., the nature and effect of which have been explained to me by Dr/Mr

....

I also consent to such further or alternative operative measures as may be found to be necessary during the course of the operation and to the administration of a general, local or other anaesthetic for any of these purposes.

No assurance has been given to me that the operation will be performed by any particular surgeon.

Date (*Signed*)..

(*Parent/Guardian*)

I confirm that I have explained to the child's parent/guardian, the nature and effect of this operation.

Date..................................... (*Signed*)...

(*Physician/Surgeon*)

FORM III. CONSENT BY PATIENT TO ELECTROPLEXY

....Hospital.

I.. of..
hereby consent to undergo the administration of electroplexy, the nature and effect of which have been explained to me by

Dr/Mr..

I also consent to the administration of an anaesthetic for this purpose.

No assurance has been given to me that the treatment will be administered by any particular practitioner.

Date.................................. (*Signed*)..
(*Patient*)

I confirm that I have explained to the patient the nature and effect of this treatment.

Date.................................. (*Signed*)..
(*Physician*)

FORM IV. THIS FORM SHOULD BE USED IN CASES OF CHILDREN SUFFERING FROM SEVERE BURNS

CONSENT BY PARENT OR GUARDIAN

....Hospital.

Patient's name ....

I.. of...,

the...of the above named, hereby

consent to the submission of my..

to a course of operative treatment to deal with the burns he/she has suffered. The purpose, nature, and effect of this treatment

have been explained to me by Dr/Mr..

I also consent to the administration of a general, local, or other anaesthetic for the purpose of rendering such treatment.

No assurance has been given to me that the treatment will be carried out by any particular surgeon.

Date..................................... (*Signed*)..
(*Parent/Guardian*)

I confirm that I have explained to the child's parent/guardian the purpose, nature and effect of this treatment.

Date..................................... (*Signed*)..
(*Physician/Surgeon*)

FORM V. THIS FORM SHOULD BE USED IN CERTAIN **MAJOR** GYNAECOLOGICAL OPERATIONS, e.g. HYSTERECTOMY AND OOPHORECTOMY IF THE PATIENT IS MARRIED AND LIVING WITH HER HUSBAND.

CONSENT BY PATIENT

....Hospital.

I.. of..

hereby consent to undergo the operation of..
the nature and effect of which have been explained to me by
Dr/Mr...

I also consent to such further or alternative operative measures as may be found to be necessary during the course of the operation and to the administration of a general, local or other anaesthetic for any of these purposes.

No assurance has been given to me that the operation will be performed by any particular surgeon.

Date.................................... (*Signed*)...
(*Patient*)

I confirm that I have explained to the patient the nature and effect of this operation.

Date.................................... (*Signed*)...
(*Physician/Surgeon*)

AGREEMENT BY HUSBAND

I.. of..

the husband of..hereby agree

to the operation of...being carried out on my wife, the nature and effect of which have been

explained to me by Dr/Mr...

Date.................................... (*Signed*)...
(*Husband*)

I confirm that I have explained to the patient's husband the nature and effect of this operation.

Date.................................... (*Signed*)...
(*Physician/Surgeon*)

N.B. If possible this form should be signed by the husband and the wife at the same time.

FORM VI. THIS FORM SHOULD BE USED IN CASES OF **PRIMARY** STERILIZATION IF THE PATIENT IS MARRIED AND LIVING WITH HIS OR HER SPOUSE.

CONSENT BY PATIENT

I.. of...

hereby consent to undergo the operation of.....................................
the nature and effect of which have been explained to me by

Dr/Mr...

I have been told that the intention of the operation is to render me sterile and incapable of parenthood. I understand that it may not be possible later to reverse the effect of the operation.

I also consent to the administration of a general or local anaesthetic.

No assurance has been given to me that the operation will be performed by any particular surgeon.

Date.................................... (*Signed*)...
(*Patient*)

I confirm that I have explained to the patient the nature and effect of this operation.

Date.................................... (*Signed*)...
(*Physician/Surgeon*)

AGREEMENT BY SPOUSE

I.. of...

the husband/wife of...

hereby agree to the operation of..
being carried out on my wife/husband, the nature and effect of

which have been explained to me by Dr/Mr.....................................

Date.................................... (*Signed*)...
(*Husband/Wife*)

I confirm that I have explained to the patient's spouse the nature and effect of this operation.

Date.................................... (*Signed*)...
(*Physician/Surgeon*)

N.B. If possible this form should be signed by the husband and the wife at the same time.

FORM VII. TERMINATION OF PREGNANCY

CONSENT BY PATIENT

....Hospital.

I.. of..

hereby consent to undergo an operation for the termination of my pregnancy. The nature of the operation has been explained

to me by Dr/Mr..

I also consent to such further operative measures as may be found to be necessary during the course of the operation, and to the administration of a general, local or other anaesthetic.

No assurance has been given to me that the operation will be carried out by any particular surgeon.

Date.............................. (*Signed*)..
(*Patient*)

I confirm that I have explained to the patient the nature of the operation.

Date.............................. (*Signed*)..
(*Physician/Surgeon*)

FORM VIII. TERMINATION OF PREGNANCY AND STERILIZATION

CONSENT BY PATIENT

....Hospital

I.. of..
hereby consent (1) to undergo an operation for the termination of my pregnancy and (2) to undergo the operation of tubal ligation. The nature and effect of these procedures have been

explained to me by Dr/Mr..
I appreciate that the intention of the tubal ligation is to render me sterile and that it may not be possible later to reverse the effect of this operation.
I also consent to such further operative measures as may be found to be necessary at operation and to the administration of a general, local or other anaesthetic.

No assurance has been given to me that these procedures will be performed by any particular surgeon.

Date.................................... (*Signed*)..
(*Patient*)

I confirm that I have explained to the patient the nature and effect of these procedures.

Date.................................... (*Signed*)..
(*Physician/Surgeon*)

AGREEMENT BY HUSBAND

I.. of..
hereby agree to the procedures as indicated above being carried out on my wife, the nature and effect of which have been explained to be my Dr/Mr..

Date.................................... (*Signed*)..
(*Husband*)

I confirm that I have explained to the patient's husband the nature and effect of these procedures.

Date.................................... (*Signed*)..
(*Physician/Surgeon*)

FORM IX. CONSENT TO **OPERATIVE** TREATMENT BY PATIENT WHO REFUSES TO HAVE A BLOOD TRANSFUSION

....Hospital.

I.. of...

hereby give my consent to the performance upon me of the

operation of..,
the nature and effect of which have been explained to me by

Dr/Mr.......................................and to the administration of a general, local or other anaesthetic. I also give my consent to the performance upon me of any other operative procedure which in the opinion of the surgeon it may be necessary to perform upon me, without having obtained my express consent, during or by reason of the said operation or anything connected with it; except that, although it has been explained to me that in the course of or by reason of the said operation it may be necessary to give me a blood transfusion so as to render the operation successful, or to prevent injury to my health, or even to preserve my life, I hereby expressly withhold my consent to and forbid the administration to me of a blood transfusion in any circumstances or for any reason whatsoever and I accordingly absolve the surgeon, the hospital and every member of the medical staff concerned from all responsibility, and from any liability to me, or to my estate, or to my dependants, for any damage or injury which may be caused to me, or to my estate, or to my dependants, in any way arising out of or connected with this my refusal to consent to any such blood transfusion.

No assurance has been given to me that the operation will be performed by any particular surgeon.

Date.................................... (*Signed*)...
(*Patient*)

Witnesses to patient's signature...
(*Surgeon*)

....
(*Witness present at interview*)

FORM X. CONSENT TO MEDICAL TREATMENT BY PATIENT WHO REFUSES TO HAVE A BLOOD TRANSFUSION

....Hospital.

I... of..

....acknowledge that I have been informed that I am or may be suffering from.......................... and that I require or may require treatment, the nature and effect of which have been explained to me by Dr......................... I hereby give my consent to the administration of such medical treatment as the physician considers necessary; except that, although it has been explained to me that in the course of the said treatment it may be necessary to give me a blood transfusion so as to enhance the effectiveness of any treatment, or even to preserve my life I hereby expressly withhold my consent to and forbid the administration to me of a blood transfusion in any circumstances or for any reason whatsoever, and I accordingly absolve the physician, the hospital and every member of the medical staff concerned, from all responsibility, and from any liability to me, or to my estate, or to my dependants, for any damage or injury which may be caused to me, or to my estate or to my dependants, in any way arising out of or connected with this my refusal to consent to any such blood transfusion.

Date.................................... (*Signed*)...
(*Patient*)

Witnesses to patient's signature:...
(*Physician*)

....
(*Witness present at interview*)

FORM XI. REFUSAL BY PARENTS TO CONSENT TO BLOOD TRANSFUSION

....Hospital.

Name of patient ....

I/We.. and..

of..

the parents of..have been informed by

Dr/Mr..that in his opinion my/our child urgently needs or may need the administration of a blood transfusion.

I/We have been informed that failure to administer a blood transfusion may endanger the life of my child.

I/We nevertheless refuse to consent to a blood transfusion being given to my/our child.

(*Signed*).. (*Signed*)..
(*Witness to parents' signatures*) (*Father*)

....
(*Mother*)

(*Date*)..

FORM XII. CONSENT BY PATIENT WHO VOLUNTEERS TO UNDERGO A CLINICAL TRIAL FOR RESEARCH

....Hospital

I... of...

hereby consent to the administration of...

Dr.. has explained that.........................
is a new drug and that it is desired to investigate its therapeutic efficacy and physiological effect. I acknowledge that the risks have been explained to me. I understand that the investigation is to be carried out solely for the purpose of medical research and I am willing to act as a volunteer for that purpose on the understanding that I shall be entitled to withdraw this consent at any time.

Date..................................... (*Signed*)...

....
(*Witness to the patient's signature*)

I confirm that I have explained to the patient the purpose and nature of this investigation and the risks involved.

Date..................................... (*Signed*)...
(*Doctor*)

Drug history enquiry form

Hospital DEPT. OF ANAESTHETICS G.803/C	*The United Sheffield Hospitals* DRUG HISTORY ENQUIRY	*Reg'd No.* *Date of Registration*

Patient's Surname.................................... Forename(s)....................................

Address.. Age....................

Consultant.. Record Number..............................

For Admission to.............................. Hospital for Operation/Investigation on..............................

All Drugs Patient taking AT PRESENT (including Dosage).

ESPECIALLY:

- Hypotensives
- Mono-amineoxidase inhibitors
- Insulin/hypoglycaemic agent
- Anti-epileptic drugs
- Anti-coagulants
- Anti-biotics and Urinary antiseptics
- Digitalis
- Barbiturates or any other sedatives

Cortico-steroids—Had patient had any in last two years? YES/NO

If YES give name of drug and duration of treatment

ANY DRUG OR OTHER SENSITIVITY?

Signature of General Medical Practitioner..............................

Date..............................

PLEASE ASK YOUR DOCTOR TO FILL IN DETAILS OF DRUG HISTORY AND BRING THIS FORM WITH YOU ON THE DAY OF ADMISSION

Appendix II Normal Values

Haematology:

Red cells

Normal values

Patient	*Hb g/100 ml*	*P.C.V. %*	*R.B.C. millions/ mm²*
Male Adults	13·5–18·0	40–54	4·5–6·5
Female Adults	11·5–16·4	36–47	3·9–5·6
Infants (cord blood)	13·6–19·6	44–62	4·0–5·6
Children, 1 year (mean)	11·2	35	4·5
Children, 10 years (mean)	12·9	37·5	4·7

Indices

Mean corpuscular volume (M.C.V.)

$$= \frac{\text{P.C.V. (\%)}}{\text{R.B.C. (mill./mm}^3\text{)}} \times 10 = 76\text{—}96\ \mu\text{m}^3$$

Mean corpuscular haemoglobin (M.C.H.)

$$= \frac{\text{Hb. (g./100 ml)}}{\text{R.B.C. (mill./mm}^3\text{)}} \times 10 = 27\text{—}32\text{ pg}$$

Mean corpuscular haemoglobin concentration (M.C.H.C.)

$$= \frac{\text{Hb. (g./100 ml)}}{\text{P.C.V. (\%)}} \times 100 = 30\text{—}35\%$$

Reticulocytes (normal) = 0·2—2·0%
E.S.R. (Westergren) = < 15 mm in 1 hour

Blood volume

Red cell volume, males = 28—35 ml/kg
females = 23—30 ml/kg
Plasma volume = 40—50 ml/kg
Total blood volume = 65—85 ml/kg

White cells

Normal values

Total white count/mm^3

Adults	= 4 000—10 000
Infants (cord blood)	= 10 000—25 000
Infants, 1 year	= 6 000—18 000
Children, 4—7 years	= 6 000—15 000
Children, 8—12 years	= 4 500—13 500

Differential while cell count:

Cell	*cells/mm*^{3}	%
Neutrophils	2500–7500	40–75
Lymphocytes	1500–3500	20–50
Monocytes	200–800	2–10
Eosinophils	40–440	1–6
Basophils	15–100	1

Clotting

Platelet count	= 150 000—400 000/mm^3
Bleeding time (Duke)	= 0—7 min
Coagulation time (Lee and White)	= 5—11 min
Prothrombin time (1-stage Quick)	= 10—14 s
Prothrombin consumption index	= 0—30%
Plasma fibrinogen	= 200—400 mg/100 ml

Biochemical values

Normal blood, plasma and serum values

Acetone, serum	= 0·3—2·0 mg/100 ml
Aldolase, serum, Male	= Less than 33 units
Female	= Less than 19 units
Ammonia, blood	= 40—70 μg/100 ml
Amylase, serum	= 80—180 Somogyi units/100 ml
Ascorbic acid, blood	= 0·4—1·5 mg/100 ml
Bilirubin, serum	
Direct	= 0·1—0·4 mg/100 ml
Total	= 0·3—1·1 mg/100 ml
Calcium, serum	= 4·5—5·5 mEq/l (9·0—11·0 mg/100 ml)
Carbon dioxide, serum	
Content	= 26—28 mEq/l

Combining power	= 24—29 mEq/l
Tension, pCO_2	= 35—45 mmHg
Chloride, serum	= 98—106 mEq/l
Cholesterol, serum	
Total	= 150—250 mg/100 ml
Esters	= 68—76% of total cholesterol
Copper, serum	= 70—140 μg/100 ml
Creatine, serum	= 0·2—0·8 mg/100 ml
Creatinine, serum	= 0·7—1·5 mg/100 ml
Fibrinogen, plasma	= 200—400 mg/100 ml
Glucose (fasting), blood	= 60—100 mg/100 ml
Iodine, protein bound, serum	= 3·5—8·0 μg/100 ml
Iron, serum	= 75—175 μg/100 ml
Iron binding capacity, total serum	= 250—410 μg/100 ml
Lactic acid, blood	= 6—16 mg/100 ml
Lactic dehydrogenase, serum	= 200—450 units/ml
Lipase, serum	= Less than 1·5 units (ml of N/20 NaOH)
Lipids, total, serum	= 450—850 mg/100 ml
Phospholipids	= 150—250 mg/100 ml
Total fatty acids	= 190—420 mg/100 ml
Neutral fat	= 0—150 mg/100 ml
Magnesium, serum	= 1·5—2·5 mEq/l
Nitrogen, nonprotein, serum	= 15—35 mg/100 ml
Osmolality, serum	= 285—295 mOsm/l
Oxygen, blood	
Tension, pO_2 Arterial	= 95—100 mmHg
pH, arterial, plasma	= 7·35—7·45
Phenylalanine, serum	= Less than 3 mg/100 ml
Phosphatase, acid, serum	= 1·0—5·0 units (King-Armstrong)
Phosphatase, alkaline, serum	= 5·0—13·0 units (King-Armstrong)
Phosphatase, inorganic, serum	= 3·0—4·5 mg/100 ml
Potassium, serum	= 3·5—4.0 mEq/l
Proteins, serum	
Total	= 6·0—8·0 g/100 ml
Albumin	= 3·5—5·5 g/100 ml
Globulin	= 2·5—3·5 g/100 ml
Gamma	= 15—25% of total
Pyruvic acid, plasma	= 1·0—2·0 mg/100 ml
Sodium, serum	= 132—142 mEq/l
Transaminase, serum	
S.G.O.T.	= 5—40 units/ml
S.G.P.T.	= 5—35 units/ml
Urea, blood	= 20—40 mg/100 ml
Urea nitrogen, blood (B.U.N.)	= 10—20 mg/100 ml
Uric acid, serum	= 3·0—6·0 mg/100 ml

Cerebrospinal fluid

Normal values

Pressure	= 70—200 mmH_2O
Volume	= 120—140 ml
Cells-lymphocytes	= 0—5/mm^3
Total proteins	= 20—45 mg/100 ml
Globulin	= 0—6 mg/100 ml
Glucose	= 50—85 mg/100 ml
Chloride (as NaCl)	= 120—130 mEq/l (700—750 mg/100 ml)
Non-protein nitrogen	= 12—30 mg/100 ml
Uric acid	= 0·3—1·5 mg/100 ml
Calcium	= 2—3 mEq/l
Phosphate	= 0·4—0·7 mEq/l
Potassium	= 3·0—4·0 mEq/l
Sodium	= 140 mEq/l

Lange curve

Normal	0000110000
First zone curve (Paretic)	5555543210
Mid zone curve (Luetic)	0123320000
End zone curve (Meningitic)	0001223531

Composition of normal urine

Specific gravity in health: 1·003–1·030.
Reaction (pH) of normal urine: 4·6–8·0 depending on diet (avg., 6·0).
Volume: Normal range = 600–2500 ml/24 hours (avg., 1200 ml).
Total solids in grams per litre: 30–70 g (avg. 50 g).
Inorganic constituents per 24 hours:

Iron	0·06–0·1 mg
Chlorides (as chloride)	6 (4–10) g (100–300 mEq) on usual diet.
Sodium (varies with intake)	4 g (170 mEq) on usual diet.
Phosphate (as phosphorous)	0·8–1·3 g
Potassium (varies with intake)	2 g (50 mEq)
Sulphur (total) as SO_3	2 (0·7–3·5) g
Calcium	0·2 (0·1–0·2) g
Magnesium	0·15 (0·05–0·3) g

Organic constituents per 24 hours:

Nitrogenous, total	25–35 g
Urea (half of total urine solids; varies with diet)	15–30 g
Creatinine	1·4 (1–1·8) g
Ammonia	0·7 (0·3–1) g
Uric acid	0·7 (0·5–1) g

Undetermined N (amino acid, etc.) 0·5 g
Protein, as such ('albumin') 0–0·1 g
Creatine, in children 10–50 mg

Glucose: 50% of people have 2–3 mg/100 ml after a heavy meal.
A diabetic can lose up to 100 g/day.

Ascorbic acid: Adults excrete 15–50 mg/24 hours; in scurvy less than 15 mg/24 hours are excreted.

Amylase (diastase): 8–32 units.

Respiratory function

Range of normals

Age and sex	*Vital capacity* (l)	*Residual volume* (l)	*Total lung volume* (l)
Age 20–39			
Male	3·45–5·90	1·13–2·32	4·80–7·92
Female	2·45–4·38	1·00–2·00	3·61–6·18
Age 40–59			
Male	2·72–5·30	1·45–2·62	4·50–7·62
Female	2·09–4·02	1·16–2·20	3·41–6·02
Age > 60			
Male	2·42–4·70	1·77–2·77	4·35–7·32
Female	1·91–3·66	1·32–2·40	3·31–5·86

Forced expiratory volume in 1 second (FEV$_1$)

This is determined spirometrically by asking the patient to breathe normally and then inspire maximally, after which he is asked to expire as much air as possible as fast as possible. From the tracing the volume of air expired in the first second (FEV$_1$) and the forced vital capacity (FVC) can be easily calculated. The FEV$_1$ is then expressed as a % of FVC.

Normal values

Sex:	*Male*			*Female*		
Age:	20–39	40–59	60	17–29	30–45	46–62
$\frac{FEV_1 \times 100}{FVC}$	76	69	73	80	81	76

As an approximation the FEV$_1$ should be more than 75% FVC.

To determine the effects of reversible airways obstruction, the estimations should be performed before and after the inhalation of isoprenaline.

Blood gases

Normal values

Arterial P_{CO_2}	= 36–44 mmHg
Arterial CO_2 content	= 21–27 mmol/l
Arterial pH	= 7·36–7·44
Arterial P_{O_2}	= 95–100 mmHg
Arterial O_2 saturation	= 93–98%
Diffusing capacity O_2	
at rest	= 20 ml/min/mmHg
exercise	= 40–80 ml/min/mmHg
Diffusing capacity CO_2 at rest	= 15 ml/min/mmHg
(Steady state method)	

Oxygen dissociation

The oxygen dissociation curve will give approximately the following values of percentage saturation at the given P_{O_2}.

P_{O_2}	100	40	20	10
% sat.	97·4	75·0	35·0	13·5

Normal standard bicarbonate	= 19–25 mEq/l
Base excess	= ±2·5 mEq/l

APGAR score

	Sign	*0*	*1*	*2*
A.	Appearance	Blue, pale	Body pink, limbs blue	All pink
P.	Pulse	Absent	Below 100	Over 100
G.	Grimace (reflex response)	None	Grimace	Cry
A.	Activity (Tone)	Limp	Some flexion	Active movements
R.	Respiration	Absent	Slow, irregular	Good strong cry

Appendix III Respiratory Nomenclature

Special symbols

— Dash above any symbol indicates a mean value.
· Dot above any symbol indicates a time derivative.

For gases

Primary symbols

(Large capital letters)

V	=	gas volume
$\dot{V}$	=	gas volume/unit time
P	=	gas pressure
$\bar{P}$	=	mean gas pressure
F	=	fractional concentration in dry gas phase
f	=	respiratory frequency (breaths/unit time)
D	=	diffusing capacity
R	=	respiratory exchange ratio

Secondary symbols

(Small capital letters)

I	=	inspired gas
E	=	expired gas
A	=	alveolar gas
T	=	tidal gas
D	=	dead space gas
B	=	barometric
STPD	=	0°C, 760 mmHg, dry
BTPS	=	body temperature and pressure saturated with water vapor
ATPS	=	ambient temperature and pressure saturated with water vapor

For blood

Primary symbols

(Large capital letters)

Q	=	volume of blood

$\dot{Q}$	=	volume flow of blood/unit time
C	=	concentration of gas in blood phase
S	=	% saturation of Hb with O_2 or CO

Secondary symbols

(small letters)

a	=	arterial blood
v	=	venous blood
c	=	capillary blood

For lung volumes

VC	=	Vital Capacity	=	maximal volume that can be expired after maximal inspiration
IC	=	Inspiratory Capacity	=	maximal volume that can be inspired from resting expiratory level
IRV	=	Inspiratory Reserve Volume	=	maximal volume that can be inspired from end-tidal inspiration
ERV	=	Expiratory Reserve Volume	=	maximal volume that can be expired from resting expiratory level
FRC	=	Functional Residual Capacity	=	volume of gas in lungs at resting expiratory level
RV	=	Residual Volume	=	volume of gas in lungs at end of maximal expiration
TLC	=	Total Lung Capacity	=	volume of gas in lungs at end of maximal inspiration

Appendix IV National Poisons Information Service

National poisons information service

Antidotes

Specific antidotes are available for a few drugs and information can be obtained about this at any time from the National Poisons Information Service:

Poisons Unit,
New Cross Hospital,
Avonley Road,
LONDON SE14
Tel: 01-407 7600

Poisons Information Centre,
Jervis Street Hospital,
DUBLIN 1. Eire.
Tel: Dublin 45588

Poisons Information Centre,
Royal Victoria Hospital,
BELFAST BT12 6BA
Tel: 0232 30503

Poisons Information Centre,
The Cardiff Royal Infirmary,
CARDIFF CF6 1SZ
Tel: 0222 33101

Scottish Poisons Information Bureau,
The Royal Infirmary,
EDINBURGH EH3 9YW
Tel: 013–229 2477

References

Ablondi, M. A., Ryan, J. F., O'Connell, G. T., Haley, R. W. 1966., 'Continuous Intercostal Nerve Blocks for Post-operative Pain Relief' *Curr. Res. Anesth. & Analg.*, **45**, 185.

Adriani, J., Morton, R. C. 1968. 'Drug dependence: Important considerations from the Anesthesiologists point of view', *Curr. Res. Anesth. & Analg.*, **47**, 472.

Apgar, V. 1953. 'A Proposal for a New Method of Evaluation of the Newborn Infant', *Curr. Res. Anesth. & Analg.*, **32**, 260.

Askrog, V., Elb, S. 1966. 'Experiments with non-rebreathing anesthesia systems during controlled ventilation', *Curr. Res. Anesth. & Analg.*, **45**, 348.

Ayre, P. 1937. 'Endotracheal anesthesia for babies with special reference to hair-lip and cleft-palate operations', *Curr. Res. Anesth. & Analg.*, **16**, 330.

Benazon, D. 1962. 'Pressor Drugs. An appraisal of their place in anaesthetic practice,' *Anaesthesia*, **17**, 344.

Bodman, R. I., Gerson, G., Smith K. 1967. 'A Simple Closed Circuit of Halothane Anaesthesia', *Anaesthesia*, **22**, 476.

Bond, A. G. 1969. 'Determination of operative blood loss (the sources of error and elimination of inaccuracy in the haemoglobin dilution technique)', *Anaesthesia*, **24**, 219.

Boulton, T. B., Cole, P. V., Hewer, C. L. 1965. 'A Reassessment of Anaesthesia by Endotracheal Insufflation', *Anaesthesia*, **20**, 442.

Boulton, T. B. 1966. 'Anaesthesia in difficult situations, 3. General Anaesthesia – Technique', *Anaesthesia*, **21**, 234.

Brice, J. G., Dowsett, D. J., Lowe, R. D. 1964. 'Haemodynamic effect of carotid artery stenosis', *Brit. Med. J.*, **2**, 1363.

Broome, B., Sellick, B. A. 1965. 'Controlled Hypercapnia in Open Heart Surgery under Hypothermia', *Lancet*, **2**, 452

Bryce-Smith, R. 1951. 'Injection of Lumbar Sympathetic Chain', *Anaesthesia*, **6**, 150.

Bullough, J. 1952. 'A T-piece technique for special inhalation anaesthesia: a safe method for reducing operative bleeding', *Brit. Med. J.*, **1**, 28.

Bullough, J. 1955. 'Non-rebreathing techniques', *Brit. J. Anaesth.*, **27**, 181.

Burton, J. D. K. 1962. 'Effects of dry anaesthetic gases on the respiratory mucous membrane', *Lancet*, **1**, 235.

Campbell, E. J. M. 1960. 'Respiratory Failure – The Relationship between Oxygen Concentrations of Inspired Air and Arterial Blood', *Lancet*, **2**, 10.

Campbell, E. J. M., Howell, J. B. L. 1960. 'Simple Rapid Methods of Estimating Arterial and Mixed Venous Carbon Dioxide Tension', *Brit. Med. J.*, **1**, 458.

Campbell, E. J. M. 1963. 'Apparatus for Oxygen Administration', *Brit. Med. J.*, **2**, 1269.

Carden, E. 1969. 'The Microvent Ventilator', *Anaesthesia*, **24**, 91.

Churchill-Davidson, H. C., Richardson, A. J. 1953. 'Neuromuscular Transmission in Myasthenia Gravis', *J. Physiol.* (*Lond.*), **122**, 252.

Churchill-Davidson, H. C. 1965. 'Anaesthesia and mono-amine oxidase inhibitors', *Brit. Med. J.*, **1**, 520.

Clutton-Brock, J. 1960. 'Some Pain Threshold Studies with Particular Reference to Thiopentone', *Anaesthesia*, **15**, 71.

Cohen, A. D. 1966. 'The Minivent', *Anaesthesia*, **21**, 563.

Cole, J. R. 1966. 'The use of ventilators and vaporizer performance', *Brit. J. Anaesth.*, **38**, 646.

Conaghan, J. P., Jacobsen, M., Rae, L., Ward-McQuaid, J. W. 1966. 'Pentazocine and Phenazocine: A Double-blind Comparison of Two Benzomorphan Derivatives in Post-operative Pain', *Brit. J. Anaesth.*, **38**, 345.

Cooper, K. 1963. 'Paracervical Block in Obstetrics', *Proc. Roy. Soc. Med.*, **56**, 1096.

Crawford, J. S. 1963. 'Paracervical Nerve Block', *Brit. Med. J.*, **2**, 119.

Crawford, J. S. 1966. 'A Comparison of Spinal Analgesia and General Anesthesia for Cesarean Section', *Amer. J. Obstet. & Gynec.*, **94**, 858.

Cuatrecasas, P., Lockwood, D. H., Caldwell, J. R. 1965. 'Lactase Deficiency in the Adult. A Common Occurrence', *Lancet*, **1**, 14.

Dawkins, M. 1964. 'Relief of Post-operative Pain', *Lancet*, **2**, 696.

Deen, L. 1963. 'Modified Ayre's T-piece', *Anaesthesia*, **18**, 838.

DeFalque, R. J., Stoelting, V. K. 1964. 'Continuous Intercostal Block', *Anesthesiology*, **25**, 237.

DeJong, R. H. 1965. 'Modified Axillary Block', *Anesthesiology*, **26**, 615.

Dingle, H. R. 1966. 'Anti-hypertensive drugs and anaesthesia', *Anaesthesia*, **21**, 151.

Dobbie, A. K. 1969. 'The Electrical Aspects of Surgical Diathermy', *Bio. Med. Eng.*, **4**, 206.

Drew, C. E., Keen, G., Benazon, D. B. 1959. 'Profound Hypothermia', *Lancet*, **1**, 745.

Dundee, J. W. 1960. 'Alterations in Response to Somatic Pain Associated with Anaesthesia: Effect of Thiopentone and Pentobarbitone', *Brit. J. Anaesth.*, **32**, 407.

Ellis, M., Blacow, N. W. 1965. 'Poison Information Bureau at Leeds: An Account of Three Years Work', *Brit. Med. J.*, **2**, 198.

Ellis, M. W., Bryce-Smith, R. 1965. 'Use of Trichloroethylene Inhalations during Physiotherapy', *Brit. Med. J.*, **2**, 1412.

Enderby, G. E. H. 1947. 'Effect of Carbon Dioxide Inhalation in the Prophylaxis of Post-operative Respiratory Complications', *Anaesthesia*, **2**, 12.

Enderby, G. E. H. 1961. 'Report on Mortality and Morbidity following 9.107 Hypotensive Anaesthetics', *Brit. J. Anaesth.*, **33**, 109.

Epstein, H. G., Hunter, A. B. 1968. 'Anaesthesia apparatus; a pictorial review of the development of the modern anaesthetic machine', *Brit. J. Anaesth.*, **40**, 636.

'Explosion Hazards: Recommendations of the Association of Anaesthetists of Great Britain and Ireland', 1971. *Anaesthesia*, **26**, 155.

Farman, J. V., Gool, R. Y., Scott, D. B. 1962. 'Intercostal Block in Abdominal Surgery: A Method for the Single-handed Surgeon', *Lancet*, **1**, 879.

Farman, J. V. 1965. 'Economical anaesthesia overseas. Air-entrainment device for use with draw-over vaporizers in children', *Brit. Med. J.*, **2**, 1428.

Fink, B. R. 1955. 'Diffusion Anoxia', *Anesthesiology*, **16**, 511.

Finnegan, P., Jones, E. S. 1969. 'Treatment of Respiratory Failure due to Chronic Lung Disease by Intermittent Positive Pressure Ventilation', *Brit. J. Anaesth.*, **41**, 856.

Fletcher, J., Langman, M. J. S., Kellock, T. D. 1965. 'Effects of Surgery on Blood Sugar Levels in Diabetes Mellitus', *Lancet*, **2**, 52.

Foëx, P., Meloche, R., Prys-Roberts, C. 1971. 'Studies of anaesthesia in relation to hypertension. III. Pulmonary gas exchange during spontaneous ventilation', *Brit J Anaesth* , **43**, 644.

Fraser, R. A. 1963. 'Hyperinsulinism under Anaesthesia in a Case of Islet Tumour of the Pancreas', *Anaesthesia*, **18**, 3.

Freeman, J. 1963. 'Physiological Effects of Haemorrhage', *Ann. Roy. Coll. Surg.*, **33**, 138.

Frostad, L. A. 1968. 'An Aid to Central Venous Pressure Measurements', *Canad. Anaesth. Soc. J.*, **15**, 501.

Gadboys, H. L., Slonim, R., Litwak, R. S. 1962. 'Homologous Blood Syndrome. 1. Preliminary Observations on its Relationship to Clinical Cardiopulmonary Bypass', *Ann. Surg.*, **156**, 793.

Geffin, B. 1964. 'Thiopentone and Post-operative Restlessness', *Anaesthesia*, **19**, 89.

Gett, P. M., Jones, E. S., Shepherd, G. F. 1971. 'Pulmonary Oedema Associated with Sodium Retention during Ventilator Treatment', *Brit. J. Anaesth.*, **43**, 460.

Gibson, G. L. 1967. 'Infection and Sterility in Intensive Care Units', *J. Roy. Coll. Surg. Irel.*, **3**, 67.

Green, R., Dawkins, M. 1966. 'Post-operative Analgesia: The Use of Continuous Drip Epidural Block', *Anaesthesia*, **21**, 372.

Guess, W. L., Stetson, J. B. 1968. 'Tissue reactions to organtin-stabilized polyvinyl chloride (P.V.C.) catheters', *J. Amer. Med. Assn.*, **204**, 580.

Hargadon, J. J., Ormston, T. O. G. 1963. 'Anaesthesia for Excision of Islet-cell Tumour of the Pancreas', *Brit. J. Anaesth.*, **35**, 807.

Harris, W. 1937. *The Facial Neuralgias*, London: Oxford University Press.

Harris, D. M., Orwin, J. M., Colqhoun, J., Schroeder, H. G. 1969. Control of Cross Infection in an Intensive Care Unit', *J. Hygiene* (*Camb.*), **67**, 525.

Harrison, G. A. 1964. 'Ayre's T-piece: A review of its modifications', *Brit. J. Anaesth.*, **36**, 115.

Hart, W. S. 1958. 'Halothane anaesthesia dripfeed administration in Neurosurgery', *Anaesthesia*, **13**, 385.

Heath, M. E., Vickers, M. D. 1968. 'An Examination of single-trace semi-automated blood volume methodology', *Anaesthesia*, **23**, 659.

Herzog, P., Norlander, O. P. 1964. 'Clinical experience with ultrasonic humidification', *Acta Anaesth. Scand. Suppl.*, **XV**, 156.

Hewitt, J. C., Hamilton, R. C., O'Donnell, J. F., Dundee, J. W. 1966. 'Clinical Studies of Induction Agents XIV: A Comparative Study of Venous Complications following Thiopentone, Methohexitone, and Propanidid', *Brit. J. Anaesth.*, **38**, 115.

Hillard, E. K. 1968. 'British Standards Relevant to Anaesthesia', *Brit. J. Anaesth.*, **40**, 702.

Jenkins, A. V. 1957. 'Modification of the standard rubber face mask for use with babies and small children', *Brit. J. Anaesth.*, **29**, 40.

Jones, E. S., Peaston, M. J. T. 1966. 'Metabolic Care during Acute Illness', *Practitioner*, **196**, 271.

Kain, M. L., Nunn, J. F. 1967. 'Fresh gas flow and rebreathing in the Magill circuit with spontaneous respiration', *Proc. Roy. Soc. Med.*, **60**, 749.

Keuskamp, D. H. G. 1963. 'Automatic ventilation in paediatric anaesthesia using a modified Ayre's T-piece with negative pressure during expiratory phase', *Anaesthesia*, **18**, 46.

Keynes, G. 1966. 'Thymectomy and Myasthenia Gravis', *Brit. Med. J.*, **1**, 106.

Klock, J. M. 1955. 'New Concepts of Nitrous Oxide Anaesthesia', *Curr. Res. Anes. & Analg.*, **34**, 379.

Kornfeld, D. S. 1969. 'Psychiatric View of the Intensive Care Unit', *Brit. Med. J.*, **1**, 108.

Kuah, E. B., Yates, M. J. 1967. 'Relief of Pain in Labour', *Lancet*, **1**, 1159.

Lee, S. 1964. 'Advantages of a combined T-piece and non-rebreathing valve', *Brit. J. Anaesth.*, **36**, 521.

Leigh, J. M. 1970. 'Variation in Performance of Oxygen Therapy Devices', *Anaesthesia*, **25**, 210.

LeVeen, H. H., Rubricius, J. L. 1958. 'Continuous Automatic Electronic Determinations of Operative Blood Loss', *Surg. Gynec. Obstet.*, **106**, 368.

Levin, J. 1958. 'Endotracheal tubes in children: A formula for the lengths', *Anaesthesia*, **13**, 40.

Loder, R. E. 1960. 'Local Anaesthetic Solution with Longer Action', *Lancet*, **2**, 346.

McClelland, R. M. A. 1965. 'Complications of Tracheostomy', *Brit. Med. J.*, **2**, 567.

McDowall, D. G. 1964. 'Anaesthesia in a Pressure Chamber', *Anaesthesia*, **19**, 321.

McIntyre, J. W. R. 1957. 'Endotracheal tubes for children', *Anaesthesia*, **12**, 94.

McMichael, H. B., Webb, J., Dawson, A. M. 1965. 'Lactase Deficiency in Adults. A Cause of "Functional" Diarrhoea', *Lancet*, **1**, 717.

Mann, F. 1973. *Acupuncture: Cure of Many Diseases*, Pan Books, London.

Mann, P. E., Hatt, S. D., Dixon, R. A., Griffin, K. D., Perks, E. R., Thornton, J. A. 1971. 'A Minimal Increment Methohexitone Technique in Conservative Dentistry', *Anaesthesia*, **26**, 3.

Mapleson, W. W. 1954. 'The elimination of rebreathing in various semi-closed anaesthetic systems', *Brit. J. Anaesth.*, **26**, 323.

Mason, A. A. 1958. *Modern Trends in Anaesthesia.* Edit. Evans, F. T. and Gray, T. C. First Edition Butterworth, London, p. 152.

Masson, A. H. B. 1964. 'Clinical Assessment of Analgesic Drugs (4): Intravenous Trial', *Brit. J. Anaesth.*, **36**, 353.

Matthew, H., Lawson, A. A. H. 1966. 'Acute Barbiturate Poisoning – A Review of Two Years Experience', *Quart. J. Med.*, **35**, 539.

Merrifield, A. J., Hill, D. W., Smith, K. 1967. 'Performance of the Portablease and the portable Fluoxair anaesthetic equipment: with reference to use under adverse conditions', *Brit. J. Anaesth.*, **39**, 50.

Mitchell, J. V., Epstein, H. G. 1966. 'A pressure operated inflating valve', *Anaesthesia*, **21**, 277.

Moffett, A. J. 1947. 'Nasal Analgesia by Postural Instillation', *Anaesthesia*, **2**, 31.

Mostert, J. W. 1958. 'Nitrous Oxide Anaesthesia without Harm', *Brit. Med. J.*, **1**, 502.

Mushin, W. W., Bendell-Baker, L., Thompson, P. W., Mapleson, W. W. 1969. *Automatic ventilation of the lungs*, Blackwell Scientific Publications, Oxford.

Nahas, R. A., Melrose, D. G., Sykes, M. K., Robinson, B. 1965. 'Post-perfusion lung syndrome', *Lancet*, **2**, 252, 254.

Nainby-Luxmore, R. C. 1967. 'Some hazards of dental gas machines', *Anaesthesia*, **22**, 545.

Nightingale, D. A., Richards, C. C., Glass, A. 1965. 'An evaluation of rebreathing in a modified T-piece system during controlled ventilation of anaesthetized children', *Brit. J. Anaesth.*, **37**, 762.

Norman, J., Adams, A. P., Sykes, M. K. 1968. 'Rebreathing with the Magill attachment', *Anaesthesia*, **23**, 75.

Nunn, J. F. 1961. 'Portable Anaesthetic Apparatus for Use in the Antarctic', *Brit. Med. J.*, **1**, 1139.

Parbrook, G. D., Rees, G. A. D., Robertson, G. S. 1964. 'Relief of Post-operative Pain: Comparison of a Mixture of 25% Nitrous Oxide and Oxygen with Morphine', *Lancet*, **2**, 480.

Peaston, M. J. 1966. 'External Metabolic Balance Studies during Naso-gastric Feeding in Serious Illnesses Requiring Intensive Care', *Brit. Med. J.*, **2**, 1367.

Peaston, M. J. 1968. 'Parenteral Nutrition in Serious Illnesses', *Hosp Med.*, **2**, 708.

Plumpton, F S., Besser, G. M., Cole, P. V. 1969. 'Corticosteroid treatment and surgery', *Anaesthesia*, **24**, 3

Pooler, H. E. 1968. 'A planned approach to the surgical patient with iatrogenic adrenocortical insufficiency', *Brit J Anaesth* , **40**, 539

Prys-Roberts, C., Meloche, R., Foëx, P. 1971a. 'Studies of anaesthesia in relation to hypertension I. Cardiovascular responses of treated and untreated patients', *Brit. J. Anaesth.*, **43**, 122.

Prys-Roberts, C., Greene, L. T., Meloche, R., Foëx, P. 1971b. 'Studies of anaesthesia in relation to hypertension. II. Haemodynamic consequences of induction and endotracheal intubation', *Brit. J. Anaesth.*, **43**, 531.

Prys-Roberts, C., Foëx, P., Greene, L. T., Waterhouse, T. D. 1972. 'Studies of anaesthesia in relation to hypertension. IV. The effects of artificial ventilation on the circulation and pulmonary gas exchanges', *Brit. J. Anaesth.*, **44**, 355.

Prys-Roberts, C., Foëx, P., Biro, G. P., Roberts, J. G. 1973. 'Studies of anaesthesia in relation to hypertension. V. Adrenergic beta-receptor blockade', *Brit. J. Anaesth.*, **45**, 671.

Rackow, H., Salanitre, E. 1968. 'A new Paediatric circle valve', *Anesthesiology*, **29**, 833.

Rees, C. J. 1950. 'Anaesthesia in the Newborn', *Brit. Med. J.*, **2**, 1419.

Relton, J. E. S., Creighton, R. E., Conn, A. W. 1968. 'Fulminant Hyperpyrexia, associated with Anaesthesia', *Anaesthesia*, **23**, 253.

Rendell-Baker, L. 1962. 'New Paediatric Face-mask and anaesthetic equipment', *Brit. Med. J.*, **1**, 1690.

Robinson, J. S. 1966. 'Control of Infection in Intensive Care Units and in the Ward Area', *J. Roy. Coll. Surg. Edin.*, **11**, 307.

Robinson, J. S. 1970. 'Physical principles of mist sterilization', *Proc. Roy. Soc. Med.*, **63**, 910.

Rollason, W. N. 1960. 'A Study of Hypotensive Anaesthesia in the Elderly', *Brit. J. Anaesth.*, **32**, 276.

Rollason, W. N., Hough, J. M. 1960. 'Is it safe to employ hypotensive anaesthesia in the elderly?', *Anaesthesia*, **15**, 69.

Ruscoe-Clarke, A., Topley, E., Flear, C. T. 1955. 'Assessment of Blood Loss in Civilian Trauma', *Lancet*, **1**, 629.

Sanger, C., Churchill-Davidson, I., Tomlinson, R. H. 1955. 'Anaesthesia for Radiotherapy under High-pressure Oxygen', *Brit. J. Anaesth.*, **27**, 436.

Saunders, C. 1967. 'The Management of Terminal Illness', *Hospital Medicine*, **1**, 4.

Schroeder, H. G., Williams, N. E. 1966. 'Anaesthesia for meningomyelocoele surgery (Some problems associated with immediate surgical closure in the neonate)', *Anaesthesia*, **21**, 57.

Schroeder, H. G. 1971. 'Psychoreactive Problems of Intensive Therapy', *Anaesthesia*, **26**, 28.

Shires, G. T., Williams, J., Brown, F. T. 1961. 'Acute Changes in Extracellular Fluid Associated with Major Surgical Procedures', *Ann. Surg.*, **154**, 803.

Simpson, B. R., Parkhouse, J., Marshall, R., Lambrechts, W. 1961. 'Extradural Analgesia and the Prevention of Post-operative Respiratory Complications', *Brit. J. Anaesth.*, **33**, 628.

Simpson, B. R., Seelye, E., Clayton, J. I., Parkhouse, J. 1962. 'Morphine Combined with Tetrahydroaminacrine for Post-operative Pain', *Brit. J. Anaesth.*, **34**, 95.

Smith, B., Omeri, M. A., Melrose, D. G., Bental, H. H., Allwork, S. 1964. 'Blood Loss after Cardio-pulmonary By-pass', *Lancet*, **2**, 273.

Spectral Requirements of Light Sources for Clinical Purposes. 1966. Med. Res. Counc. Memo. No. 43. H.M.S.O.

Steen, N. S., Chen, S. L. 1963. 'Automatic non-rebreathing valve circuits. Some principles and modifications', *Brit. J. Anaesth.*, **36**, 379.

Stephens, K. F. 1965. 'Transportable apparatus for Halothane anaesthesia', *Brit. J. Anaesth.*, **37**, 67.

Stewart, H. C. 1963. 'The Pharmacology of Anti-emetic Drugs', *Brit. J. Anaesth.*, **35**, 174.

Sullivan, S. F., Patterson, R. W. 1968. 'Posthyperventilation Hypoxia: Theoretical Considerations in Man', *Anesthesiology*, **19**, 98.

Sykes, M. K. 1959. 'Non-rebreathing valves', *Brit. J. Anaesth.*, **31**, 450.

Sykes, M. K. 1963. 'Venous Pressure as a Clinical Indication of the Adequacy of Transfusion', *Ann. Roy. Coll. Surg.*, **33**, 163.

Sykes, M. K. 1964. 'Sterilizing Mechanical Ventilators', *Brit. Med. J.*, **1**, 561.

Sykes, M. K. 1968. 'Rebreathing circuits: a review', *Brit. J. Anaesth.*, **40**, 666.

Tatjeen, C. H., Freedman, H. L., Harris, H. 1966. 'A System of Continuous Paracervical Block Anesthesia', *Amer. J. Obstet. & Gynec.*, **94**, 854.

Taylor, G., Pryce-Davis, J. 1966. 'The Prophylactic Use of Antacids in the Prevention of the Acid-pulmonary-aspiration Syndrome', *Lancet*, **1**, 288.

Thornton, J. A., Saynor, R., Schroeder, H. G., Taylor, D. G., Verel, D. 1963. 'Estimation of Blood Loss with Particular Reference to Cardiac Surgery: Description of a Method', *Brit. J. Anaesth.*, **35**, 91.

Thornton, J. A. 1971. 'Assessment of Fluid Loss in Trauma and Operation and its Replacement', *General Anaesthesia*, 3rd Edit. eds. T. C. Gray and J. F. Nunn. Butterworth, London.

Tom, A. 1956. 'An Innovation in Technique for Dental Gas', *Brit. Med. J.*, **1**, 1085.

Vale, R. J. 1958. 'A modified semi-open system for children's anaesthesia', *Brit. J. Anaesth.*, **30**, 182.

Vale, R. J. 1959. 'Modified angle piece for children's anaesthesia', *Brit. J. Anaesth.*, **31**, 558.

Voss, T. J. V. 1963. 'Deadspace in Paediatric Anaesthetic Apparatus', *Brit. J. Anaesth.*, **35**, 452.

Wallace, A. B. 1951. 'The Exposure Treatment of Burns', *Lancet*, **1**, 501.

Waters, D. J. 1961. 'A composite semi-closed anaesthetic system for spontaneous respiration', *Brit. J. Anaesth.*, **33**, 417.

Waters, D. J., Mapleson, W. W. 1961. 'Rebreathing during controlled respiration with various semi-closed systems', *Brit. J. Anaesth.*, **33**, 374.

Waters, D. J. 1967. 'Use and misuse of a pressure-limiting bag', *Anaesthesia*, **22**, 322.

Waters, R. M. 1926. 'Advantages and technique of Carbon Dioxide filtration with inhalation anaesthesia', *Curr. Res Anesth & Analg* , **5**, 160

Whitby, J L. 1970. 'Sterilization of pulmonary ventilators', *Proc. Roy. Soc. Med.*, **63**, 909.

Winters, R. W. 1967. 'Studies of Acid-base Disturbances', *Paediatrics*, **39**, 700.

Wood, J. B., Frankland, A. W., James, V. H. T., Landon, J. 1965. 'A rapid test for adrenocortical function', *Lancet*, **1**, 243.

Working Party on Anaesthetic Explosions. 1956. Association of Anaesthetists Great Britain and Ireland.

Wulfsohn, N. L., Politzer, W. M. 1962. '5-Hydroxytryptamine in Anaesthesia', *Anaesthesia*, **17**, 64.

Index